Trauma and Infection Control in Revision Hip and Knee Arthroplasty

Richard S. Yoon • Jaclyn Jankowski
Frank Liporace
Editors

Trauma and Infection Control in Revision Hip and Knee Arthroplasty

A Case-Based Approach

Springer

Editors
Richard S. Yoon
Orthopedic Surgery
Rutgers - RWJBH
Jersey City, NJ, USA

Jaclyn Jankowski
Orthopedic Surgery
Rutgers - RWJBH
Jersey City, NJ, USA

Frank Liporace
Orthopedic Surgery
Rutgers - RWJBH
Jersey City, NJ, USA

ISBN 978-3-031-71970-7   ISBN 978-3-031-71971-4 (eBook)
https://doi.org/10.1007/978-3-031-71971-4

This Springer imprint is published by the registered company Springer Nature Switzerland AG
The registered company address is: Gewerbestrasse 11, 6330 Cham, Switzerland

Preface

Around the globe, the number of primary total hip and knee arthroplasty being performed continues to increase exponentially. Concurrently, with advancing technology, younger patients are being indicated, while total joint recipients stay healthier and get older. This combination allows for a unique scenario where the number of complications, specifically infections and periprosthetic fractures, also will see a concurrent rise in incidence, especially in older patients who are sicker and with poor bone stock.

This scenario was the basis of the purpose for this book, where a concise, yet comprehensive guide would allow for facile work-up, implementation and execution of operative techniques to maximize outcomes in total joint patients sustaining periprosthetic fractures and infections. Here, we asked world-renowned experts in the field to contribute their own experiences into concise, case-based, chapters that will be directly referenced and utilized by you, our reader.

Our target audience includes the community orthopaedic surgeon who wants a guide and update in the latest techniques in treating patients with these difficult clinical scenarios. Our patients need our help, and whether you are in a busy urban setting or in a desolate rural place, we hope that our book will act as a quick reference, clinical guide that can aid in delivering excellent patient care.

Our expert authors start out by helping you to formulate the proper approach in obtaining the correct diagnosis in both revision hip and knee arthroplasty, especially when considering the presence of infection. Salient points and literature, with case examples help guide the reader into concise and prudent management.

Along these lines, Chap. 3 outlines the importance points in working up periprosthetic hip and knee fractures, including the importance of obtaining a proper medical and radiographic history and planning for the surgery; here, the importance of imaging and ruling out infection is also discussed.

Chapter 4 delves into the nuances of aseptic revision surgery in hip arthroplasty, specifically on the femoral side. We discuss the options available on the femoral side and provide tips and tricks in avoiding pitfalls even in the most daunting clinical scenarios, which often include severe bone loss. Additionally, options and timing for modular, revision stems as well as proximal femoral replacements are also discussed in a case-based fashion.

Chapters 5, 6 and 7 move on to discuss the management of periprosthetic fractures in the acetabulum, proximal femur and distal femur. Highlighting the importance of proper diagnosis and assessment of implant stability and bone stock/quality, our authors provide a case-based synopsis of several techniques and treatment algorithms that allow for appropriate operative care.

In Chap. 8, our infection expert tackles the difficult problem of revision total hip arthroplasty and includes anatomic approaches and strategies for both two-stage treatment for chronic cases, as well as appropriate timing for acute cases.

Moving onto the knee, salient pearls regarding revision knee arthroplasty is discussed in Chap. 9, where specific tips in implant selection and technique can be extremely useful in creating the appropriate, stable, bone void filling construct, in even the most severe bone loss scenario.

In Chap. 10, treating an extensor mechanism disruption can be an extremely challenging task, but our authors offer their expert insight and technique in achieving an optimal clinical outcome.

In Chap. 11, our authors discuss the options for fixation versus revision in fractures around total knee arthroplasty. Focusing on identifying implant stability and bone stock, case-based techniques and tips for success will help you immediately apply them to your own practice and cases.

Finally, in Chap. 12, another expert in infection joint management discusses again the specific details of the work-up, along with proper technique (including two-stage), that can help one efficiently eradicate the infection and salvage the limb.

By summarizing these important points in the world of hip and knee arthroplasty, we hope that this book creates a concise, quick-reference, case-based guide in treating patients presenting with these difficult clinical problems. Immediately applying these techniques and strategies will hopefully improve your own outcomes, as they have improved ours.

We hope you find this book helpful in achieving your goals and taking care of our patients, an ever-growing population of people who want to continue to stay mobile and functional, in spite of these devastating injuries.

Frank A. Liporace
Jaclyn Jankowski
Richard S. Yoon

Contents

Contributors

Obinna O. Adigweme Rothman Orthopedic Institute, Orlando, FL, USA

Thomas L. Bernasek Florida Orthopaedic Institute, Tampa, FL, USA

Marcelo Batista Bonadio University of São Paulo, São Paulo, Brazil

Cory A. Collinge Harris Methodist Hospital Fort Worth, Fort Worth, TX, USA

Brian M. Culp Department of Orthopedic Surgery, Rush University Medical Center, Chicago, IL, USA

Edward M. DelSole Department of Orthopaedic Surgery, Tower Health, Keystone Spine and Pain Management, Wyomissing, PA, USA

Derek J. Donegan University of Pennsylvania, Philadelphia, PA, USA

George J. Haidukewych Department of Orthopedic Surgery, Orlando Health, Orlando, FL, USA

John S. Hwang Department of Orthopaedic Surgery, Rutgers, The State University of New Jersey, New Jersey Medical School, Newark, NJ, USA

Stephen Johnstone Department of Orthopaedic Surgery, Columbia University, New York, NY, USA

John Kampa Department of Orthopaedic Surgery, Hennepin Healthcare, Minneapolis, MN, USA

Erik N. Kubiak UMC/UNLV Department of Orthopedic Surgery, University Medical Center of Southern Nevada, Las Vegas, NV, USA

University of Nevada Las Vegas, Las Vegas, NV, USA

Richard Kyle Department of Orthopaedic Surgery, Hennepin Healthcare, Minneapolis, MN, USA

Brett R. Levine Department of Orthopedic Surgery, Rush University Medical Center, Chicago, IL, USA

Frank A. Liporace Division of Orthopaedic Trauma and Complex Adult Reconstruction, Department of Orthopaedic Surgery, Cooperman Barnabas/Jersey City Medical Center- RWJBH, Livingston/Jersey City, Jersey City, NJ, USA

Department of Orthopedic Surgery, Rutgers - RWJBH, Jersey City, NJ, USA

Raphael S. F. Longobardi Department of Orthopaedic Surgery, RWJ Barnabas Health, Jersey City, NJ, USA

Department of Orthopaedic Surgery, NYU Langone Health, NYU Grossman School of Medicine, New York, NY, USA

Steven T. Lyons Florida Orthopaedic Institute, Tampa, FL, USA

William B. Macaulay Department of Orthopaedic Surgery, Columbia University, New York, NY, USA

Kendall M. Masada University of Pennsylvania, Philadelphia, PA, USA

Brian T. Palumbo Florida Orthopaedic Institute, Tampa, FL, USA

Aldo M. Riesgo Division of Adult Reconstruction, Department of Orthopaedic Surgery, Baptist Health, Miami, FL, USA

Robert A. Sershon Department of Orthopedic Surgery, Rush University Medical Center, Chicago, IL, USA

Roshan P. Shah Department of Orthopaedic Surgery, Columbia University, New York, NY, USA

Neil P. Sheth University of Pennsylvania, Philadelphia, PA, USA

James D. Slover Zucker School of Medicine at Hofstra/Northwell, Hempstead, NY, USA

Lenox Hill Hospital, New York, NY, USA

T. Kyle Stoops Florida Orthopaedic Institute, Tampa, FL, USA

Li Sun Division of Orthopaedic Trauma and Complex Adult Reconstruction, Department of Orthopaedic Surgery, Cooperman Barnabas/Jersey City Medical Center-RWJBH, Livingston/Jersey City, Jersey City, NJ, USA

Richard S. Yoon Division of Orthopaedic Trauma and Complex Adult Reconstruction, Department of Orthopaedic Surgery, Cooperman Barnabas/Jersey City Medical Center-RWJBH, Livingston/Jersey City, Jersey City, NJ, USA

Department of Orthopedic Surgery, Rutgers - RWJBH, Jersey City, NJ, USA

1 Getting the Diagnosis and Planning in Revision Hip Arthroplasty: Infected or Not?

Stephen Johnstone, William B. Macaulay, and Roshan P. Shah

Introduction

Periprosthetic joint infections are a dreaded complication for both patients and doctors alike. The extensive surgical and medical interventions needed to clear an infection cause major disruption for patients' lives physically and emotionally, not to mention the potential for medical sequelae beyond the infection. Because of this, diagnosing a true infection becomes paramount. However, it can be difficult due to the lack of reliable tests both clinically and in the laboratory. In some cases, the marginal specificity and sensitivity of tests may never turn a suspected infection into a confirmed infection. The desired diagnostic gold standard is a simple, cheap, non-invasive, sensitive, and specific test that has yet to be accepted. As such, the diagnosis of infection is a synthesis of clinical suspicion guided by a collection of preoperative and intraoperative laboratory, pathology, and microbiology values. All of these tests and data points have their strengths and weaknesses and must be interpreted together alongside the surgeon's experience. And yet, it must be stated that many cases of infection are clear and treatment decisions can be made rapidly. We aim to discuss strategies for the diagnosis of periprosthetic joint infections (PJI), which are based on the current consensus literature as well as newer developments.

S. Johnstone · W. B. Macaulay · R. P. Shah (✉)
Department of Orthopaedic Surgery, Columbia University, New York, NY, USA
e-mail: William.Macaulay@nyulangone.org

Background

The diagnosis of a prosthetic joint infection remains a consensus [1–4]. Over the last several years, the definition of a true periprosthetic infection has been debated. An accepted definition is critical until a true gold standard can be found. In 2011, the Musculoskeletal Infection Society developed the following criteria for diagnosing an infected prosthetic joint:

MSIS Definition

1. A sinus tract communicating with the prosthesis
2. A pathogen is isolated by culture from two separate tissue or fluid samples obtained from the affected prosthetic joint
3. Four of the following six criteria exist:
   (a) Elevated serum erythrocyte sedimentation rate (ESR) or serum C-reactive protein (CRP) concentration
   (b) Elevated synovial white blood cell (WBC) count
   (c) Elevated synovial neutrophil percentage (PMN%)
   (d) Presence of purulence in the affected joint

R. S. Yoon et al. (eds.), *Trauma and Infection Control in Revision Hip and Knee Arthroplasty*,
https://doi.org/10.1007/978-3-031-71971-4_1

(e) Isolation of microorganism in one culture of periprosthetic tissue or fluid
(f) Greater than five neutrophils per high-power field in five high-power fields observed from histologic analysis of periprosthetic tissue at 400× magnification

An international consensus group dedicated to providing a comprehensive set of recommendations for approaching periprosthetic joint infections [2] modified these criteria slightly in 2014 and again in 2018:

International consensus 2014 preoperative diagnostic criteria	
One major criteria	
1. Two positive periprosthetic cultures with phenotypically identical organisms	
2. A sinus tract communicating with the joint or visualization of the prosthesis	
Or four out of five minor criteria	
1. Elevated serum C-reactive protein (CRP) and erythrocyte sedimentation rate (ESR)	
2. Elevated synovial fluid white blood cell (WBC) count or ++change on leukocyte esterase test strip	
3. Elevated synovial fluid polymorphonuclear neutrophil percentage (PMN%)	
4. Positive histological analysis of periprosthetic tissue.	
5. A single positive culture	
International consensus 2018	
Preoperative diagnosis	
One major criteria	
1. Two positive periprosthetic cultures with phenotypically identical organisms	
2. A sinus tract communicating with the joint or visualization of the prosthesis	
Minor criteria	Score
Elevated serum CRP *or* D-Dimer	2
Elevated serum ESR	1
Elevated synovial WBC *or* leukocyte esterase	3
Elevated synovial PMN %	2
Elevated synovial CRP	1
Positive alpha-defensin	3
Decision:	>/=6 infected
	2–5 possibly infected
	0–1 not infected
Intraoperative diagnosis	
Positive histology	3
Positive purulence	3
Single positive culture	2
[International consensus Group]	

In 2014, the international consensus group repealed the presence of purulence, citing recent evidence that purulence was subjective and was inadequate in isolation as diagnostic criteria [3, 5]. The second alteration required that both ESR and CRP be elevated rather than one of the two. Lastly, they added the infrequently used leukocyte esterase litmus test strip as part of the list of minor criteria and treated it as synonymous with synovial fluid white blood cell count.

In 2018, while the Major Criteria remained consistent, refinements were made to the weight of each minor criteria. Instead of a binary system of positive or negative a scoring system was developed and validated. If preoperative diagnostic criteria were inconclusive and surgical management was elected, the 2018 criteria reincluded purulence with a score of 3 recognizing its importance despite subjectivity.

Regardless of the modifications, both acknowledged the difficulty in achieving certainty by following these criteria. This definition performs well for infections that are obvious: sinus tracts, purulent aspirates, swift bacterial growth on cultures, or grossly elevated lab values with no confounding medical conditions. While it provides some guidance for equivocal cases, many times the diagnosis remains elusive, particularly with subclinical infections, and culture negative infections that may involve biofilms with only periodic bacterial shedding. Cultures may be difficult to grow, require longer incubation such as *P. acnes*, or may not even be able to be cultured [6, 7]. Laboratory studies can be discordant or hover around cutoff values, which can be inconsistent in the literature [8–10]. Moreover, a diagnosis would ideally be obtained prior to surgical intervention; yet, the final criterion is only satisfied once surgery has been committed. Though research into laboratory tests continues, the 2013 consensus emphasizes, "Clinical judgment should not be outweighed by use of the diagnostic algorithm or any one individual test. A preoperative aseptic diagnosis using this algorithm should not eliminate suspicion for PJI" [6]. The clinical exam and patients' concomitant medical profile should retain high value in diagnosing a PJI.

Clinical Presentation and Physical Examination

Infection has traditionally been classified into three types based on Fitzgerald's description in 1977 [11, 12]. They are based on the presumed mechanism and timing of presentation. A fourth type has been proposed by Tsukayama in 1996 [13]. Modified from the original paper, Type I is denoted an acute infection, presenting fewer than 6 weeks (originally 3 months) after surgery. Bacterial seeding is thought to be from the immediate perioperative period. Type II is a chronic infection presenting more than 6 weeks (originally 26 months) after surgery. Types III, usually presenting well after 6 weeks, is defined as an infection that presents acutely after a previously well-functioning joint. These are thought to occur secondary to hematologic seeding from a distant site—urinary tract, remote abscess, dental infection, and the like. The final type, Type IV, describes a scenario in which a presumed joint without infection yields a positive intraoperative culture soon after surgery.

The presentation of early versus late infection can be different. Late infections often present with insidious pain, discomfort, and swelling. They frequently, but not always, have incisions that remain free of erythema or drainage. Infections within the first 6 weeks to 3 months may display other signs. A retrospective study from Australia noted the following symptomatic frequencies: pain 42%, fever 38%, wound erythema wound 42%, swelling 25%, purulent discharge 72%, sinus tract 5%, and hypotension (systolic less than 90 mmHg) 6%. Some suggest methicillin-resistant staph aureus (MRSA) presents more readily as a pyogenic infection [14, 15]. Decreased range of motion in a previously well-functioning joint suggests a joint effusion which may be due to infection. Infrequently, patients present with sepsis. The most frequent presenting symptom that creates suspicion for a PJI is a painful joint [8, 15, 16]. Pain characteristics can vary from rapid onset and unremitting pain to mild sensations of discomfort. Although a history of a postoperative pain-free interval can suggest infection, pain, or discomfort in a joint should place infection high within the differential that must be excluded.

Beyond joint specific clinical signs and symptoms, patients' health and comorbidities are relevant to the diagnosis of infection. Several risk factors have been described that increase a patient's risk of PJI, particularly in the early postoperative period. Congestive heart failure, chronic pulmonary disease, anemia, diabetes, depression, renal disease, pulmonary circulation disorders, liver disease (hepatitis B and C), coagulopathy, malignancy, obesity with BMI above 40, diabetes, stroke, dementia, urinary tract infections, rheumatoid arthritis, and electrolyte disturbance (Na+, K+) all have been associated with infection [17–22]. There is not yet clear understanding of the relative importance of these risk factors. Surgical factors that are associated with the risk of infection include hematomas, postoperative drainage, and extended surgical times [17–22]. A general rule of thumb is to include infection in the differential diagnosis of every arthroplasty complaint and planned revision surgery.

Imaging

Several standard and nuclear image-based strategies—plain radiographs, CT, MRI, technetium 99m polyclonal IgG, Gallium-67, Indium-111, and FDG-PET—have been examined for their diagnostic potential [8, 23–32]. In general, their ability to rule out an infection is better than their ability to distinguish an infection from other active metabolic processes. Prior to any advanced workup, X-rays are use l to assess the state of the bone and prosthesis. Their utility lies in preoperative planning. Fractures, malalignment, and periprosthetic lucencies can all be seen. Obvious infectious signs such as sequestrum or periosteal reactions may also be observed. Notably, aseptic loosening, healing fractures, and fracture due to infection can all display similar features [8]. CT scans and MRIs are difficult to use for the diagnosis of infection due to metal artifact interference with the image processor [6, 8, 29]. Nonetheless, they have utility in revealing fluid collections, joint distention, and periprosthetic tissue signs of infection. They can also illuminate other differential diagnoses of a painful joint such as ALVAL or malrotation. Although X-rays are recommended as a rapid inexpensive surgery of the joint, CT scans and MRI scans are not recommended by the international consensus as part of the diagnostic workup for infection [6].

In some regions, nuclear medicine has an important role in the diagnosis of PJI. Several generations and multiple tracer permutations of nuclear imaging exist. Three-phase bone scintigraphy with Technetium 99m +/− gallium was the first generation of nuclear imaging. Over the last 15 years, leukocyte-labeled Indium-111m scans combined with T99m sulfur colloid marrow scintigraphy has replaced it to become the gold standard of periprosthetic imaging. FDG-PET scans have emerged as the most recent nuclear imaging modality for diagnosing PJI [23, 26]. Conflicting evidence exists that can either support or argue against the use of these modalities. Nagoya et al. used triple phase bone scans with T99m to obtain a sensitivity of 88%, specificity of 90%, and accuracy of 89%. Positive predictive value (PPV) and negative predictive value were 83% and 93%, respectively [28]. Reinartz et al. found triple phase bone scan to be inferior to PET scan with a sensitivity of 79%, specificity of 88%, NPV of 88%, and positive predictive value of 79%, and accuracy of 85% [33]. Other studies have failed to reach these values. Levitsky et al. reported a sensitivity of 33%, specificity of 85%, PPV 30%, and NPV 88% [34, 35]. In the nuclear medicine literature, Love et al. noted its limitations, finding accuracies of 50–70%; combining T99m with Gallium elevated it only slightly to 65–80% [27]. Three-phase bone scan is a relatively inexpensive, widely available test. Criticism stems from its inability to distinguish infection from inflammation and aseptic loosening. Moreover, it can lead to false positives for up to 2 years after surgery, which is often the period of interest. It might be best employed as a screening test [26, 36]. When negative, the diagnosis of infection is less likely.

Leukocyte-labeled Indium-111m combined with T99m sulfur colloid has improved on the positive predictive value and specificity of nuclear scanning. Alone, Indium-111m did not perform as well. The theorized basis is that neutrophils are usually absent in aseptic loosening and thus show little activity in sterile cases. Furthermore, infection stimulates uptake of leukocytes but suppresses uptake of sulfur colloid giving a spatial incongruency in the images [24]. Combined, Joseph et al. found 100% specificity and PPV [25]. However, many false negatives occurred with 66% sensitivity and 89% negative predictive value. Accuracy was 90%. Love et al. echoed these results with improved sensitivity and NPV: 100% sensitivity, 91% specificity, 82% PPV for hips, 100% PPV for knees, and 100% NPV for both hips and knees [37]. Attractive from a diagnostic perspective, the process is expensive, adds additional radiation, is inconvenient and requires experienced radiologists. Though not perfect, this combination has been considered the standard for nuclear radiography for PJI.

Other investigations have shifted towards FDG-PET scans as a means of improving diagnosis and also spatial resolution, something that triple phase bone scans, leukocyte scintigraphy, and bone marrow scintigraphy lack. Results from a 2008 study reported 85% sensitivity, 93% specificity, PPV of 80%, and NPV of 95%. Accuracy reached 91% [23]. A meta-analysis found a wide range of results. Sensitivity ranged from 22% to 100% with specificity ranging from 73% to 100% [26]. This methodology performs better for hips as its spatial patterns and interpretation have been better delineated. Overall, there is no clear advantage of FDG-PET scans over leukocyte labeled Indium-111m with T99m sulfur colloid scans.

Controversy has recently emerged between the orthopedic literature and the nuclear medicine literature. Diaz-Ledezma et al. employed a quality measurement tool for critical appraisal and bias [36]. It cast doubt on the existing literature for nuclear medicine in the diagnosis of periprosthetic infections, suggesting that there was enough bias and variation among studies to proceed with caution and selectivity when using nuclear medicine as a means of diagnosing a total joint infection. Rebuttal suggested that the current state of clear medicine, when proper protocols and interpretations are followed, can achieve a diagnostic accuracy of 93%. Drawbacks remain, however, with expense, convenience, inaccuracy before 2 years, distinguishing between infection and inflammation, and availability of trained experienced radiologists for definitive interpretations. The international consensus acknowledged the effectiveness of nuclear imaging but stated that the optimal imaging modality had yet to be elucidated. Moreover, given more cost-effective techniques, there is currently no definitive utility for nuclear imaging [6].

Laboratory Analysis

The simple first line workhorse for diagnosing periprosthetic infections has been erythrocyte sedimentation rate (ESR) and C-reactive protein (CRP) [6, 8, 9, 12, 34, 38–42]. Both are genetic markers of inflammation, rising in disease states but also postoperatively. ESR tends to rise more slowly than does CRP and remains elevated for up to 6 months [8]. CRP by contrast rises rapidly postoperatively and declines to normal levels within approximately 3 weeks [41]. Current accepted limits are 30 mm/h for ESR and 10 mg/L for CRP.

Erythrocyte Sedimentation Rate

The Westergren Erythrocyte Sedimentation Rate test was developed in 1897 by Edmund Biernacki and confirmed in 1918 by Robert Sanno Fahraeus and Alf Vilhelm Albertsson. ESR measures the rate of red blood cell settlement over a period of an hour. In states of inflammation, more fibrinogen is present causing red blood cells to form rouleaux and thus fall faster [43]. Thus, it is a genetic marker of inflammation of which infection is only one source. Others include rheumatologic diseases, temporal arteritis, some cardiac conditions such as heart failure and neoplasms. ESR also varies with age and gender. For women greater than 50 years old, normal ESR is 30 mm/h or less. For men greater than 50 years old, normal ESR is 20 mm/h. For those under 50, the values drop to 20 mm/h in women and 15 mm/h for men [43]. Typically age and gender are not addressed in the lab and a standard threshold of 30 mm/h is used. As a generic marker of inflammation, ESR is useful but its sensitivity and specificity for infection do not perform up to desired expectations. Levitsky et al. showed better results for ESR > 30 mm/h than triple phase bone scan but still only showed a sensitivity of 60%, specificity of 65%, PPV of 25%, and NPV of 90% [34]. Spangehl et al. found opposite values in his prospective analysis of revision hips. ESR sensitivity was 82%, specificity 85%, NPV 58%, and PPV 95% [12, 34, 44]. Della Valle et al. reported values somewhere in between: sensitivity 90.2%, specificity 66%, NPV 89.7%, and PPV 67.3% [39]. A meta-analysis of laboratory values by Berbari et al. provided pooled data for ESR of 88% sensitivity and 70% specificity [9]. ESR is not effective in isolation.

C-Reactive Protein

The 1980s saw the gradual use of CRP as a means of supplementing bone scans, radiographs, and ESR for diagnostic tests [42]. CRP is one of a number of acute-phase reactant proteins that rapidly rise in concentration in response to inflammation, inflammatory diseases, trauma, infection, malignancy, and cardiac diseases among others [45]. It is produced by hepatocytes under transcriptional direction of interleukin-6. A benefit to CRP and several other markers such as IL-6 and alpha defense is the relative rapid rise and fall of values. CRP peaks slightly earlier than ESR, thus acute symptom evaluation may result in lower ESR values but high CRP levels. Normal levels of CRP can begin to normalize after 3 weeks, while ESR can remain elevated for longer [8, 41].

Not only does it minimize the postoperative elevation period, but it has a better diagnostic performance profile. Multiple studies over the past several decades have recorded sensitivities and specificities with an optimal threshold value of >10 mg/L as highly suspicious for infection. Sensitivity has a tight range of 94–100%, specificity from 75.5% to 97%, PPV 59% to 75%, and NPV 95.2% to 97% [9, 12, 38–41, 44, 46]. Bingham et al. in an analysis of alpha-defensin-1 published lower performance of CRP: 79% sensitivity and 66% specificity [47].

Further, the quandary of concomitant diseases or conditions such as heterotopic ossification obfuscates increased values in CRP. Historically, inflammatory arthritides have been a cause of elevated CRP and ESR after total joint arthroplasty, and studies often exclude these patients [48, 49]. A study by Cipriano et al., however, found that CRP and ESR still have diagnostic value in detecting infection in patients with inflammatory arthritis [50]. Optimal thresholds were only slightly altered, and sensitivity, specificity, PPV, and NPV were within narrow ranges. It would stand to reason that aseptic loosening, a process that stimulates macrophages, would also have elevated inflammatory markers. However, Nilsdotter-Augustinsson et al. showed inflammatory markers in this group are well below thresholds [46]. CRP levels have yet to be fully evaluated in the context of total joints for other conditions such as hepatic diseases, poor nutrition, end stage renal disease, or cardiac conditions that may falsely elevate or depress CRP levels.

Given the possible influence of other medical factors in serum CRP values, synovial CRP has been investigated for its diagnostic potential. Multiple studies concluded that while synovial CRP correlates strongly with serum CRP, its diagnostic strength and accuracy was no different from serum CRP [51–54]. Though reaching the same conclusions that no advantage was to be had with synovial CRP, three studies had somewhat differing cutoff values for infection: 2.8, 6.6, and 9.5 mg/L [51, 52, 54].

Combinations of these tests perform better than one alone. This is reflected in the International Consensus diagnosis criteria, whereas the corresponding MSIS criterion was satisfied if just one was elevated. Sanzen et al. noted that ESR and CRP do not always correlate [42]. Nilsdotter-Augustinsson et al. give the ranges of inflammatory markers for both infections and aseptic revisions, and each range includes values above and below the threshold level regardless of the diagnosis of infection [46].

McArthur set out to describe the percent of infections in which one or both ESR and CRP are negative [55]. Twenty-three percent of infected THA's had a normal ESR or CRP, while 16% had a normal ESR and 4% had a normal CRP but elevated ESR. In aggregate, only 4% of infected joints in their registry were found to have both normal ESR and CRP. Notably 18% of this subset of patients had been exposed to antibiotics. Aspirate cell counts, % PMNs, and positive cultures were used to diagnose infection. Austin et al. reinforces the reliability of combining ESR and CRP in clinical practice. Of 116 patients classified as infected, only five had normal ESR and CRP. Because infection continued to be suspected clinically, cultures were obtained preoperatively or intraoperatively and four out of five were positive [38]. It is important to note that normal inflammatory markers can be found with infection.

Synovial White Blood Cell Count and Differential

ESR and CRP are ordered initially in our diagnostic workup for infection. Should these be equivocal or unquestionably positive, we aspirate the synovial fluid for analysis of white blood cell count and percentage of neutrophils. While serum measurements of white blood cell count have minimal diagnostic value, synovial measurements have high diagnostic value [56, 57]. Yet the threshold is not clearly delineated and has fluctuated from 1100 to 4000 white blood cells [6, 9, 10, 39, 50, 57–60]. Moreover the reported units often vary and do not seem reconcilable. Bauer et al. noted that when converted to cells/uL, reported thresholds were 50,000, 2, 2.5, and

1700 cell/μL for infection [8]. They ultimately considered the threshold to be greater than 500 cells/uL. Modification of the threshold does little to change the sensitivities and specificities of cell count. Ghanem et al., using a cutoff of 1100 cells, produced a sensitivity of 90.7%, specificity of 88.1% [60]. A cutoff of 64% neutrophils held a sensitivity of 95% and specificity of 94%. Dinneen et al. had a higher cutoff of 1590 cells/μL and demonstrated a lower sensitivity and specificity: 89.5% and 91.3% [59]. Increasing the threshold to 4200 cells/mL resulted in lowering of the sensitivity to 84% and specificity increased to 93% [10]. The International Consensus settled at 3000 cells/μL and PMN% of >80% as thresholds for chronic infection.

There are few observations about the aspiration technique and quality of the fluid. A dry tap does not disfavor infection as significant scar tissue may compromise the tap or secure pockets of fluid. When fluid is obtained, the quality and appearance can inform suspicion for infection. However, purulent appearing fluid may be of crystalline origin [61]. Metallosis, particularly in hips with metal on metal wear and trunnionosis should also be considered when murky fluid is encountered. Finally, test results may need adjustments if the synovial fluid contains excessive red blood cells. Bloody taps can introduce more WBCs in the aspiration [57]. When dealing with thresholds as low as 1100, this can be significant. We use the following formula [62]:

$$WBC_{corrected} = WBC_{observed} - \left(WBC_{serum} \times RBC_{fluid} / RBC_{serum}\right)$$

IL-6 and Alpha-Defensin

For over a decade, the orthopedic infection literature has strengthened the diagnostic reputation of various biomarkers like synovial IL-6 and alpha-defensin. Deirmengian et al. screened 43 biomarkers from synovial fluid [62]. Five biomarkers had perfect scores with sensitivity of 100% and specificity of 100%: alpha-defensin 1 3 (alpha-defensin), neutrophil elastase-2 (ELA-2), bactericidal/permeability-increasing protein (BPI), and neutrophil gelatinase-associated lipocalin (NGAL). Area under the curve values for eight other markers was over 0.9 (IL-6, IL-1beta, IL-10, IL-1alpha, IL-8, CRP, resistin, and thrombospondin). Of these, IL-6 and alpha-defensin have supportive evidence for their diagnostic use.

IL-6, produced by macrophages and monocytes, is an upstream signaling molecule of hepatocyte producing acute-phase reactants including CRP. Some reports demonstrate a more precise and better diagnostic profile than CRP. IL-6 has been investigated as an infection sentinel [9, 48, 49, 51, 63, 64]. DiCesare et al. reported a case-control study of 58 infected and non infected patients [48] ESR, CRP, and IL-6 were all elevated with infected cases; but IL-6 predictive values were higher than the other markers. Using a threshold of 10 pg/mL, sensitivity was 100%, specificity 95%, PPV 89%, NPV 100%, accuracy 97%. Moreover, the authors note that Il-6 is useful because it does not loiter like ESR and CRP. In terms of surgery, it peaks 6 to 12 h postoperatively and returns to its basal rate 48–72 h after. Another study comparing ESR, CRP, IL-6, procalcitonin, and TNF-alpha in chronic infections from 2007 found that IL-6 and CRP were the best diagnostic indicators for infection. IL-6 (threshold < 12.0 pg/mL) did not perform as well as CRP in this study, with a sensitivity for IL-6 95%, specificity 87%, PPF 74%, NPV 98%, and accuracy of 89% compared to CRP (<3.2 mg/dL) results of 95%, 96%, 91%, 98%, and 96% accuracy [64]. The authors stressed the recurrent principle that combination of these two markers identified every single infected case. Lenski et al. investigated synovial IL-6 and also found a correlation with infection [49]. 10,000 pg/mL, a much greater concentration than serum values, proved an optimal threshold for diagnosing infection. Sensitivity was 90.9%, specificity 94.7%, and the likelihood ratio was 17.27. IL-6 outperformed the other synovial investigative markers lactate dehydrogenase, glucose, and white blood cells. Similar to CRP, synovial and serum IL-6 appear to contain the same ability to diagnose joint infection [65]. Despite consistently high sensitivity and specificity, contextualization and caution must be utilized. As multiple authors note, IL-6 can be elevated during chronic inflammatory states, menstruation, trauma, malignancy, Paget's disease, and multiple sclerosis [34, 48, 64].

Alpha defensin is a more recent biomarker that has garnered attention and is being used clinically to test for infection. It is an antimicrobial peptide released by neutrophils. It depolarizes the bacterium's cell membrane causing a rapid demise [66, 67]. Deirmengian et al. reported synovial alpha-defensin as an appealing marker because it had an excellent diagnostic profile and little change in the setting of inflammatory arthropathies or antibiotics [67]. They identified 112 aseptic patients and 37 infected patients according to the MSIS definition and determined synovial alpha-defensin and CRP levels. The presence of alpha-defensin alone displayed a sensitivity of 97.3% and specificity of 95.5%. 143 of 149 patients were correctly identified. The authors developed an algorithm combining alpha-defensin data with CRP data using a 3 mg/dL threshold. If alpha-defensin was positive, then CRP was analyzed. If CRP was positive, then infection was confirmed. If negative, then an aseptic diagnosis was given. This was because CRP has a much better sensitivity; if negative, it is unlikely to be infected. Together, alpha-defensin and CRP produced a sensitivity of 97.3% and specificity of 100%. This algorithm also suggests that alpha-defensin should be an initial marker rather than a confirmatory marker.

As mentioned, this study noted success with alpha-defensin in two other subgroups: inflammatory arthritic patients and those receiving antibiotics. There were no significant differences in the values of alpha-defensin in those with and without inflammatory arthropathies. This supports the prior findings of Cipriano et al. that ESR, CRP, and synovial white blood cells can be used in patients with inflammatory disease. In patients who had received antibiotics, surprisingly, the threshold for alpha-defensin rose. In contrast, CRP, ESR, and synovial white blood cells all decreased in the context of antibiotic treatment.

Bingham et al. support these conclusions [68]. In 55 painful joints, alpha-defensin outperformed ESR, CRP, and synovial white blood cell count. It achieved a sensitivity of 100% and specificity 95%. In time, alpha-defensin may become a key element to the consensus criteria for the diagnosis of PJI.

Other markers have been evaluated such as IL-4, procalcitonin, and TNF-alpha with underwhelming results. IL-4 has a similar profile to IL-6 but has not been incorporated yet as an infection marker [69]. One simple and quite literal litmus test has been investigated: synovial leukocyte esterase litmus paper test [66, 70, 71]. It offers the benefit of being quick, inexpensive, and widely available as urine dip sticks. More technically intricate solutions though molecular diagnostics and biofilm extraction—Polymerase Chain Reaction (PCR) and Sonication—are being developed. At the current time, however, they are not widely used.

Serum and Synovial Studies in the Acute Perioperative Period

The boundary between acute infection and chronic infection occurs at 6 weeks, by convention. CRP can remain elevated for 3 or more weeks postoperatively while ESR can remain abnormal with diurnal variation for 6 weeks to 3 months [8]. Therefore, thresholds must be adjusted for use in the acute perioperative period of 6 weeks. Bedair et al. found in acute perioperative total knee infections that ESR and CRP were of little value while synovial white blood cell count was most useful. They proposed optimal cutoffs of 27,800 cell/μL, 89% PMNs, and CRP 95 mg/L [72].

Yi et al. performed a similar analysis for acute hip infections [73]. 6033 hips were reviewed of which 73 (1.2%) underwent reoperation. Of those, 36 were diagnosed as infection by the MSIS criteria. Patients who had received antibiotics prior to aspiration were eliminated from the study. As expected, ESR, CRP, synovial white blood cell count, and %PMNs were all elevated compared to the non-infected group. Optimal cutoffs for acute infection were: ESR 44 mm/h, CRP 93 mg/L, synovial WBC 12,800 cells/μL, and 89% PMN. Sensitivities and specificities were as follows: ESR sensitivity 92%, specificity 53%, PPV 76%, NPV 80%; CRP sensitivity 88%, specificity 100%, PPV 100%, NPV 83%; synovial WBC sensitivity 89%, specificity 100%, PPV 100%, NPV 88%, PMN's sensitivity 81%, specificity 90%, PPV 91%, NPV 79%. They recommended use of synovial WBC as the best test for diagnosing infection. For both hips and knees, the international consensus group recommended thresholds of >100 mg/L for CRP, >10,000 cells/μL for synovial WBC, and % PMNs >90%. ESR was not recommended. We routinely use these modified threshold levels for diagnosing infection in the acute period.

Synovial Fluid Cultures

Biomarkers are surrogates for infection, and the elusive gold standard remains direct identification of the pathogen. Culturing aspirated fluid from the joint is the best method for identification of the organism. However, culturing organisms remains a challenge. First, a large enough number of living organisms must be obtained via aspiration. One obstacle to this is the quiescence of bacteria within biofilms [74, 75]. Second, culture methods vary by species, and the correct medium must be employed for the offending pathogen [7]. For some, like mycobacterium and *propionibacterium acnes*, the necessary duration of culture is prolonged beyond the institutional laboratory standard. Third, patients on antibiotic treatment prior to aspiration may have a lower yield.

William Wade commented that "we are grossly ignorant of bacterial life on earth" [76]. Less than 2% of bacteria can be cultured in the lab. The ability to culture 50% of oral flora is actually quite high, when colonic flora are predominantly unable to be cultured [76]. Also, some bacteria can enter a non-culturable state [74]. Since many bacteria living in humans cannot be cultured, efforts are underway to characterize traces of their presence without culture. Genetic polymorphisms render identification difficult; Sendi et al. showed that *E. coli* obtained from synovial fluid differed morphologically from those cultured from biofilms obtained via sonication [75].

By contemporary practices, although culture guides antibiotic treatment, it may not be the defining factor for diagnosis of a hip infection. Furthermore, every painful hip should include infection as part of the differential, but not every painful hip requires aspiration without positive preliminary tests. Barrack et al. aspirated 270 hips before revision surgery to determine whether infection was also present [77]. They determined only six to be infected. Additionally, 32 hips had false-positive results. Their PPV was 6% though NPV 99%. Given these numbers, they recommended aspiration only for those hips with a high pre-test probability of infection. Thus, current recommendations test ESR and CRP first before suggesting hip aspiration in the diagnostic workup of infection.

MSIS requires growth of the same organism from two or more separate specimens for a positive aspiration. The sensitivity of aspiration has been reported over a wide range from 50% to 89%. Its specificity had a more precise range from 81% to 100% with the majority being at the upper end of the range. PPV was 6% to 100% and NPV 35% to 99% [78–81].

Blood culture medium is beneficial for processing the aspirated fluid [80, 82, 83]. Using blood culture medium, Font-Vizcarra et al. found a sensitivity for acute infection of 91%, specificity 100%, PPV 100%, NPV 93%, and for chronic infection it was 79%, 100%, 100%, and 88%, respectively [80]. Geller et al. confirmed the enhancement of positive culture acquisition with 41 positive cultures from blood culture bottles compared to 19 with standard swab techniques [82]. Levine et al. found that the improvement afforded by blood culture medium led to less morbidity and more cost-effectiveness [83]. We routinely send all joint aspiration fluid to the laboratory in blood culture medium.

At most centers, culture results are finalized as early as after 48 to 72 h. Schaefer et al. examined culture results for 14 days [7]. They obtained 10 specimens from each of 284 late revision hip and knee arthroplasties. 110 patients were deemed infected (38.7%), with the majority having identical isolated organisms in two or more specimens. Median time to diagnosis was 4 days by culture. By 7 days, only 73.6% of all infections were identified. After 7 days, infections from *coryneform* species, *peptostreptococcus* species, and *Propionibacterium acnes* became evident. Thus, orthopedic surgeons must know and guide the laboratory protocols at their institutions. When we suspect indolent bacteria or previously had a negative culture from aspiration, we make a special request of our laboratory to monitor cultures longer than the standard protocol of 5 days.

In light of the challenges to diagnosis by aspiration and the variations in culture protocols, Parvisi et al. stated cultures should be viewed as confirmatory tests and be used to guide antibiotic treatment rather than as the gold standard of diagnosis [2]. While patients should not be on a course of antibiotics at the time of aspiration, there is no obstruction to positive culture from normal preoperative antibiotics [84, 85]. Thus we do not hold preoperative antibiotics when obtaining intraoperative culture to guide antibiotic treatment.

Culture Negative Infections

In the setting of high clinical suspicion and positive serological testing, negative cultures may nonetheless indicate a difficult to identify pathogen. Culture negative infections occur in up to 30% of symptomatic joints [29]. These may occur when patients receive prior antibiotic treatment courses, when biofilms sequester bacteria, inadequate laboratory incubation times, when the pathogen is recalcitrant to growth on standard media, or when dealing with unusually fastidious organisms [9]. Berbari et al. reported on the treatment of 60 culture negative infections out of 897 total infections. Many had sinus tracks or findings of purulence. At 5 years, patients treated with two-stage debridement and reimplantation had better outcomes than irrigation, debridement, and poly-exchange with component retention.

Choi et al. found that 40 (23%) of 175 confirmed PJI cases were culture negative [86]. They found no association with age, gender, host condition, and laboratory data. Twenty-seven (68%) of these had undergone recent antibiotic treatment as compared to 53 (42%) of 135 in the positive culture group. They also found an association with a history of resection arthroplasty and a lower ESR. Interestingly, the culture negative group showed a lower rate of treatment failure of 15% recurrent infection compared to 39% in the culture positive group. We recommend a 2-week holiday from all antibiotics prior to aspiration, and repeat aspiration with blood culture media and longer incubation when faced with culture negativity in the setting of high pre-test suspicion for infection.

Atypical Bacterial and Fungal Infections

When suspicion remains high and when cultures remain negative, one should entertain the possibility for an atypical bacteria or fungal infection. There are rare case reports and small series in the literature [87–90]. The true incidence of these types of infections has not been determined. Currently, based on low incidence and expense, fungal and AFB panels are not recommended for routine culture [6, 89]. These tests, instead, may have more value in the setting of high suspicion, failure of medical and surgical treatments, and persistent negative cultures [91]. Comorbid conditions and complex treatment histories increase the risk for this type of infection. Diabetes, autoimmune diseases, immunosuppression, prior periprosthetic infections with prolonged antibiotics, malignancies, HIV, cardiac disease, and hepatic disease all increase the possibility of an atypical infection [87–89]. Fungal cultures should be monitored for up to 4 weeks [88]. Despite the international consensus recommendations, we use AFB panels and fungal cultures for all cultures to increase our yield and in acknowledgment that more than one pathogen may co-exist in an infection.

Intraoperative Frozen Section Histology

The consensus statement defines a minor criterion of infection to be at least five WBC per high powered field in at least five high powered fields at 400-times magnification. The utility of frozen section histology in detecting acute inflammation depends heavily on the skills of the surgical pathologist and varies by institution. Many studies have questioned the performance of histology. Della Valle et al. found that frozen section was helpful for ruling out infection (NPV 95%) but had a poor positive predictive value (PPV 50%) [92].

Despite its inclusion in the international consensus, the use of histology is diminishing [93]. In addition to unreliable performance, other reasons for this include the desire for a diagnosis prior to surgery and the importance of sending appropriate tissue. For example, white blood cells normally exist and can be entrapped in fibrinous tissue around an implant or attached marginally to epithelial cells. This tissue must not be used for frozen section analysis [8, 94]. We have a strong partnership with our musculoskeletal pathologists and a history of reliable results. Thus we routinely obtain histology as one additional datum in the diagnosis of infection.

Sonication

Sonication of explanted hardware has been proposed to increase the yield of cultures [68, 95–99]. Sonication is a method of extracting bacteria from biofilms adherent to prosthetic implants. Because explantation is required, sonication is less a diagnostic tool than a refinement of an already diagnosed infection or presumed infection. Sonication may have value in identifying a specific microbe in culture negative infections or in polymicrobial infections. Newer technologies are emerging that can sonicate hardware in real time and identify the presence of bacteria.

Sonication involves placing the prosthesis first in a sealed container in the operating room. A solution is then added; either Ringer's solution is added in the operating room or Thioglycolate broth is added in the microbiology lab. The prosthesis is then vortexed anywhere from 30 s to 1 min followed by ultrasonication for 5 min. Small 0.5 mL aliquots of the supernatant are then plated onto standard aerobic and anaerobic agar plates and incubated. This process is designed to separate the biofilm from the prosthesis, thus enabling viable bacteria to grow on the agars [98, 99].

Tunney et al. found 26 positive cultures out of 120 hip implants and prepared with sonication [99]. Only five of these showed positive cultures by conventional techniques. Trampuz et al. found a sensitivity of 79% with sonication versus 60.8% with conventional culture [98]. Sonication has greater sensitivity with polymicrobial infections as well. Janz et al. found 12 polymicrobial infections out of 41 infections as compared to six with standard culture [95]. Portillo et al. found 9% polymicrobial infections compared to 4% using standard culture [100]. Sonication can speed the time to positive result as well. Portillo et al. found positive results in 48% of cultures on day two compared to 26% with standard tissue culture. Sonication of antibiotic spacers may guide antibiotic treatment and duration following the second stage. Sori et al. found that 20% of 55 spacers were positive for bacteria at the time of second stage reimplantation, and 63% of those failed by 12 months, compared to 25% of patients with negative sonication cultures [101].

Several issues remain with sonication. First, an institutional infrastructure must be created for sonication of implants and spacers. The laboratory must have access to sonicators. Strict protocols must be followed so that false positives do not result from environmental contamination. It is likely that a commercial sonication technology will be optimized for arthroplasty surgery. At this time, we do not make use of sonication technology but would employ it for revision surgery and second-stage reimplantation surgery if it were available.

Polymerase Chain Reaction (PCR)

Polymerase chain reaction (PCR), bypasses culturing as a method of identifying bacteria is a potential powerful means for detecting pathogens. It amplifies bacterial DNA using primers, and then analyzes those strands using electrophoresis. Not only does

PCR allow for identification of non-culturable bacteria, it avoids the delays of culturing slow growing pathogens such as mycobacterium. Developed as early as the 1970s, its use in identifying periprosthetic infections began to pick up in the 1990s. Synovial fluid from 50 knees were assessed using standard synovial fluid culture, intraoperative culture, and PCR. Six infections were identified with synovial fluid cultures and nine additional infections were identified with intraoperative cultures. PCR, on the other hand, found 32 infections with no false positives from the control group [102]. Panousis et al. found similar results from intraoperative synovial fluid with 12 out of 92 joints diagnosed as infected by culture and 32 cases diagnosed as infected by PCR [103]. They found a 92% sensitivity, 74% specificity, PPV 34%, and NPV 98%. The increase in PCR positive cases were considered false positives. Another study used PCR to identify 17 of 18 culture positive joints and 4 of 5 culture negative infections. It also found organisms in 50 of 57 presumed negative cases [91].

The potential power of PCR has not been found in every study. Using cultures from synovial fluid, biopsy, and sonicate fluid from 366 hip and knee prostheses, Gomez et al. found equivalent sensitivities and specificities for cultures and PCR with no statistical significance differentiating them [104]. On balance, however, studies show that PCR can detect more bacterial species than traditional cultures. It remains questionable whether the identified bacterial nucleic acid is a false positive or an actual symptomatic infection. Ince et al. compared PCR and culture for patients with presumed aseptic acetabular loosening and found that neither identified hidden microorganisms [105]. Ultimately, PCR was not recommended by the international consensus group because of its false-positive variance. We do not utilize this diagnostic test currently.

Case Presentations

Issues, Controversies, Problems

The MSIS criteria and International Consensus offer significant clarity and guidance. Yet when the diagnosis is needed before surgery, the guidelines have been criticized for requiring surgical data, including histology and even aspiration of hip synovial fluid, which is often first performed prior to arthrotomy. Figure 1.1 shows a right hip X-ray taken 17 months after the primary THA. The patient is 78 years old with controlled diabetes (HgA1c: 5.9%), asthma, hypertension, and obesity with BMI of 40 kg/m^2. She presented to the emergency room after experiencing purulent drainage from the inferior aspect of the wound but without systemic symptoms of fevers, chills, or sweats. One week prior, she developed a bulge and blister in the location of the drainage. She reports a recent sinusitis that was treated with a course of antibiotics. She has had worsening of her persistent trochanteric bursitis since the index surgery, without and new development of groin pain. The prior surgeon performed an abductor repair using a suture anchor.

On exam, she did not demonstrate micromotion tenderness with hip movement and had a normal range of motion. She had a 2 cm × 3 cm × 2.5 cm deep wound located at the inferior aspect of her incision, with copious purulent drainage. Serology revealed a CRP of 9.0 mg/L (normal less than

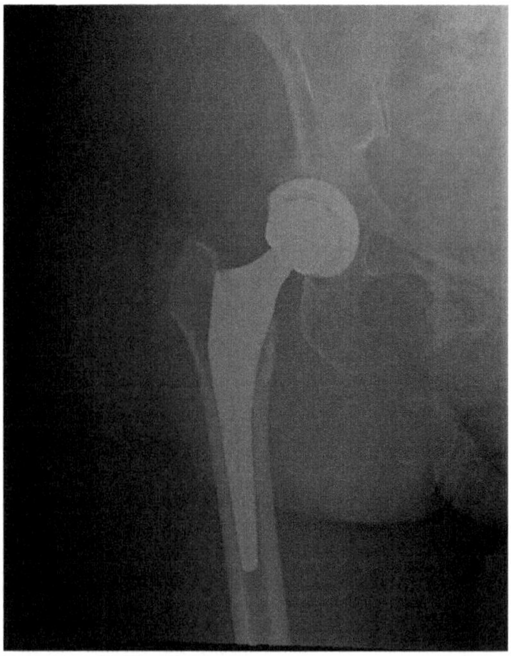

Fig. 1.1 78F presenting 17 months after primary THA with new purulent drainage

10 mg/L) and ESR of 76 mm/h (normal less than 20 mm/h). Though we had little doubt an infection was present, whether the implant was involved remained questionable in setting of abductor repair with suture anchor, persistent bursitis symptoms, and no groin pain, pain with range of motion, and no systemic signs. By the MSIS and International consensus criteria, drainage communicating with the joint would be a sufficient condition for PJI. However, by exploratory probing, the drainage tract had an endpoint. ESR was elevated, but CRP within normal limits. There was no aspiration performed, and thus the diagnosis of infection was deferred until after operative treatment.

Intraoperatively, purulence was encountered outside of the IT band fascia and this communicated to a fluid collection deep to the IT band. There was no apparent communication with the joint space. The transosseous external rotator repair was well healed, as was the abductor tendon repair using suture anchor. No areas of purulence or necrosis were found in the greater trochanter. Upon aspiration of the joint fluid, prior to arthrotomy, purulence was encountered; this showed 360,000 WBC with 99% segmented neutrophils. Histology was not performed. Multiple cultures grew MSSA. Thus the diagnosis of infection was u imately supported by both definitions though neither aspiration results nor cultures were available at the time of surgery due to our institutional testing durations.

This patient was successfully with thorough debridement, irrigation, and exchange of the head and liner, followed by 6 weeks of oxacillin. ESR and CRP at 6 months were normalized, and at 1 year following this surgery, she had no symptoms in the hip.

The reliance of surgical data may lead to delays in diagnosis and even over-treatment of infection. Figure 1.2 is an AP pelvis of a 73-year-old female obtained incidentally 1 year prior to the image in Fig. 1.3. In the intervening year, she suffered urosepsis from *E. coli* with extended spectrum beta-lactamase production. During her hospitalization and treatment, she suffered right hip pain, but no specific evaluation or treatment for it. She lives and was treated abroad in Latin America. She presented with pain and disability

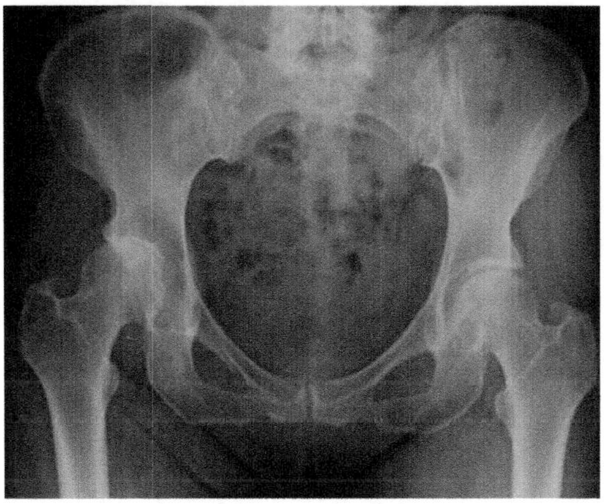

Fig. 1.2 73F with AP pelvis in a 74F

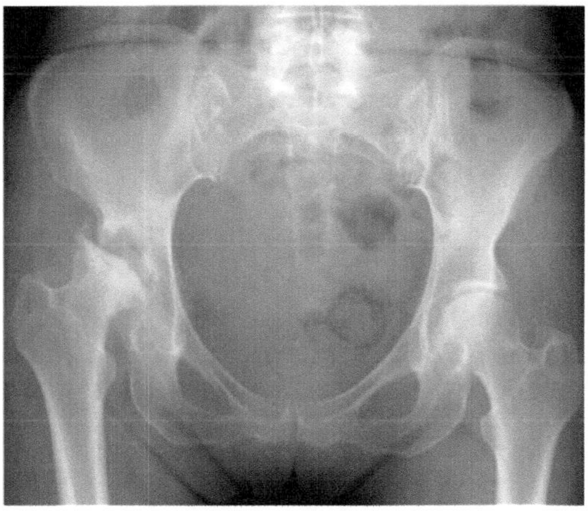

Fig. 1.3 Same patient 1 year later with right hip destruction

but without systemic signs of fevers, chills, or sweats. Her physical exam showed severe pain with range of motion but no swelling, erythema, or drainage. ESR was normal at 19 mm/h, CRP was normal at less than 5 mg/L. We decided to treat conservatively with two-staged replacement due to the recent history suggestive of septic destructive arthritis. Intraoperatively, there was insufficient synovial fluid aspirated through the capsule. Histology revealed fewer than two neutrophils per high powered field seen in multiple samples of tissue. Multiply obtained cultures, including fungal and AFB, were negative. There was a Paprosky 2b acetabular defect. She was successfully treated with debridement, irrigation, a static antibiotic spacer, and 6 weeks of IV antibiotics, followed by reconstruction (Figs. 1.4 and 1.5). At 2 years postoperatively, she had normal ESR, CRP, and resolution of her symptoms.

By criteria, the diagnosis of infection was not supported in this case. We entertained a differential diagnosis that included AVN and rapidly destructive osteoarthritis of the hip. However, the history, prior management in a less medically sophisticated country, presence of bone loss on both sides of the joint, and moth-eaten, segmental appearance of the acetabular bone loss, all lead us to prefer a diagnosis of recently active septic arthritis. At the time of surgery, her presumed infection may have been cured, indolent, culture negative, or incorrectly diagnosed. Nonetheless, the treatment was successful and demonstrated the importance of shared decision-making and fully informed consent.

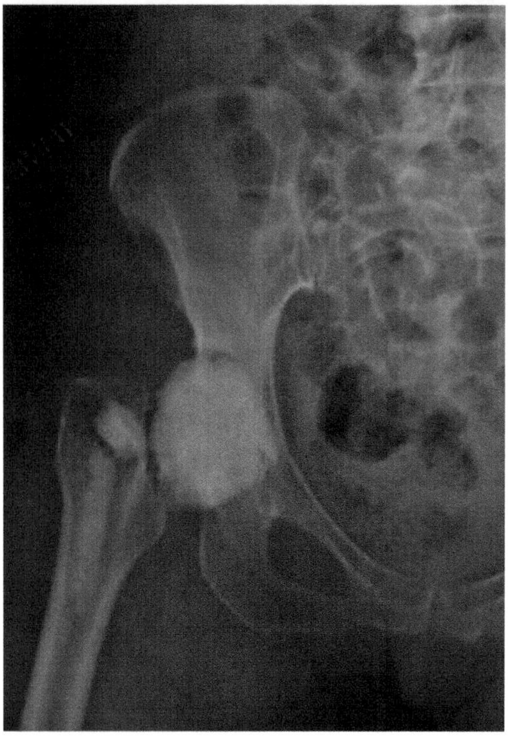

Fig. 1.4 Antibiotic spacer

Similarly, Figs. 1.6, 1.7, and 1.8 show images for a 60-year-old female with uncontrolled diabetes, osteoporosis, and hypertension who presented to the emergency room with acute pain and inability to walk. Two years prior, she was vacationing in Nicaragua and suffered an associated both column fracture from a low energy fall. She was treated locally with dual-column plating through a single Kocher-Langenbeck exposure. One year later, also while vacationing in Nicaragua, she suffered a femoral fracture after a low energy fall and was treated locally with tension band wiring. She was found to have ESR of 86 mm/h, CRP of 136 mg/L (normal less than 10 mg/L) and HgA1c of 12.1%. Intraoperatively, there was no purulence encountered. Synovial fluid was aspirated and periarticular tissues were sent for histology, however in this community hospital neither cell counts nor histology are available and samples must be

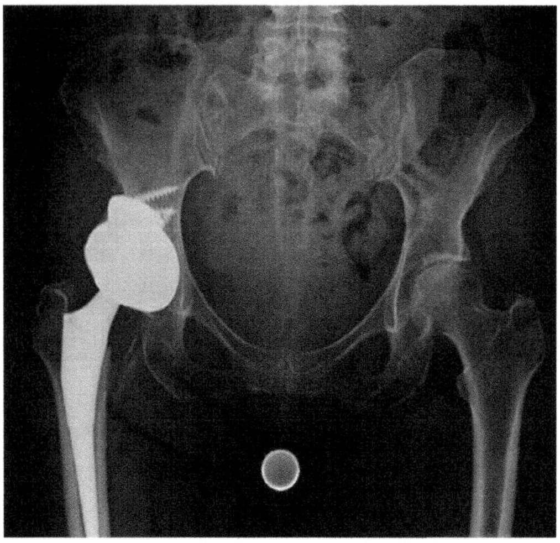

Fig. 1.5 After reconstruction

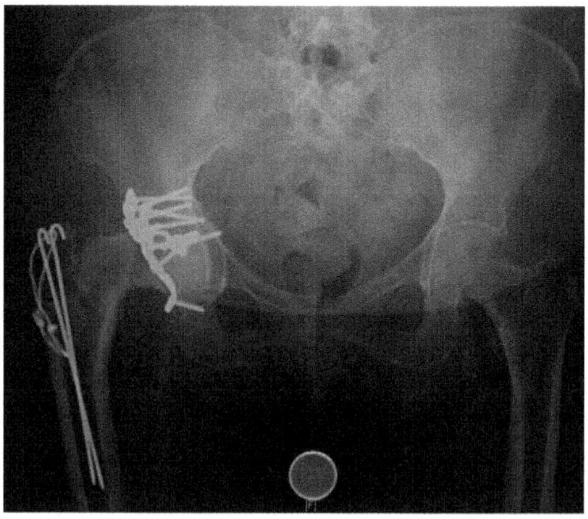

Fig. 1.6 60F with acute R hip pain

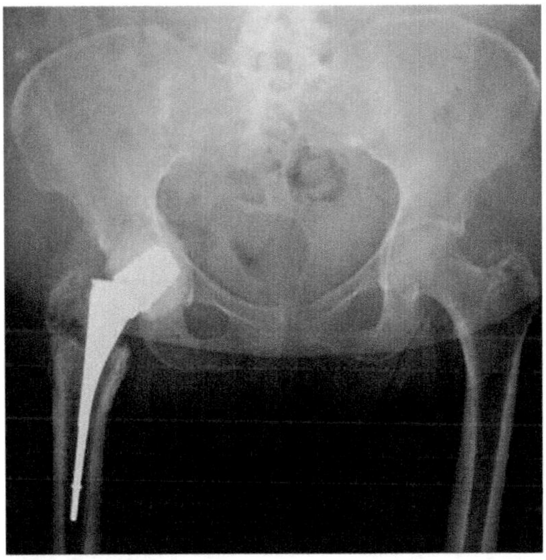

Fig. 1.7 Spacer

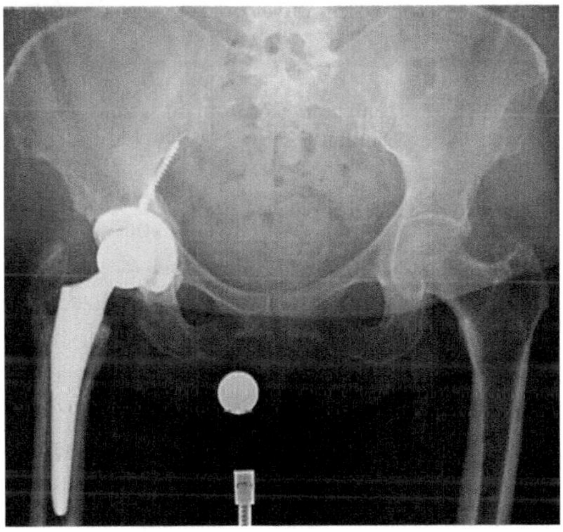

Fig. 1.8 Reconstruction

sent to the university hospital downtown. She had a nonunion of her greater trochanter. Thus, in line with the patient's preferences, an antibiotic spacer was placed after removal of hardware. She received antibiotics for 6 weeks while her diabetes was tightly controlled. When her HgA1c reached a level of 7.8%, and with normalizing trends for her ESR and CRP, she was reconstructed using a primary type of femoral stem. Her inflammatory labs have normalized and her symptoms have resolved at last follow-up of 1 year.

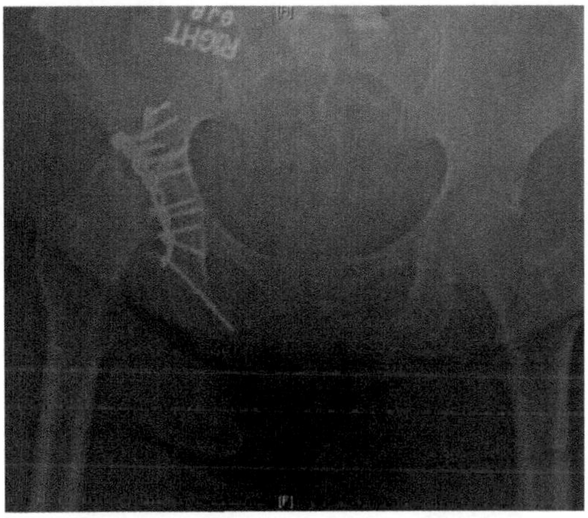

Fig. 1.9 70F after ORIF with *enterococcus* and *proteus*

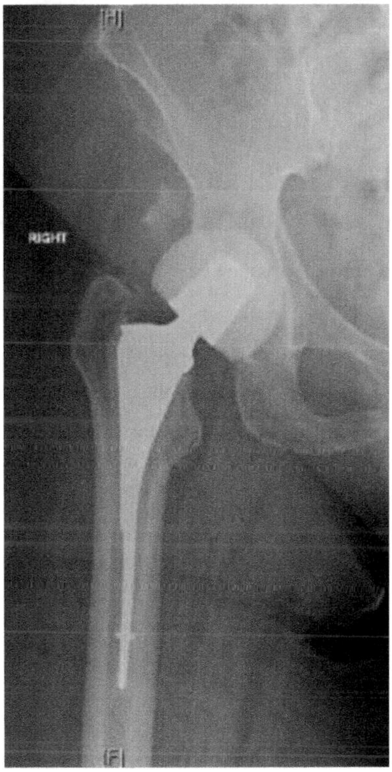

Fig. 1.10 Spacer made with tailored antibiotics

Figures 1.9, 1.10, and 1.11 show a 70-year-old female who presented 18 months after right posterior column and posterior wall fracture following a motor vehicle accident. She has a BMI of 43 kg/m^2 and her post-fracture surgery was complicated by persistent drainage and outside wound cultures

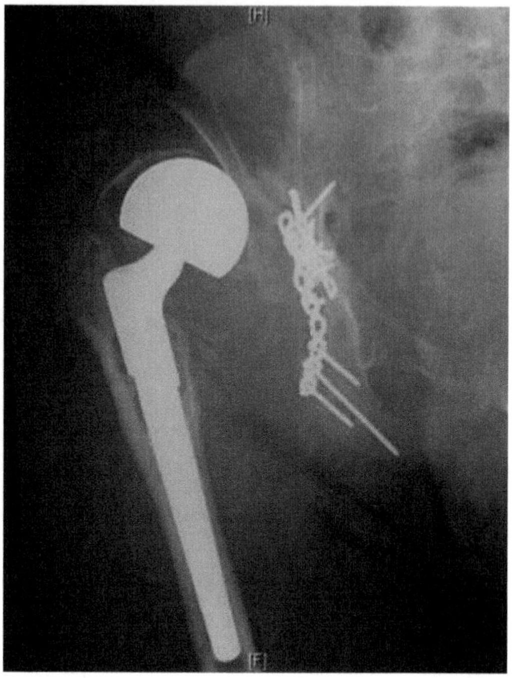

Fig. 1.12 64 M with purulence from his wound and deficient posterior wall after ORIF

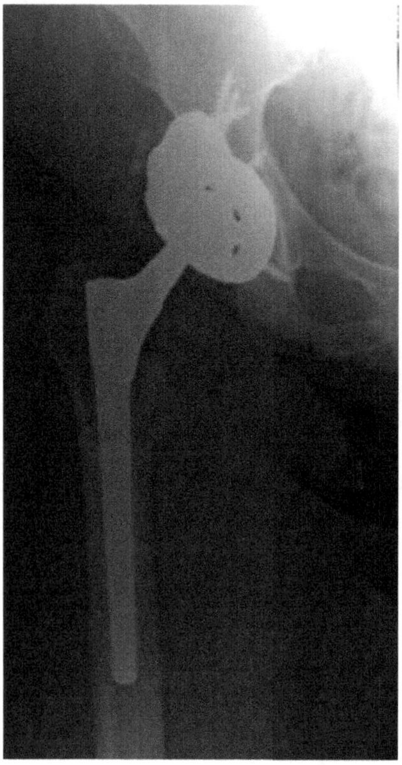

Fig. 1.11 Reconstruction with acetabular augmentation

showing proteus and enterococcus. She had several courses of oral antibiotics prior to presentation. On exam, she had inability to weight bear and pain with all range of motion. Her wound was healed with no drainage or erythema. Her ESR was 61 mm/h and her CRP was 48.1 mg/L. Preoperative aspiration by our radiologist obtained 1 cm^3 of sanguineous fluid that was sent only for aerobic and anaerobic culture and grew nothing. Intraoperatively, she was found to have a large mature capsule 2 in deep to skin and superficial to the fascia. This contained nearly 1 L of seroma fluid. Aspiration of this showed 155 WBC with 3% segmented neutrophils. There was minimal intra-articular fluid. However, histology showed greater than 10 neutrophils/high powered field. Multiple cultures were negative, including AFB and fungal cultures.

By the MSIS criteria and by the International Consensus, the diagnosis of infection was not supported. However, she had multiple courses of antibiotics prior to presentation and the risk of culture negative infection was high. We decided to treat it with an antibiotic spacer and 6 weeks of vancomycin. Once her inflammatory labs normalized, she was reconstructed with a metadiaphyseal fitting stem and acetabular augment to replace the posterior wall and superiolateral bone lost after the fracture. At one 18 months following surgery, she was found to have normalized inflammatory labs and mild symptoms of trochanteric bursitis.

Figures 1.12 and 1.13 show a 64-year-old male who presented to the emergency room with purulent drainage from his right hip incision. He initially had a posterior column fixation after an auto versus bicycle accident 14 years before. He suffers from bipolar disorder, diabetes, atrial fibrillation, and hypertension. He was noncompliant with weight-bearing orders following that surgery and had displacement of his posterior wall with dislocation of his hip. He was treated with closed reduction. Then, 2 years prior to presentation, he was treated elsewhere with a hemiarthroplasty for persistent pain using a size 62 head. This dislocated shortly after surgery and was left dislocated. He had persistent drainage

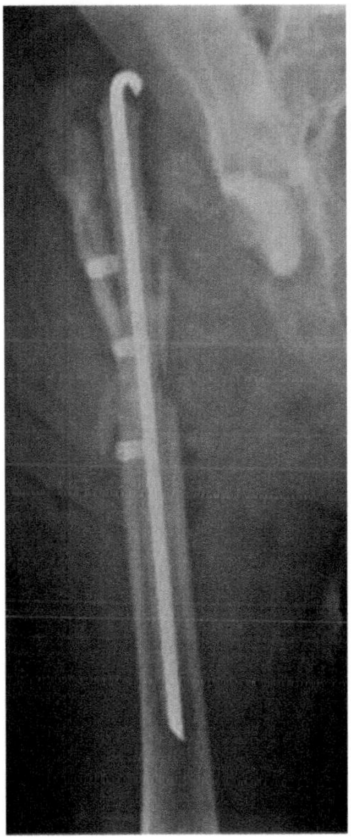

Fig. 1.13 Spacer with tailored antibiotics

and multiple cultures from his wound showing MRSA. He had been on chronic suppressive oral antibiotics. He was able to ambulate with crutches or walker, but spent most of his time in a wheelchair. Exam showed a purulent blister that was not actively draining. His right leg was shortened, but had no pain with range of motion.

Inflammatory labs revealed an ESR of 128 mm/h and CRP of 136 mg/L. With a chronic draining sinus tract that communicated with the implant, he met the diagnostic criteria for infection. Furthermore, he had positive histology and cultures that grew MRSA. He was treated with removal of hardware, extended trochanteric osteotomy, and static antibiotic spacer. He was given 6 weeks of vancomycin. His pain improved and he was satisfied with his level of function which was similar to is preoperative level with a dislocated hemiarthroplasty. Despite our recommendation to undergo reconstruction, he opted to maintain his hip spacer. At 1 year, he is satisfied and without signs of infection.

Tips, Tricks, and Avoiding Pitfalls

As these cases show, getting to a diagnosis of infection in revision hip arthroplasty can be tricky. It is important to consider infection in every differential diagnosis and to obtain serology studies with the standard preoperative workup. Serum ESR and CRP are effective screening tests. When synovial fluid is available, for example, if fluoroscopy or ultrasound guidance is available in the office setting, it too should be analyzed if infection is suspected. Emerging tests, like alpha-defensin, may prove to be effective for diagnosis. For the time being, the MSIS criteria and the International Consensus can be helpful to guide the diagnosis of infection.

When the diagnosis of infection is not clear prior to surgery, it is critical that a thorough discussion with the patient covers the possibility of infection. A missed diagnosis may mean multiple revision surgeries with high comorbidity. Oftentimes, the patient's preference will help steer the operative management of the revision surgery. While unindicated surgery is never advocated, the high incidence of culture negative infections supports the notion of erring on the side of temporary antibiotic spacer.

We recommend sending tissue cultures and fluid samples in odd numbers, preferably 3 or 5. This will help prevent "ties" and concerns for contamination or unreliable results. We recommend using blood culture medium for all fluid cultures. Furthermore, on a technical note, we recommend sterilizing the top of the culture bottles with an alcohol swab and changing the needle prior to puncture of the blood culture tubes. When the amount of fluid obtained is insufficient for multiple studies, we preferentially send the cell count, followed by culture, and lastly, crystal analysis.

Authors' Preferred Method

- Our preferred diagnostic framework follows the MSIS and International Consensus closely. However, as the prior cases demonstrate, we will frequently augment the guidelines with our clinical judgment and err towards treating a possible infection. Without a robust gold standard for the diagnosis of infection, it is important to take in all data and synthesize an overall pre-test probability of infection. Furthermore, we incorporate alpha-defensin into our implementation of the guidelines when we have synovial fluid for analysis. We do not routinely employ nuclear imaging, IL-6, sonication, or PCR in our diagnosis of hip infection.

Take-Home Points

- Consider infection in every differential diagnosis prior to revision THA.
- Obtain ESR and CRP as part of every preoperative workup prior to revision arthroplasty.
- If either is elevated, consider aspiration of the synovial fluid for alpha-defensin, cell count and differential, culture, and crystal analysis.
- Histology is a helpful adjunct. If you do not currently have reliable pathology partners, consider working with them to develop their reliability.
- Do not send fibrinous periprosthetic tissue for histology, which is less reliable than synovial tissue.
- Always send an odd number of cultures, either 3 or 5, from multiple sites around the hip.
- Culture negative infections are common. Cultures are not a gold standard for diagnosing infection and negative cultures do not rule infection out.
- While the morbidity of an unnecessary two-stage revision is far from trivial, for many patients it may be preferable to the risk of a later two-stage revision.
- Thoroughly discuss the possibility of infection with patients when the diagnosis is unclear. Their risk tolerance will help guide the optimal treatment when the diagnosis is unclear.
- There is an unmet need for a gold standard test to diagnose infection, and tests with better performance will be introduced in the coming years.

References

1. Hozack WJ, Parvizi J. New definition for periprosthetic joint infection. J Arthroplast. 2011;26(8):1135.
2. Parvizi J. New definition for periprosthetic joint infection. Am J Orthop. 2011;40(12):614.
3. Parvizi J, Zmistowski B, Berbari EF, Bauer TW, Springer BD, Della Valle CJ, Garvin KL, Mont MA, Wongworawat MD, Zalavras CG. New definition for periprosthetic joint infection: from the Workgroup of the Musculoskeletal Infection Society. Clin Orthop Relat Res. 2011;469(11):2992.
4. Workgroup Convened by the Musculoskeletal Infection Society. New definition for periprosthetic joint infection. J Arthroplasty. 2011;26(8):1136.
5. Alijanipour P, Adeli B, Hansen EN, Chen AF, Parvizi J. Intraoperative purulence is not reliable for diagnosing periprosthetic joint infection. J Arthroplast. 2015;30(8):1403.
6. Cats-Baril W, Gehrke T, Huff K, Kendoff D, Maltenfort M, Parvizi J. International consensus on periprosthetic joint infection: description of the consensus process. Clin Orthop Relat Res. 2013;471(12):4065.
7. Schäfer P, Fink B, Sandow D, Margull A, Berger I, Frommelt L. Prolonged bacterial culture to identify late periprosthetic joint infection: a promising strategy. Clin Infect Dis. 2008;47(11):1403.
8. Bauer TW, Parvizi J, Kobayashi N, Krebs V. Diagnosis of periprosthetic infection. J Bone Joint Surg. 2006;88(4):869.
9. Berbari E, Mabry T, Tsaras G, Spangehl M, Erwin PJ, Murad MH, Steckelberg J, Osmon D. Inflammatory blood laboratory levels as markers of prosthetic joint infection: a systematic review and meta-analysis. J Bone Joint Surg Am. 2010;92(11):2102–9.
10. Schinsky MF. Perioperative testing for joint infection in patients undergoing revision total hip arthroplasty. J Bone Joint Surg Am. 2008;90(9):1869.
11. Fitzgerald RH Jr, Nolan DR, Ilstrup DM, Van Scoy RE, Washington JA 2nd, Coventry MB. Deep wound sepsis following total hip arthroplasty. J Bone Joint Surg Am. 1977;59(7):847.
12. Spangehl MJ, Younger AS, Masri BA, Duncan CP. Diagnosis of infection following total hip arthroplasty. Instr Course Lect. 1998;47:285.
13. Tsukayama DT, Estrada R, Gustilo RB. Infection after total hip arthroplasty. A study of the treatment of one hundred and six infections. J Bone Joint Surg Am. 1996;78(4):512.
14. Barrett L, Atkins B. The clinical presentation of prosthetic joint infection. J Antimicrob Chemother. 2014;69(Suppl 1):i25.
15. Peel TN, Cheng AC, Buising KL, Choong PFM. Microbiological aetiology, epidemiology, and clinical profile of prosthetic joint infections: are current antibiotic prophylaxis guidelines effective? Antimicrob Agents Chemother. 2012;56(5):2386.

16. Virolainen P, Lahteenmaki H, Hiltunen A, Sipola E, Meurman O, Nelimarkka O. The reliability of diagnosis of infection during revision arthroplasties. Scand J Surg. 2002;91(2):178.
17. Everhart JS, Altneu E, Calhoun JH. Medical comorbidities are independent preoperative risk factors for surgical infection after total joint arthroplasty. Clin Orthop Relat Res. 2013;471(10):3112.
18. Kurtz SM, Lau E, Schmier J, Ong KL, Zhao K, Parvizi J. Infection burden for hip and knee arthroplasty in the United States. J Arthroplast. 2008;23(7):984.
19. Kurtz SM, Ong KL, Lau E, Bozic KJ, Berry D, Parvizi J. Prosthetic joint infection risk after TKA in the medicare population. Clin Orthop Relat Res. 2009;468(1):52.
20. Pugely AJ, Martin CT, Gao Y, Schweizer ML, Callaghan JJ. The incidence of and risk factors for 30-day surgical site infections following primary and revision total joint arthroplasty. J Arthroplast. 2015;30(9):47.
21. Pulido L, Ghanem E, Joshi A, Purtill JJ, Parvizi J. Periprosthetic joint infection: the incidence, timing, and predisposing factors. Clin Orthop Relat Res. 1710;466(7):2008.
22. Urquhart DM, Hanna FS, Brennan SL, Wluka AE, Leder K, Cameron PA, Graves SE, Cicuttini FM. Incidence and risk factors for deep surgical site infection after primary total hip arthroplasty: a systematic review. J Arthroplast. 2010;25(8):1216.
23. Chryssikos T, Parvizi J, Ghanem E, Newberg A, Zhuang H, Alavi A. FDG-PET imaging can diagnose periprosthetic infection of the hip. Clin Orthop Relat Res. 2008;466(6):1338.
24. Gemmel F, Van den Wyngaert H, Love C, Welling MM, Gemmel P, Palestro CJ. Prosthetic joint infections: radionuclide state-of-the-art imaging. Eur J Nucl Med Mol Imaging. 2012;39(5):892.
25. Joseph TN, Mujtaba M, Chen AL, Maurer SL, Zuckerman JD, Maldjian C, Di Cesare PE. Efficacy of combined technetium-99m sulfur colloid/indium-111 leukocyte scans to detect infected total hip and knee arthroplasties. J Arthroplast. 2001;16(6):753.
26. Kwee TC, Kwee RM, Alavi A. FDG-PET for diagnosing prosthetic joint infection: systematic review and metaanalysis. Eur J Nucl Med Mol Imaging. 2008;35(11):2122.
27. Love C, Marwin SE, Palestro CJ. Nuclear medicine and the infected joint replacement. Semin Nucl Med. 2009;39(1):66.
28. Nagoya S, Kaya M, Sasaki M, Tateda K, Yamashita T. Diagnosis of peri-prosthetic infection at the hip using triple-phase bone scintigraphy. J Bone Joint Surg Br Vol. 2008;90-B(2):140.
29. Nodzo SR, Bauer T, Pottinger PS, Garrigues GE, Bedair H, Deirmengian CA, Segreti J, Blount KJ, Omar IM, Parvizi J. Conventional diagnostic challenges in periprosthetic joint infection. J Am Acad Orthop Surg. 2015;23:S18.
30. Palestro CJ, Love C, Tronco GG, Tomas MB, Rini JN. Combined labeled leukocyte and technetium 99m sulfur colloid bone marrow imaging for diagnosing musculoskeletal infection. Radiographics. 2006;26(3):859.
31. Scher DM, Pak K, Lonner JH, Finkel JE, Zuckerman JD, Di Cesare PE. The predictive value of indium-III leukocyte scans in the diagnosis of infected total hip, knee, or resection arthroplasties. J Arthroplast. 2000;15(3):295.
32. van der Bruggen W, Bleeker-Rovers CP, Boerman OC, Gotthardt M, Oyen WJG. PET and SPECT in osteomyelitis and prosthetic bone and joint infections: a systematic review. Semin Nucl Med. 2010;40(1):3.
33. Reinartz P, Mumme T, Hermanns B, Cremerius U, Wirtz DC, Schaefer WM, Niethard F-U, Buell U. Radionuclide imaging of the painful hip arthroplasty: positron-emission tomography versus triple-phase bone scanning. J Bone Joint Surg Br. 2005;87-B(4):465.
34. Levitsky KA, Hozack WJ, Balderston RA, Rothman RH, Gluckman SJ, Maslack MM, Booth RE. Evaluation of the painful prosthetic joint. J Arthroplast. 1991;6(3):237.
35. Pill SG, Parvizi J, Tang PH, Garino JP, Nelson C, Zhuang H, Alavi A. Comparison of fluorodeoxyglucose positron emission tomography and 111Indium–white blood cell imaging in the diagnosis of periprosthetic infection of the hip. J Arthroplast. 2006;21(6):91.
36. Diaz-Ledezma C, Lamberton C, Lichstein P, Parvizi J. Diagnosis of periprosthetic joint infection: the role of nuclear medicine may be overestimated. J Arthroplast. 2015;30(6):1044.
37. Love C, Marwin SE, Tomas MB, Krauss ES, Tronco GG, Bhargava KK, Nichols KJ, Palestro CJ. Diagnosing infection in the failed joint replacement: a comparison of coincidence detection 18F-FDG and 111In-labeled leukocyte/99mTc-sulfur colloid marrow imaging. J Nucl Med. 1864;45(11):2004.
38. Austin MS, Ghanem E, Joshi A, Lindsay A, Parvizi J. A simple, cost-effective screening protocol to rule out periprosthetic infection. J Arthroplasty. 2008;23(1):65.
39. Della Valle CJ, Sporer SM, Jacobs JJ, Berger RA, Rosenberg AG, Paprosky WG. Preoperative testing for sepsis before revision total knee arthroplasty. J Arthroplast. 2007;22(6):90.
40. Greidanus NV. Use of erythrocyte sedimentation rate and C-reactive protein level to diagnose infection before revision total knee arthroplasty. A prospective evaluation. J Bone Joint Surg Am. 2007;89(7):1409.
41. Larsson S, Thelander ULF, Friberg S. C-reactive protein (CRP) levels after elective orthopedic surgery. Clin Orthop Relat Res. 1992;275:237–42.
42. Sanzen L, Carlsson AS. The diagnostic value of C-reactive protein in infected total hip arthroplasties. J Bone Joint Surg Br. 1989;71(4):638.

43. Krzysztof Bochen AK, Milaniuk S, Kulczyńska M, Prystupa A, Dzida G. Erythrocyte sedimentation rate—an old marker with new applications. J Pre Clin Clin Res. 2011;5(2):50.
44. Spangehl MJ, Masri BA, O'Connell JX, Duncan CP. Prospective analysis of preoperative and intraoperative investigations for the diagnosis of infection at the sites of two hundred and two revision total hip arthroplasties. J Bone Joint Surg Am. 1999;81(5):672.
45. Pepys MB, Hirschfield GM. C-reactive protein: a critical update. J Clin Investig. 1805;111(12):2003.
46. Nilsdotter-Augustinsson Å, Briheim G, Herder A, Ljunghusen O, Wahlström O, Öhman L. Inflammatory response in 85 patients with loosened hip prostheses: a prospective study comparing inflammatory markers in patients with aseptic and septic prosthetic loosening. Acta Orthop. 2007;78(5):629.
47. Bingham J, Clarke H, Spangehl M, Schwartz A, Beauchamp C, Goldberg B. The alpha defensin-1 biomarker assay can be used to evaluate the potentially infected total joint arthroplasty. Clin Orthop Relat Res. 2014;472(12):4006.
48. Di Cesare PE. Serum interleukin-6 as a marker of periprosthetic infection following total hip and knee arthroplasty. J Bone Joint Surg Am. 2005;87(9):1921.
49. Lenski M, Scherer MA. Synovial IL-6 AS inflammatory marker in periprosthetic joint infections. J Arthroplast. 2014;29(6):1105.
50. Cipriano CA, Brown NM, Michael AM, Moric M, Sporer SM, Della Valle CJ. Serum and synovial fluid analysis for diagnosing chronic periprosthetic infection in patients with inflammatory arthritis. J Bone Joint Surg Am. 2012;94(7):594–600.
51. Jacovides CL, Parvizi J, Adeli B, Jung KA. Molecular markers for diagnosis of periprosthetic joint infection. J Arthroplast. 2011;26(6):99.
52. Parvizi J, Jacovides C, Adeli B, Jung KA, Hozack WJ, Mark B. Coventry award: synovial C-reactive protein: a prospective evaluation of a molecular marker for periprosthetic knee joint infection. Clin Orthop Relat Res. 2011;470(1):54.
53. Tetreault MW, Wetters NG, Moric M, Gross CE, Della Valle CJ. Is synovial C-reactive protein a useful marker for periprosthetic joint infection? Clin Orthop Relat Res. 2014;472(12):3997.
54. Vanderstappen C, Verhoeven N, Stuyck J, Bellemans J. Intra-articular versus serum C-reactive protein analysis in suspected periprosthetic knee joint infection. Acta Orthop Belg. 2013;79(3):326.
55. McArthur BA, Abdel MP, Taunton MJ, Osmon DR, Hanssen AD. Seronegative infections in hip and knee arthroplasty: periprosthetic infections with normal erythrocyte sedimentation rate and C-reactive protein level. Bone Joint J. 2015;97-B(7):939.
56. Toossi N, Adeli B, Rasouli MR, Huang R, Parvizi J. Serum white blood cell count and differential do not have a role in the diagnosis of periprosthetic joint infection. J Arthroplast. 2012;27(8):51.
57. Zmistowski B, Restrepo C, Huang R, Hozack WJ, Parvizi J. Periprosthetic joint infection diagnosis. J Arthroplast. 2012;27(9):1589.
58. Bar J, MacDonald SJ, Bourne RB. Preoperative evaluations in revision total knee arthroplasty. Clin Orthop Relat Res. 2006;446:40.
59. Dinneen A, Guyot A, Clements J, Bradley N. Synovial fluid white cell and differential count in the diagnosis or exclusion of prosthetic joint infection. Bone Joint J. 2013;95-B(4):554.
60. Ghanem E. Cell count and differential of aspirated fluid in the diagnosis of infection at the site of total knee arthroplasty. J Bone Joint Surg Am. 2008;90(8):1637.
61. Freehill MT, McCarthy EF, Khanuja HS. Total knee arthroplasty failure and gouty arthropathy. J Arthroplasty. 2010;25(4):658.e7.
62. Shah RP, Sheth NP, Gray C, Alosh H, Garino JP. Periprosthetic fractures around loose femoral components. J Am Acad Orthop Surg. 2014;22(8):482.
63. Deirmengian C, Kardos K, Kilmartin P, Cameron A, Schiller K, Parvizi J. Diagnosing periprosthetic joint infection: has the era of the biomarker arrived? Clin Orthop Relat Res. 2014;472(11):3254.
64. Bottner F, Wegner A, Winkelmann W, Becker K, Erren M, Gotze C. Interleukin-6, procalcitonin and TNF-: markers of peri-prosthetic infection following total joint replacement. J Bone Joint Surg Br Vol. 2007;89-B(1):94.
65. Randau TM, Friedrich MJ, Wimmer MD, Reichert B, Kuberra D, Stoffel-Wagner B, Limmer A, Wirtz DC, Gravius S. Interleukin-6 in serum and in synovial fluid enhances the differentiation between periprosthetic joint infection and aseptic loosening. PLoS One. 2014;9(2):e89045.
66. Deirmengian C, Kardos K, Kilmartin P, Cameron A, Schiller K, Booth RE, Parvizi J. The alpha-defensin test for periprosthetic joint infection outperforms the leukocyte esterase test strip. Clin Orthop Relat Res. 2014;473(1):198.
67. Deirmengian C, Kardos K, Kilmartin P, Cameron A, Schiller K, Parvizi J. Combined measurement of synovial fluid—defensin and C-reactive protein levels: highly accurate for diagnosing periprosthetic joint infection. J Bone Joint Surg. 2014;96(17):1439.
68. Achermann Y, Vogt M, Leunig M, Wust J, Trampuz A. Improved diagnosis of periprosthetic joint infection by multiplex PCR of sonication fluid from removed implants. J Clin Microbiol. 2010;48(4):1208.
69. Gollwitzer H, Dombrowski Y, Prodinger PM, Peric M, Summer B, Hapfelmeier A, Saldamli B, Pankow F, von Eisenhart-Rothe R, Imhoff AB, Schauber J, Thomas P, Burgkart R, Banke IJ. Antimicrobial peptides and proinflammatory cytokines in periprosthetic joint infection. J Bone Joint Surg Am. 2013;95(7):644.
70. Parvizi J, Jacovides C, Antoci V, Ghanem E. Diagnosis of periprosthetic joint infection: the

utility of a simple yet unappreciated enzyme. J Bone Joint Surg Am. 2011;93(24):2242–8.
71. Wetters NG, Berend KR, Lombardi AV, Morris MJ, Tucker TL, Della Valle CJ. Leukocyte esterase reagent strips for the rapid diagnosis of periprosthetic joint infection. J Arthroplast. 2012;27(8):8.
72. Bedair H, Ting N, Jacovides C, Saxena A, Moric M, Parvizi J, Della Valle CJ. The Mark Coventry award: diagnosis of early postoperative TKA infection using synovial fluid analysis. Clin Orthop Relat Res. 2010;469(1):34.
73. Yi PH, Cross MB, Moric M, Sporer SM, Berger RA, Della Valle CJ. The 2013 Frank Stinchfield award: diagnosis of infection in the early postoperative period after total hip arthroplasty. Clin Orthop Relat Res. 2013;472(2):424.
74. Oliver JD. The viable but nonculturable state in bacteria. J Microbiol. 2005;43 Spec No:93.
75. Sendi P, Frei R, Maurer TB, Trampuz A, Zimmerli W, Graber P. Escherichia coli variants in periprosthetic joint infection: diagnostic challenges with sessile bacteria and sonication. J Clin Microbiol. 1720;48(5):2010.
76. Wade W. Unculturable bacteria—the uncharacterized organisms that cause oral infections. JRSM. 2002;95(2):81.
77. Barrack RL, Harris WH. The value of preoperative aspiration in revision total hip replacement surgery. J Arthroplast. 1993;8(1):101.
78. Fehring TK, Cohen B. Aspiration as a guide to sepsis in revision total hip arthroplasty. J Arthroplast. 1996;11(5):543.
79. Fink B, Makowiak C, Fuerst M, Berger I, Schafer P, Frommelt L. The value of synovial biopsy, joint aspiration and C-reactive protein in the diagnosis of late peri-prosthetic infection of total knee replacements. J Bone Joint Surg Br Vol. 2008;90-B(7):874.
80. Font-Vizcarra L, García S, Martínez-Pastor JC, Sierra JM, Soriano A. Blood culture flasks for culturing synovial fluid in prosthetic joint infections. Clin Orthop Relat Res. 2010;468(8):2238.
81. Somme D, Ziza J-M, Desplaces N, Chicheportiche V, Chazerain P, Leonard P, Lhotellier L, Jacquenod P, Mamoudy P. Contribution of routine joint aspiration to the diagnosis of infection before hip revision surgery. Joint Bone Spine. 2003;70(6):489.
82. Geller JA, MacCallum KP, Murtaugh TS, Patrick DA, Liabaud B, Jonna VK. Prospective comparison of blood culture bottles and conventional swabs for microbial identification of suspected periprosthetic joint infection. J Arthroplasty. 2016;31(8):1779–83.
83. Levine BR, Evans BG. Use of blood culture vial specimens in intraoperative detection of infection. Clin Orthop Relat Res. 2001;382:222.
84. Burnett RSJ, Aggarwal A, Givens SA, McClure JT, Morgan PM, Barrack RL. Prophylactic antibiotics do not affect cultures in the treatment of an infected TKA: a prospective trial. Clin Orthop Relat Res 2009;468(1):127.
85. Tetreault MW, Wetters NG, Aggarwal V, Mont M, Parvizi J, Della Valle CJ. The Chitranjan Ranawat Award: should prophylactic antibiotics be withheld before revision surgery to obtain appropriate cultures? Clin Orthop Relat Res. 2013;472(1):52.
86. Choi H-R, Kwon Y-M, Freiberg AA, Nelson SB, Malchau H. Periprosthetic joint infection with negative culture results: clinical characteristics and treatment outcome. J Arthroplast. 2013;28(6):899.
87. Anagnostakos K, Kelm J, Schmitt E, Jung J. Fungal periprosthetic hip and knee joint infections. J Arthroplast. 2012;27(2):293.
88. Azzam K. Microbiological, clinical, and surgical features of fungal prosthetic joint infections: a multi-institutional experience. J Bone Joint Surg Am. 2009;91(Suppl_6):142.
89. Gebauer M, Frommelt L, Achan P, Board TN, Conway J, Griffin W, Heidari N, Kerr G, McLaren A, Nelson SB, Nijhof M, Zahar A. Management of fungal or atypical periprosthetic joint infections. J Arthroplast. 2014;29(2):112.
90. Hwang BH, Yoon JY, Nam CH, Jung KA, Lee SC, Han CD, Moon SH. Fungal peri-prosthetic joint infection after primary total knee replacement. Bone Joint J. 2012;94-B(5):656.
91. Jacovides CL, Kreft R, Adeli B, Hozack B, Ehrlich GD, Parvizi J. Successful identification of pathogens by polymerase chain reaction (PCR)-based electron spray ionization time-of-flight mass spectrometry (ESI-TOF-MS) in culture-negative periprosthetic joint infection. J Bone Joint Surg Am. 2012;94(24):2247.
92. Della Valle CJ, Bogner E, Desai P, Lonner JH, Adler E, Zuckerman JD, Di Cesare PE. Analysis of frozen sections of intraoperative specimens obtained at the time of reoperation after hip or knee resection arthroplasty for the treatment of infection. J Bone Joint Surg Am. 1999;81(5):684.
93. Parvizi J, Adeli B, Zmistowski B, Restrepo C, Greenwald AS. Management of periprosthetic joint infection: the current knowledge. J Bone Joint Surg Am. 2012;94(14):e104 1.
94. Athanasou NA, Pandey R, de Steiger R, Crook D, Smith PM. Diagnosis of infection by frozen section during revision arthroplasty. J Bone Joint Surg Br. 1995;77(1):28.
95. Janz V, Wassilew GI, Kribus M, Trampuz A, Perka C. Improved identification of polymicrobial infection in total knee arthroplasty through sonicate fluid cultures. Arch Orthop Trauma Surg. 2015;135(10):1453.
96. Puig-Verdie L, Alentorn-Geli E, Gonzalez-Cuevas A, Sorli L, Salvado M, Alier A, Pelfort X, Portillo ME, Horcajada JP. Implant sonication increases the diagnostic accuracy of infection in patients with delayed, but not early, orthopaedic implant failure. Bone Joint J. 2013;95-B(2):244.
97. Shen H, Tang J, Wang Q, Jiang Y, Zhang X. Sonication of explanted prosthesis combined with incubation in BD Bactec bottles for pathogen-

based diagnosis of prosthetic joint infection. J Clin Microbiol. 2014;53(3):777.
98. Trampuz A, Piper KE, Jacobson MJ, Hanssen AD, Unni KK, Osmon DR, Mandrekar JN, Cockerill FR, Steckelberg JM, Greenleaf JF, Patel R. Sonication of removed hip and knee prostheses for diagnosis of infection. N Engl J Med. 2007;357(7):654.
99. Tunney MM, Patrick S, Gorman SP, Nixon JR, Anderson N, Davis RI, Hanna D, Ramage G. Improved detection of infection in hip replacements: a currently underestimated problem. J Bone Joint Surg. 1998;80(4):568.
100. Portillo ME, Salvadó M, Sorli L, Alier A, Martínez S, Trampuz A, Gómez J, Puig L, Horcajada JP. Multiplex PCR of sonication fluid accurately differentiates between prosthetic joint infection and aseptic failure. J Infect. 2012;65(6):541.
101. Sorli L, Puig L, Torres-Claramunt R, Gonzalez A, Alier A, Knobel H, Salvado M, Horcajada JP. The relationship between microbiology results in the second of a two-stage exchange procedure using cement spacers and the outcome after revision total joint replacement for infection: the use of sonication to aid bacteriological analysis. Bone Joint J. 2012;94-B(2):249.
102. Mariani BD, Martin DS, Levine MJ, Booth RE, Tuan RS. Polymerase chain reaction detection of bacterial infection in total knee arthroplasty. Clin Orthop Relat Res. 1996;331:11.
103. Panousis K, Grigoris P, Butcher I, Rana B, Reilly JH, Hamblen DL. Poor predictive value of broad-range PCR for the detection of arthroplasty infection in 92 cases. Acta Orthop. 2005;76(3):341.
104. Gomez E, Cazanave C, Cunningham SA, Greenwood-Quaintance KE, Steckelberg JM, Uhl JR, Hanssen AD, Karau MJ, Schmidt SM, Osmon DR, Berbari EF, Mandrekar J, Patel R. Prosthetic joint infection diagnosis using broad-range PCR of biofilms dislodged from knee and hip arthroplasty surfaces using sonication. J Clin Microbiol. 2012;50(11):3501.
105. Ince A, Rupp J, Frommelt L, Katzer A, Gille J, Lohr JF. Is "aseptic" loosening of the prosthetic cup after total hip replacement due to nonculturable bacterial pathogens in patients with low-grade infection? Clin Infect Dis. 2004;39(11):1599.

The Infected Prosthetic Knee

2

Raphael S. F. Longobardi

Introduction

> From this I conclude that the best education for the situations of actual life consists of the experience we acquire from the study of serious history. For it is history alone which without causing us harm enables us to judge what is the best course in any situation or circumstance. (Polybius, The Rise of the Roman Empire, 264 B.C. [1])

Our responsibility, as physicians, lies in our ability to diagnosis and to treat various disease processes. There are few conditions and processes more debilitating and potentially more catastrophic, than an infected prosthetic joint. The diagnosis of this condition is fraught with challenges, as we still await a single diagnostic test with 100% specificity and sensitivity. Until that time when one is available, we physicians must rely on our clinical acumen and suspicions, along with understanding the patient's clinical history, for ascertaining this diagnosis. The goals of this chapter are to review the conditions and clinical landscape that surround this diagnosis; review the current literature regarding the diagnosis and treatment; discuss a step-wise algorithm for identification of this condition, and review technical procedures for resolving this debilitating complication.

R. S. F. Longobardi (✉)
Department of Orthopaedic Surgery, RWJ Barnabas Health, Jersey City, NJ, USA

Department of Orthopaedic Surgery, NYU Langone Health, NYU Grossman School of Medicine, New York, NY, USA

Incidence

Total knee arthroplasty is a remarkable clinically successful procedure and the number performed in younger and more active patients is increasing every year. As patients outlive the longevity of their implants, the expected volume of revisions is expected to increase. In a review of ICD-9 codes of 51,345 patients, the most common causes of revision total hip arthroplasty were instability/dislocation (22.5%), mechanical loosening (19.7%), and infection (14.8%) [2]. In a similar study of 60,355 patients, the most common causes of revision total knee arthroplasty were an infection (25.2%) and implant loosening (16.1%) [3].

Aside from the psychological and physical morbidity of peri-prosthetic joint infections, they have a substantial financial burden on the healthcare industry. The length of stay of an infected total joint was 1.87–2.21 times longer than reported for an uninfected total joint [4, 5]. Similarly, hospital charges were 1.5–1.7 times higher in infected total joints although costs of treatment depend on the causative organism. The total cost of treatment of a prosthetic joint infection due to methicillin-resistant *Staphylococcus aureus* (MRSA) is estimated at $107,264 compared to MSSA at $68,053. Cost differences are also seen when treating a case of prosthetic joint infection compared to a case of revision due to aseptic loosening. That number was 2.8 times higher in the infected case [4].

R. S. Yoon et al. (eds.), *Trauma and Infection Control in Revision Hip and Knee Arthroplasty*,
https://doi.org/10.1007/978-3-031-71971-4_2

Pathogenesis

There are two main mechanisms to explain the pathogenesis of prosthetic joint infection. The first is locally introduced and often related to operative contamination. Contamination can be introduced via local skin flora from the patient or from air-borne bacteria in the operating room from hair, skin, or nares of the operating room staff. These usually manifest as surgical site infections and present as delayed wound healing, infected wound hematomas, or even suture abscesses. Bone or prosthetic surface colonization can occur with this mechanism as well but less likely [6].

The second mechanism is hematogenous seeding. Any bacteremic episode postoperatively can seed a prosthetic joint. These commonly manifest after genitourinary infections, dentogingival, and gastrointestinal infections occurring following dental and gastrointestinal procedures. Dentogingival infections are associated with strep viridians and anaerobes while genitourinary and gastrointestinal infections are associated with Gram-negative bacteria and anaerobes [6].

The most common bacteria responsible for orthopedic device-related infections are *Staphylococcus aureus* and *Staphylococcus epidermidis* and their prevalence is related to their presence of normal skin flora and their ability to form a biofilm (see Table 2.1).

Biofilm is defined as "a community of bacterial cells that is adherent to a surface interface or each other and encased in a self-produced polymeric matrix" [7]. Biofilm formation allows for bacterial survival during suboptimal periods of growth and environmental stress. They behave differently from planktonic bacteria. The classic planktonic model is described as bacteria that are free floating in cells without substantial extracellular polymeric substances [8]. They usually occur immediately after surgery and manifest as superficial infections that can be treated with oral and or intravenous antibiotics. In the biofilm model, bacteria are commonly polymicrobial and have extracellular polymeric substances. They can bind not only fluids, like in the planktonic model but also to tissues and device surfaces (see Fig. 2.1). They can manifest acutely or colonize and continue to grow and become indolent and manifest months to years after surgery. They form micro-colonies and can sense and communicate with one another by phenomena known as

Table 2.1 Common biofilm bacterial species

Staphylococcus Aureus
Staphylococcus Epidermidis
Pseudomonas Aeruginosa
Actinomyces Israeli
Candida Albicans
Escherichia Coli
Haemophilus Influenzae
Group A streptococcus
Streptococcus viridians

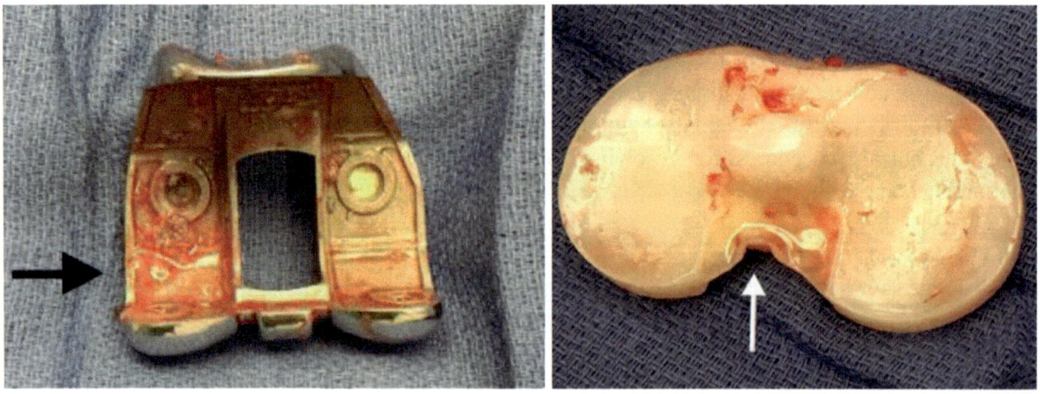

Fig. 2.1 In an infected knee prosthesis, Biofilm remnants (black and white arrow) surrounding an explanted femoral component and polyethylene

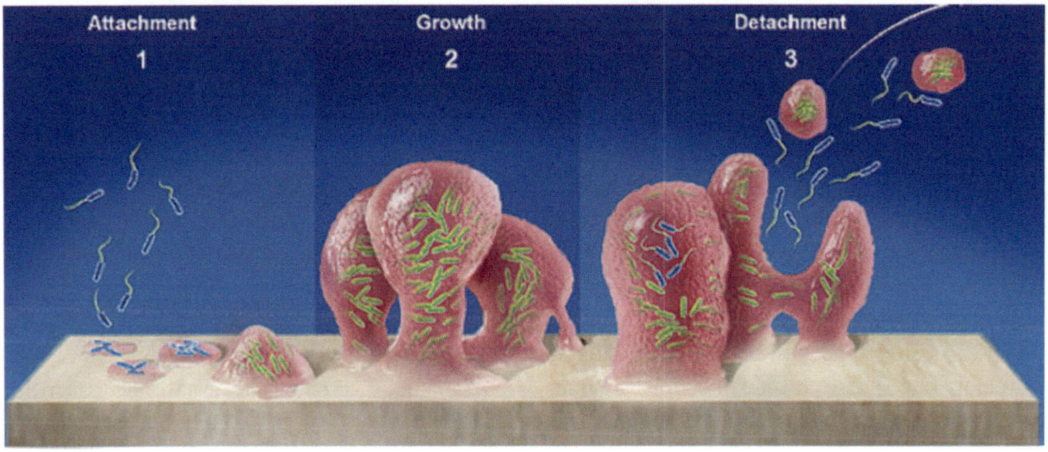

Fig. 2.2 Life cycle of Biofilm

quorum sensing. This occurs in high microbial densities that facilitates cell-to-cell signaling and enables gene activation responsible for biofilm formation [9].

Infection of biofilm bacteria occurs when the bacteria bind to the surface of implants, evading or defeating the host response and begin the biofilm life cycle. The life cycle (Fig. 2.2) starts with attachment. After the bacteria attach, they form a slimy matrix that encapsulates them in which they can grow and replicate, developing complex communities of multicellular organisms. When they have used all the available resources, they begin the final stage of the life cycle known as detachment or shedding. These free agent bacteria can spread and attach to other surfaces that have the sustenance they need to begin the life cycle again.

Once a biofilm is established, the hosts' immune response has little to no effect on these bacteria. Even intravenous antimicrobial therapy is unsuccessful on this distinct and protected environment. These bacteria exist in a stationary phase of growth and are not active metabolically unlike other rapidly growing and dividing bacteria [10, 11]. This characteristic reduces the effect of antibiotics, which are only effective against rapidly dividing bacteria. The slow growing nature of these bacteria also gives them the ability to be present subclinically for months to years and may not cause implant loosening and infection until several years later [10, 11].

Identification and Classification of the Infected Prosthetic Joint

Peri-prosthetic joint infections can be very challenging to diagnose, and since there is no single widely accepting diagnostic criteria, it adds to the challenge. The current, most common classification system utilized for infected prosthetic joints is one which categorizes these infections into either an acute or chronic condition. This contrasts to the former classification system, originally espoused by Coventry in 1970's, which divided the infections appearance predominantly based on time. Stage I, occurred in the acute postoperative setting; Stage II were those infections that occurred from 6 to 24 months postoperatively; Stage III were those greater than 24 months postoperatively [12].

Spangehl recently describes each of these with two subdivisions within those relative groups [13].The first of the acute are those infections that occur within the first 4 weeks postoperatively. These occur as a result of intraoperative contamination. The second type within the acute category is those in which a normal, well-functioning joint which becomes infected [13]. This is believed to be due to hematogenous contamination from a bacterial source somewhere within the body but at a remote site away from the joint.

Regarding chronic infections, there are similarly two subdivisions. There is a chronic type, which is thought to occur from the time of surgery [13]. These are believed to be a result of organisms of low virulence or small bacterial load. These also occur at a time greater than the first 4 weeks post-operatively. They often result in being the source of persistent knee pain, months following surgery, in an otherwise well-functioning and radiographically intact knee. Their discovery is typically related to the diagnostic evaluation for the painful postoperative knee arthroplasty.

The second type of chronic infection is extremely rare. These chronic infections are diagnosed as a result of routine intraoperative cultures at the time of aseptic revision arthroplasty [13, 14]. It is important to interpret these findings relative to the entirety of the patient's preoperative course and diagnostic studies leading toward the revision procedure. Otherwise, the diagnosis of an infected joint may be erroneously diagnosed.

In August of 2011, the Musculoskeletal Infection Society (MSIS) analyzed the available evidence to propose a new way of defining peri-prosthetic joint infections and create a universally adopted definition consisting of major and minor criteria [15] (Table 2.2). The two major criteria, in which when the presence of either one would indicate a prosthetic joint infection, and six minor criteria, when the presence of four or more would indicate a prosthetic joint infection. The major criteria include a sinus tract communicating with the joint and two positive peri-prosthetic cultures with phenotypically identical organisms. The first of the six minor criteria is an elevated serum CRP of >10 mg/L and an elevated ESR >30 mm/h, both of which need to be elevated.

The second two criteria are elevated synovial WBC count and elevated synovial neutrophil percentage (PMN%). Multiple studies have looked at the levels of synovial cell count and PMN%. Results have ranged from 1100 to 3500 cells/mm with a %PMN of 64–80%. These studies are summarized in Table 2.4. These values also depend on the acuteness of symptoms. Acute infection is within 4–6 weeks, and international consensus recommends synovial fluid WBC of >10,000 cells/mm, 90% PMNs, and CRP greater than 100 mg/L [16]. ESR is not a reliable marker postoperatively because it can be elevated up to 42 days, and in some studies 1 year after surgery, whereas CRP can normalize after 7 days [17].

Table 2.2 Criteria for the diagnosis of peri-prosthetic infections

Major	• Two positive peri-prosthetic cultures with phenotypically identical organisms
	• A sinus tract communicating with the joint
Minor (3 of 5 required)	• Elevated serum CRP >10 mg/L AND ESR >30 mm/h
	• Elevated synovial fluid white blood cell (WBC) count OR + 2 change on leukocyte esterase test strip
	• Elevated synovial fluid %PMN
	• Positive histological analysis of peri-prosthetic tissue of >5 neutrophils per high-power field at 400× magnification
	• A single positive culture

The fourth minor criterion is the presence of purulence in the affected joint (Fig. 2.3). This, however, is not specific to infection and can be found in adverse local tissue reaction and corrosion reactions from metal on metal implants [18]. The next criterion is the isolation of a microorganism in the culture of peri-prosthetic tissue or fluid. (This will be discussed in more detail later in the chapter.) The last criterion is a histologic analysis of peri-prosthetic tissue with greater than five neutrophils per high-power field at a magnification of 400 times. This criterion is operator dependent, and levels can be elevated in the presence of inflammatory arthropathies or peri-prosthetic fractures due to the acute inflammation from the fracture [16].

Diagnosis

Prosthetic joint infections, and specifically the subject of this chapter, prosthetic knee infections, remain the bane of the involved patients' and orthopedists' existences. The classic signs of inflammation have been well documented since the Roman physicians Celsus (38 B.C.), and later Galen (130 A.D.), first noted them [19]. Redness (rubor), swelling (tumor), warmth/heat (calor), pain (dolor), and loss of function (functio laesa)

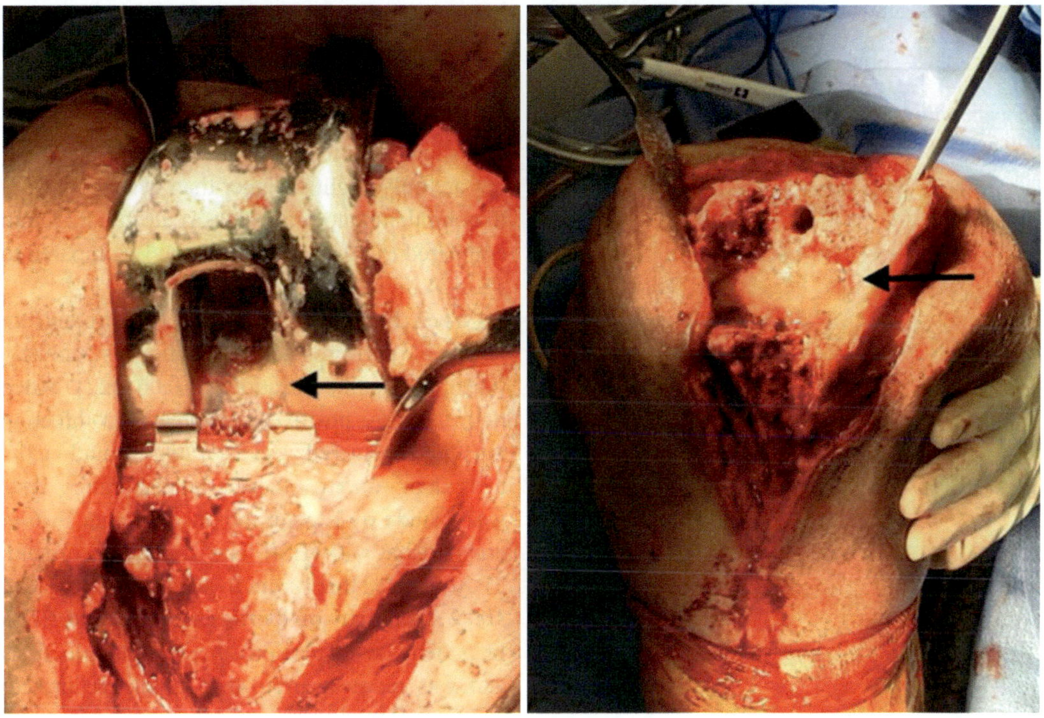

Fig. 2.3 Arrows are pointing to intra-articular purulence in an infected total knee replacement

are all part of a constellation of signs that point toward a compromised joint (Fig. 2.4) [19]. Patients who present with all these signs and symptoms typically are found to have joint infections. The diagnostic dilemmas occur with those patients with more recalcitrant symptoms, or only the complaint of pain. How we identify those individuals accurately and in expeditious fashion is dependent upon the utilization of our evidence-based knowledge regarding this topic.

Despite the wide array of testing, history and physical exam remain the most crucial in diagnosing prosthetic joint infection. Every patient with a painful total knee should have a high suspicion for prosthetic joint infection until proven otherwise. History should include a review of symptomatology consistent with infection as discussed above as well as a review of the risk factors that increase the risk of peri-prosthetic joint infection (Table 2.3) [20].

These risks may include a recent history of prior infection or recent bacteremic event, for example, an upper respiratory infection, a gastrointestinal infection, or recent surgery. Other risks include diabetes, smoking, obesity, malnutrition, and systemic inflammatory diseases. Details of complications of the initial surgery can raise red flags of current infections. These include prolonged operative time, excessive wound drainage, or wound healing issues postoperatively.

The timing of onset of the pain, as well as the severity and character of the pain, is important. Location of the pain should also be asked to rule out other sources of referred pain such as knee pain from the hip or hip pain from the knee, as well as pain referred from the lumbar spine. Proper examination and imaging of the lumbar spine should be performed if the diagnosis is questionable.

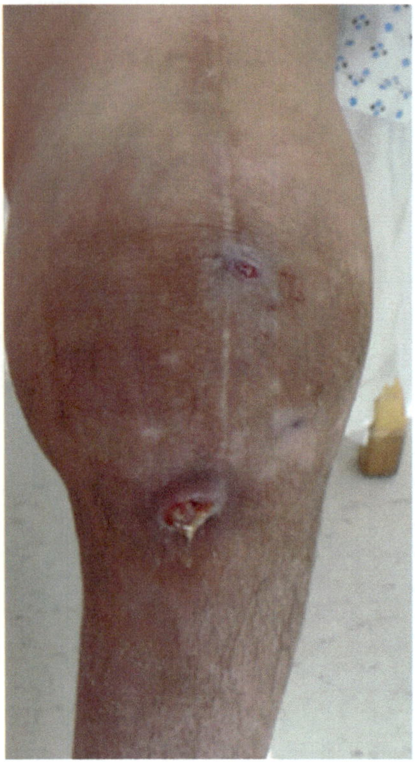

Fig. 2.4 Prosthetic joint infection with classic signs of inflammation and draining sinus tract

Table 2.3 Risk factors for prosthetic joint infection

Factors that increase the risk of PJI	
Uncontrolled diabetes	IV drug use
Morbid obesity	Extended stay in rehabilitation facility
Chronic renal disease	Recent hospitalization
Active liver disease	Previous surgery in the affected joint
Smoking	Male gender
Alcohol use	

Laboratory Tests

In all cases of suspected prosthetic joint infection, erythrocyte sedimentation rate (ESR) and c-reactive protein (CRP) levels should be obtained as an initial screening tool. However, other inflammatory conditions that can lead to elevation of these inflammatory markers. The liver produces c-reactive protein as an acute phase reactant, and elevated levels are seen in cases of both systemic infection in inflammatory arthritis and noninfectious inflammatory arthritis. Regardless of inflammatory arthritis, ESR and c-reactive protein are useful in the diagnosis of chronic peri-prosthetic infection in this setting. It was shown that the optimal cutoffs for these values are only slightly higher than when compared to noninflammatory arthritis, a cutoff of 32 mm/h compared to 30 mm/h and 17 mg/L compared to 15 mg/L, respectively [21].

When both ESR and c-reactive protein are negative, peri-prosthetic infection is unlikely (negative likelihood ratio 0 to 0.06) [22]. When both tests are positive, peri-prosthetic infection must be considered, and aspiration should be the next step. Among other serum laboratory tests was a study by Elgeidi looking at serum IL-6 in comparison with ESR and c-reactive protein. They reported that serum IL-6 had a sensitivity of 100%, specificity of 90.9%, and an NPV of 100% in patients with peri-prosthetic joint infections and was more accurate than c-reactive protein and ESR alone [23].

If only one of the two markers are high and the other is normal than proceeding with aspiration should be performed, if the patient has not had antibiotics within 2 weeks. If the patient was taking antibiotics at the time of office visit, then it is advised to hold antibiotics and wait at least two more weeks to aspirate. This is because of the higher false-negative rate in patients who received antibiotics within 2 weeks of aspiration [24]. False negatives are also seen in cases of subclinical infection, as in the biofilm model. In these cases, the c-reactive protein can be normal despite the peri-prosthetic infection ensuing. Because of this problem studies have looked at measuring synovial c-reactive protein as a more accurate way of diagnosing infection that serum c-reactive protein. Zamani et al. examined synovial c-reactive protein levels and found that it is a method of differentiating inflammatory and noninflammatory arthritis [25].

Parvizi et al. took it another step further to analyze synovial c-reactive protein in peri-prosthetic joint infections and found it to have a sensitivity of 70% and specificity of 100% and a promising means of diagnosing prosthetic joint infection [26].

Table 2.4 Comparisons of inflammatory cells concentrations in joint fluid

Year	Author	Journal	Cutoff (cells/mm)	Sensitivity/specificity
2013	Dinneen et al.	JBJS	1590	90%/91%
2012	Zimistowski et al.	JOA	3000	93%/94%
2010	Shukla et al.	JOA	3528	78%/96%
2008	Ghanem et al.	JBJS	1100	91%/88%
2007	Nilsdotter et al.	Acta Ortho	1700	86%/92%
2004	Trampuz et al.	Am J Med	1700	94%/88%

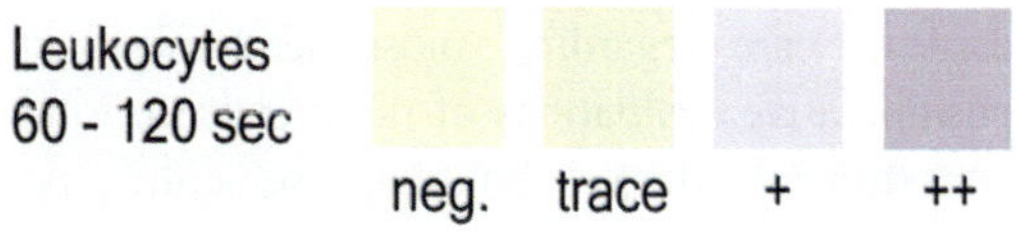

Fig. 2.5 Leukocyte esterase detection

Synovial fluid WBC count is another commonly studied test in the setting of PJI. The optimal cutoff of this test has varied over the years regarding chronic PJI. A summary table of studies determining chronic synovial WBC values can be seen in Table 2.4. In the acute setting, within 6 weeks, however, these values are much different because it can be difficult to differentiate whether the white count value is due to the expected inflammation from the surgical incision or an acute prosthetic joint infection. Studies have looked at different thresholds for white blood cell count and found that at 10,700 cells/uL the sensitivity, specificity, PPV, and NPV were 95%, 91%, 62%, and 99%, respectively. With the threshold set at 27,800 cells/μL the sensitivity, specificity, PPV, and NPV were 84%, 99%, 94%, and 98%, respectively. Based on the observations of this study by Bedair et al., they suggest that synovial count greater than 27,800 cells/μL is the single best predictor of PJI in the early postoperative period [27].

A more recent method of diagnosing periprosthetic infection is leukocyte esterase test strips. Leukocyte esterase is an enzyme secreted by activated neutrophils that have been recruited to areas of infection. It is detectable by colorimetric strip tests through reactions that result in a color change and that vary according to the type of strip used. This simple test requires the application of synovial fluid to a urine test strip with subsequent attention to leukocyte esterase. It is a fast and easy tool that can be done right in the office (Fig. 2.5).

The presence of leukocyte esterase in the synovial fluid has recently been proposed as a marker for prosthetic joint infection and added to the modified MSIS definition as a minor criterion if ++ results were seen [28]. Parvizi et al. demonstrated that the leukocyte esterase strip test yielded a sensitivity of 80.6% and a specificity of 100% for a ++ result [29]. Similarly, Wetters et al. found the strip test valuable with a sensitivity of up to 100% and a specificity of up to 88% for detection of prosthetic joint infection [30].

Alpha-defensin has also been recently studied in the analysis of synovial fluid for prosthetic joint infection. It is a natural occurring antimicrobial peptide produced by neutrophils, part of the innate immune response. In recent studies, it was shown that its mean synovial fluid level was not affected by concurrent antibiotic treatment or in the presence of systemic inflammatory disease. Deimengian et al. studied alpha-defensin alone and in combination with synovial c-reactive protein and found that the sensitivity of alpha-defensin alone is 97% with a specificity of 96%. When tested in combination with synovial c-reactive protein the specificity went up to 100% with a sensitivity of 97% [31]. Several other biomarkers are being studied to aid in diagnosis but in a study by Deirmengian et al., five biomarkers had the most promise. These five markers (human alpha-defensin 1–3, neutrophil elastase 2, bactericidal/permeability-increasing protein, neutrophil gelatinase-associated lipocalin, and lactoferrin) predicted prosthetic joint infection with 100% specificity and sensitivity even when including patients with systemic inflammatory disease and those receiving antibiotic treatment. This study, among others, show that synovial biomarkers do show promise as a valuable tool in diagnosing prosthetic joint infection [32].

Plain Radiographs

The staple of orthopedic diagnostic testing has always been the plain radiograph. Typically, following prosthetic knee implantation, radiographic documentation of the position and alignment of the components are made and act as a baseline assessment of the joint replacement. Consequently, radiologic assessment is the standard of care regarding subsequent follow-up postoperative evaluations of the prosthetic joint. Unfortunately, these radiographs are neither specific nor sensitive for the diagnosis of prosthetic joint infection [33]. In the setting of acute infection, they may be able to detect soft tissue swelling, or rarely, in extreme circumstances, evidence of intra-articular gas. This should not be confused with intra-articular air that may be found on postoperative radiographs within the first 24 h following surgery. Rather the value of plain radiographs comes with the serial evaluation of the joint over time, where subtle changes and progression of radiolucencies may occur [33]. In many instances, infected prosthetic joints have a normal appearance on plain radiographs.

Regarding radiolucencies on postoperative follow-up radiographs, it is important to understand normal changes. The development of a <2 mm thin radiolucency at the bone-cement or bone component interface, within the first 6 months of a cemented component [or during the first year of a press-fit component] is considered normal, provided it does not progress [34]. This typically is seen as a lucency at the prosthesis interface that may or may not have sclerosis of the underlying bone. Another normal radiographic finding is related to component stress shielding of the distal femur. On lateral radiographs, in the intercondylar notch region, there may develop a normal radiolucency in this area of relative non-weight-bearing portion of the distal metaphysis [34]. This contrasts to areas of radiodensity seen juxtaposed to the weight-bearing portion of the prosthesis (Figs. 2.6 and 2.7). Radiographic findings related to infection often take 3 to 6 months to become manifest. Radiolucency and periosteal

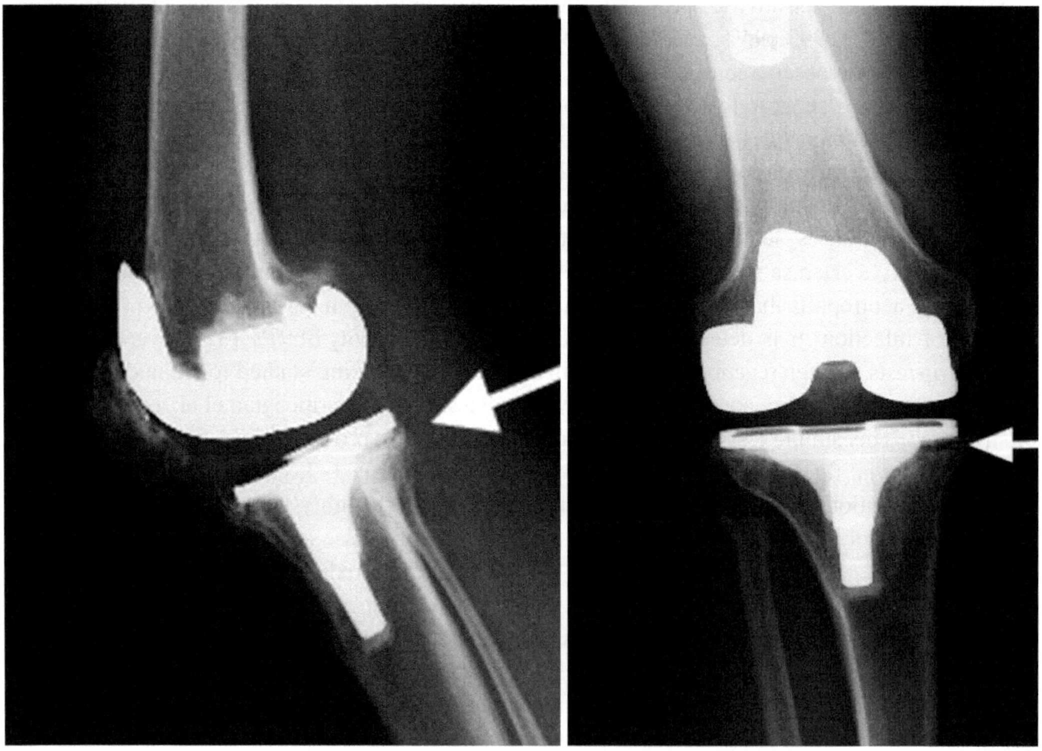

Fig. 2.6 Radiographic signs of loosening

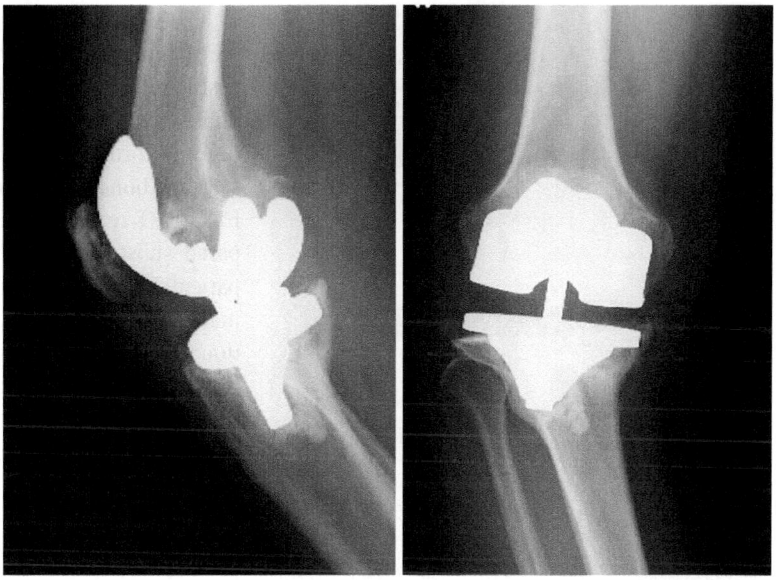

Fig. 2.7 Radiographic signs of loosening

bone reaction can be associated with infection, but not isolated to this etiology. Endosteal scalloping, bone erosion, articular destruction and collapse, and late occurrence of intra-articular gas are more specific findings associated with infection [35]. The presence of radiodense sequestrum with surrounding radiolucent bone abscess is a more classic indication of infection [35].

Plain radiographs continue to be the "work horse" for orthopedic diagnostic imaging. It provides an inexpensive, fast and reliable tool in the evaluation of the postoperative knee replacement. It also provides a valuable radiographic study to compare to more advanced imaging, such as computed tomography (CT), magnetic resonance imaging (MRI), or nuclear scintigraphy without image distortion due to metal artifact.

Computed Tomography

The routine use of computed tomography (CT) has not been a routine part of the diagnostic pathway for the detection of infected prosthetic joints. CT scans have a greater ability to differentiate tissue plains than conventional radiography, but its utility is limited due to the presence of metal prostheses causing beam deflection artifact. This results in distortion of the anatomy and thereby limits the scans ability to detect the subtle signs of infection. CT can effectively detect osteolytic lesions associated with infection, even in the presence of metal prostheses [28]. Likewise, it can also be effective in the detection of loculations, complex effusions, sinus tracts, fistulae, and abscesses [36]. CT is most helpful in cases of painful prosthetic knees with normal or equivocal plain radiographs. CT continues to have the ability to detail peri-prosthetic radiolucencies not visualized with plain radiographs (Fig. 2.8). In these cases, CT can detect rotational malalignments and subtle peri-prosthetic fractures and loosening [36].

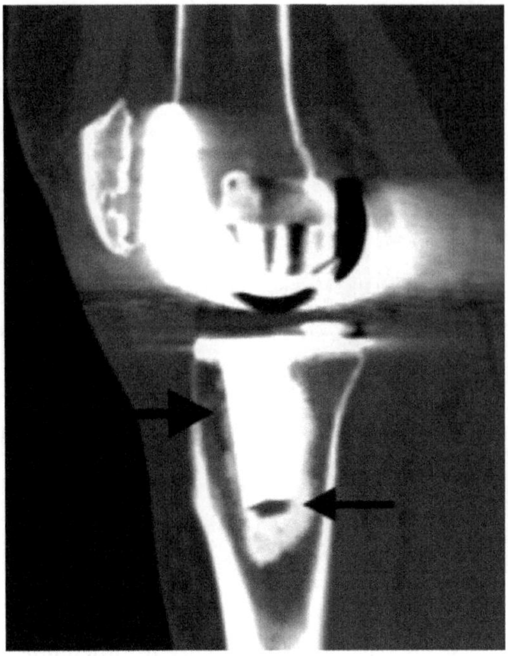

Fig. 2.8 Arrows indicating areas of lucency around the tibial component

Fluorodeoxyglucose Positron Emission Tomography and Positron Emission Tomography with CT

The development of positron emission tomography (PET) in medicine has led to its application in musculoskeletal conditions and imaging. Fluorodeoxyglucose-positron emission tomography (FDG-PET) is a tomographic imaging technique that produces images of superior resolution when compared to other functional imaging techniques [37]. The increased metabolic requirements of inflammatory cells related to infection (i.e., neutrophils and macrophages) require the increase utilization of the labeled glucose moiety, fluorodeoxyglucose (FDG). FDG-PET scans theoretically can detect preferentially the accumulation of these metabolically active inflammatory cells [38]. Due to the overlap of these inflammatory cells activity in more benign processes, such as synovitis or even aseptic loosening, FDG-PET has similarly increased uptake that may result in a false-positive study when the diagnosis of prosthetic infection is sought [39, 40].

There are multiple benefits of FDG-PET in the diagnosis of prosthetic joint infection. The first is related to the relative speed of the procedure; it takes a shorter time to perform than the time performing a combined labeled-white cell scan and bone marrow scintigraphy [38]. Second, FDG-PET requires a single injection of the prepared substrate; there is no preparation of the patients' blood for re-infusion [41]. Third, normal bone marrow has standard glucose utilization profiles. The advantage of FDG-PET scan is the extremely low uptake in normal bone marrow which, thereby, increases its sensitivity to detect low-grade infections that show milder, increase uptake [42].

The greatest disadvantages of FDG-PET scan is the relative availability of the testing to be performed and the greater expense of performing this procedure [41]. These factors aside, the true benefit of FDG-PET comes in the capacity to accurately diagnosis infection of prosthetic joints. There have been few studies that compare the efficacy of FDG-PET to traditional nuclear medicine studies utilized for prosthetic joint infection. Chryssikos et al., reported an 85% sensitivity, 93% specificity, and 91% accuracy in the use of FDG-PET [37]. In contrast, Love and Marwin published findings on their comparison of FDG-PET to the combination of indium-111-labeled leukocyte and 99mTc sulfur colloid marrow scanning. Their study substantiated the use of that combination [of indium-111-labeled leukocyte and 99mTc sulfur colloid marrow scanning] as the gold standard for diagnosing prosthetic joint infections. They reported a 100% sensitivity, and 100% specificity with this combination of test; their results for FDG-PET were similar to prior singular studies [39]. In contrast to this, Pill et al. in 2006, reached different findings in their study, with lesser values of sensitivity and specificity for combined indium-111-labeled leukocyte and 99mTc sulfur colloid marrow scanning and, yet again, similar values of sensitivity and specificity for FDG-PET [43]. As such, FDG-PET cannot be recommended currently as a replacement for indium-111-labeled leukocyte and 99mTc sulfur colloid marrow scanning, in the diagnostic evaluation for prosthetic joint infection. It has been recommended for the use of distinguishing prosthetic infection from synovitis and aseptic loosening, but the routine combined use of these three diagnostic studies is not recommended [40].

The final application of FDG-PET scan is in combination with computed tomography. This technique has had limited scientific studies related to efficacy in diagnosis prosthetic joint infections. It currently is still considered investigational and not an approved imaging technique for the diagnosis of prosthetic joint infection and/or inflammation, here in the United States [41].

Magnetic Resonance Imaging

The routine use of magnetic resonance imaging (MRI) in the diagnosis of prosthetic joint infection is both rare and limited. The main utility for MRI is its ability to discriminate differences and gradations of soft tissues, such as ligament, tendon, muscle, articular cartilage, and meniscus. Bone and joint imaging is typically performed utilizing T1, long T2, and fat-suppressed T2 images, in multiple orthogonal planes. The greatest deficiency MRI has in the diagnosis of prosthetic joint infections is the distortion of the magnetic field caused by the metallic prosthesis, with consequential distortion of the surrounding tissues imaging. Stainless steel implants contain more iron and, therefore, cause greater magnetic distortion. Titanium implants, have significantly less iron, have been reported to result in less image distortion with MRI [44]. Newer imaging techniques aid in the ability to minimize metallic susceptibility artifact. For example, STIR (short tau inversion recovery) sequences have shortened echo times (TE) which result in diminished metal artifact distortion, as well as, slightly diminished resolution when compared to fat suppression modes [45].

MRI continues to be useful in the diagnosis of infection related soft tissue conditions. MRI can accurately diagnosis soft periarticular pathologies such as swelling/cellulitis, sinus tracts and fistulae, abscesses, and even osteomyelitis. Infection is demonstrated on MRI by a hyperintense signal on short T2 or STIR sequences, with the corresponding hypointense signal on T1 sequences [46]. The use of intravenous gadolinium enhances inflammatory and neoplastic processes identification with the characteristic hyperintense signal. Post-contrast fat-suppressed sequences help aid in distinguishing abscesses from hematomas/seromas; the abscess will have a characteristic enhancing rim on the post-contrast sequences while the hematoma/seroma will not [46]. Osteomyelitis may be detected utilizing MRI, even in the presence of prosthetic components. Cortical destruction and sequestrum can be identified by the loss of the normal low/no-signal intensity that typifies cortical bone on MRI. Similarly, subcortical edema or enhancement (if gadolinium is utilized), along with periosteal reactivity, as noted by linear hyperintense signal, can be identified along the cortical surfaces on T2 or STIR sequences [46]. Sequestrum, like cortical bone, has a typical low/no-signal intensity, but due to the inflammatory process surrounding it, the hyperintense signal is found juxtaposed [46].

Radionuclide Imaging

Radionuclide imaging is currently the imaging modality of choice for the detection of prosthetic joint infection. It allows for imaging of prosthetic joints surrounding bone and soft tissues without being limited by metal/prosthetic hardware-related artifact. Over the past three decades, there has evolved multiple scintigraphy tests with various radiotracers being utilized. The following analysis services as part of an evidence-based option for the evaluation of prosthetic joint infections.

Technetium-99m Imaging

The technetium bone scan that is a widely available and easily performed test is extremely sensitive in detecting bone remodeling changes around prosthetic joints [47]. The scan can be performed at different sequential time points following injection of the radiotracer technetium-99 methylene-diphosphate; thus a single-phase or triple-phase scan [48]. A single delayed-phase scan occurs approximately 4 h after injection of radiotracer; this phase reflects areas of bone mineral metabolism, with either new bone formation or bone resorption. The triple phase consists of an immediate flow-phase scan at the time of tracer administration (Figs. 2.9, 2.10, 2.11, 2.12, 2.13, 2.14, 2.15, 2.16, 2.17, 2.18, 2.19, 2.20, and 2.21). A blood-pool phase to display areas of increased vascularity, which consists of a scan approximately 15 min following tracer administration (Figs. 2.10, 2.11, 2.12, 2.13, 2.14, 2.15, 2.16, 2.17, 2.18, 2.19, 2.20, 2.21, and 2.22). Finally, the delayed phase, which is approximately 4 h following administration [48] (Fig. 2.23). The delayed-phase displays areas of increase bone turnover as a result of multiple conditions, besides infection. For example, in total knee replacements, over the course of the first year, there are variable peri-prosthetic patterns of uptake on technetium scans. At 1 year, technetium scan may show more than 60% of femoral components, and nearly 90% of tibial components with demonstrably increased radiotracer accumulation [49].

Peri-prosthetic loosening, by either septic or aseptic reasons, will show increased radiotracer concentrations about the component; thus the presence of this is a non-specific finding for potential loosening. The absence of radiotracer uptake though is stronger evidence against infection. Studies by both Palestro (1991) and Love (2009), both concluded, though, that technetium bone scan was neither sensitive nor specific for diagnosing the infected prosthetic knee [50, 51]. With the overall accuracy of technetium bone scintigraphy being only 50–70% in the diagnostic evaluation of painful prosthetic joints, its clinical efficacy as an isolated test would only be suitable as a screening test. Its efficacy improves when performed in conjunction with another radionuclide test, such as labeled leukocyte imaging [51].

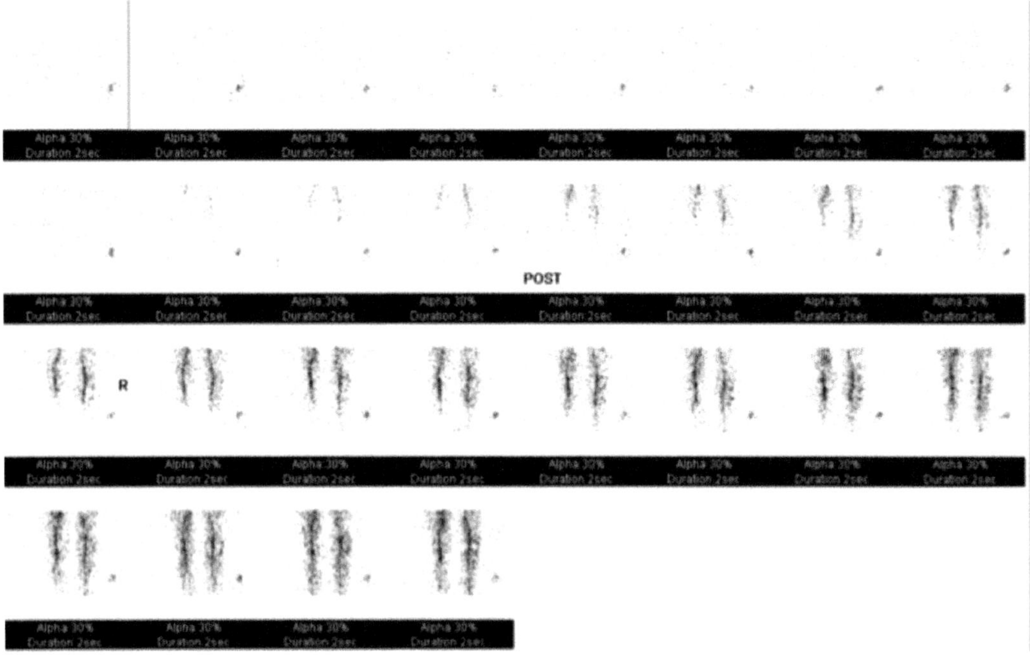

Fig. 2.9 Technetium-99m Scan acute flow phase

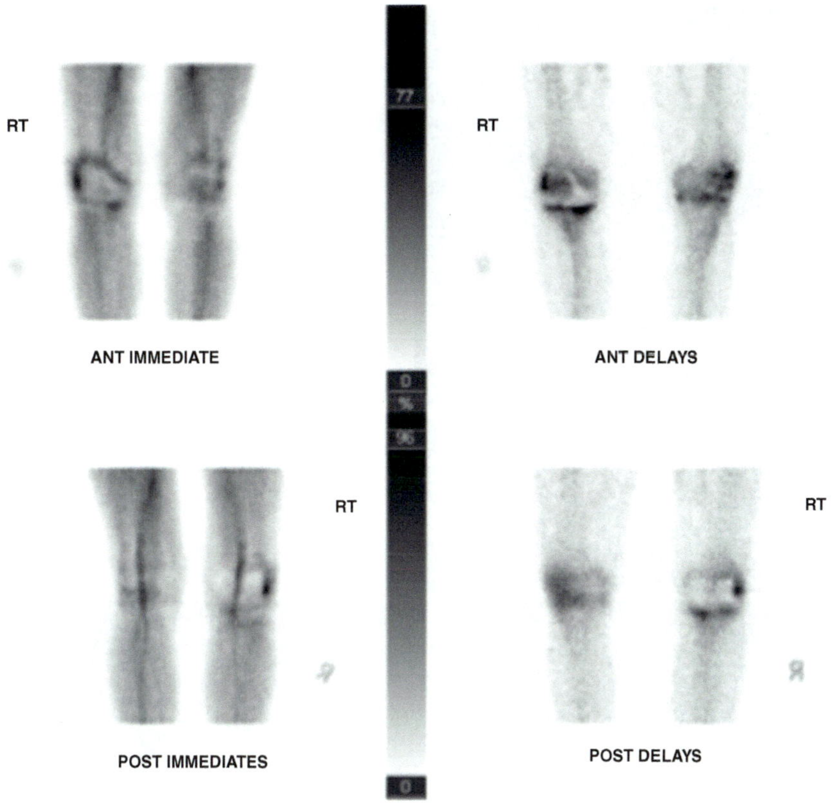

Fig. 2.10 Technetium-99 Scan is showing immediate and delayed-phase evidence for prosthetic loosening of right knee arthroplasty

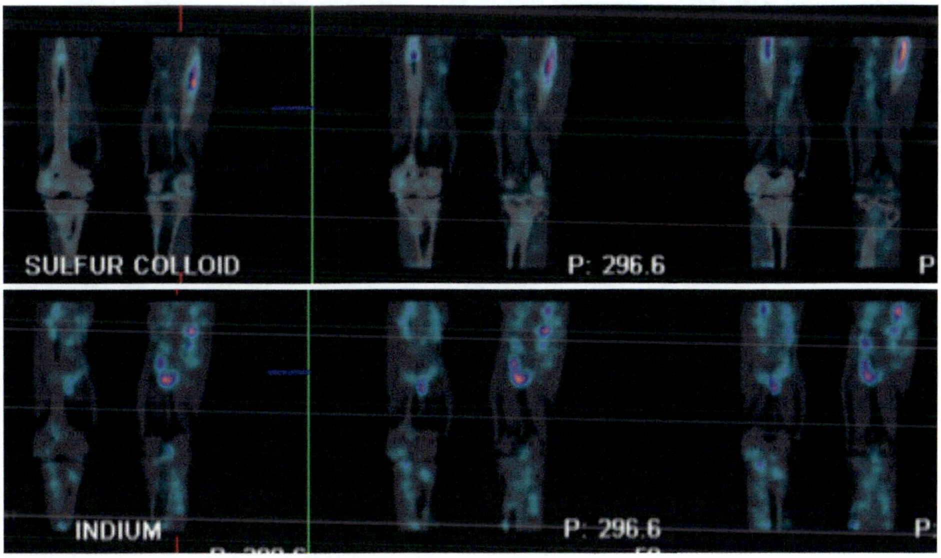

Fig. 2.11 Indium Scan and Sulfur-Colloid Scan: This is a differential test showing the absence of uptake in the sulfur-colloid scan in the intercondylar region versus the presence of uptake in that same area in the indium scan. This is positive for infection

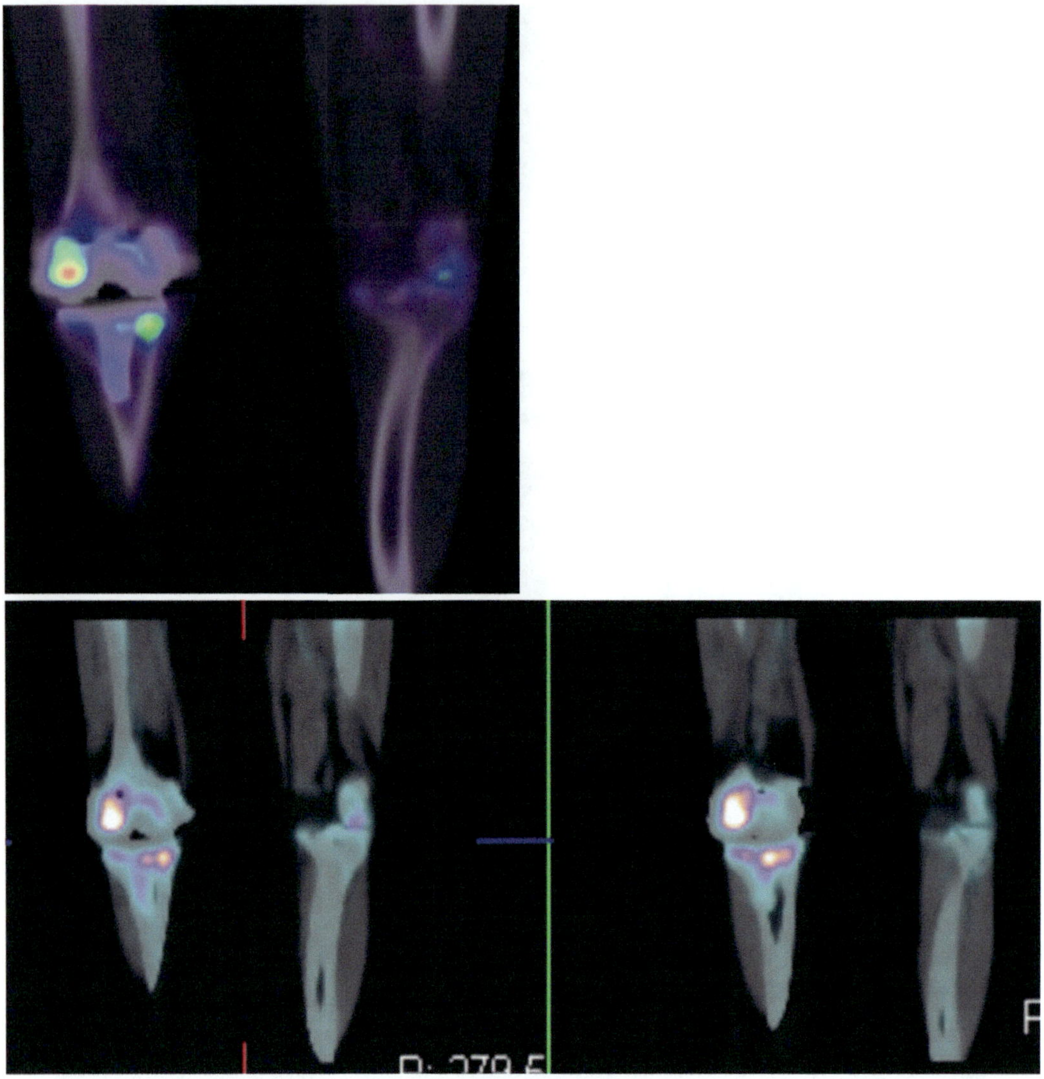

Fig. 2.12 Indium Scan with significant uptake within distal femur and proximal tibia indicative of infection. Comparative sulfur-colloid scan not shown

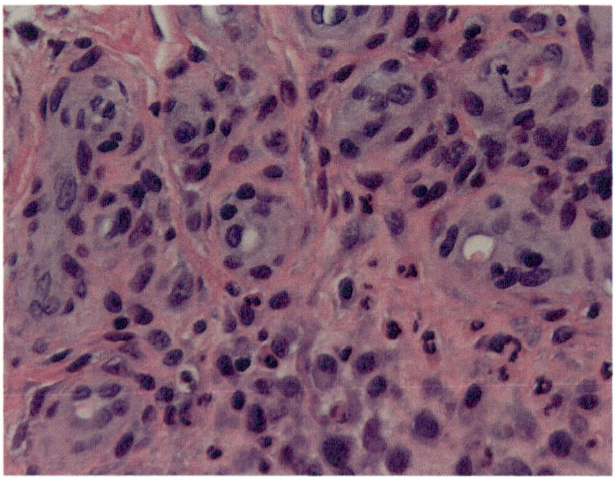

Fig. 2.13 Knee joint synovium with >10 cells per HPF. Hematoxylin and eosin stain, 400×

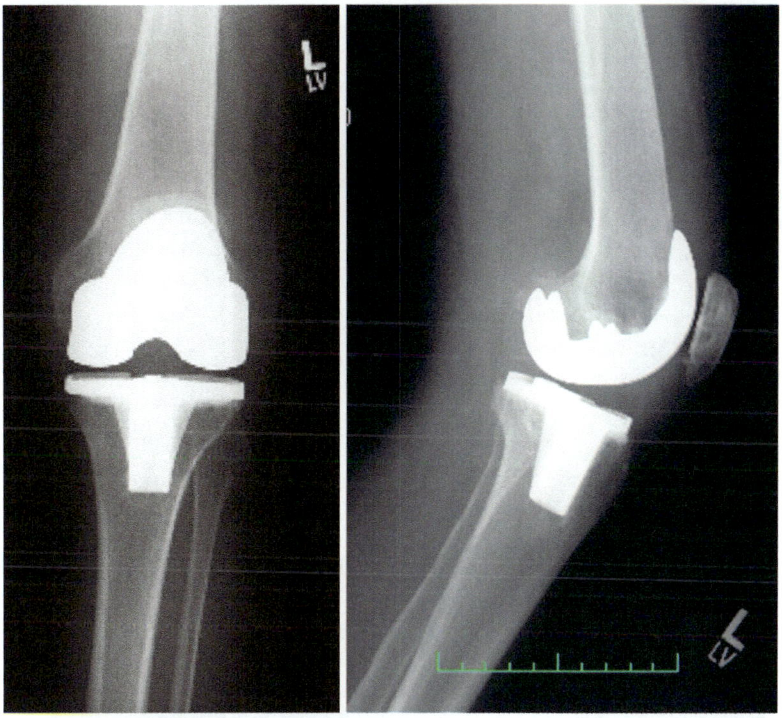

Fig. 2.14 6 years postoperative total knee arthroplasty; seen at the time of acute infection

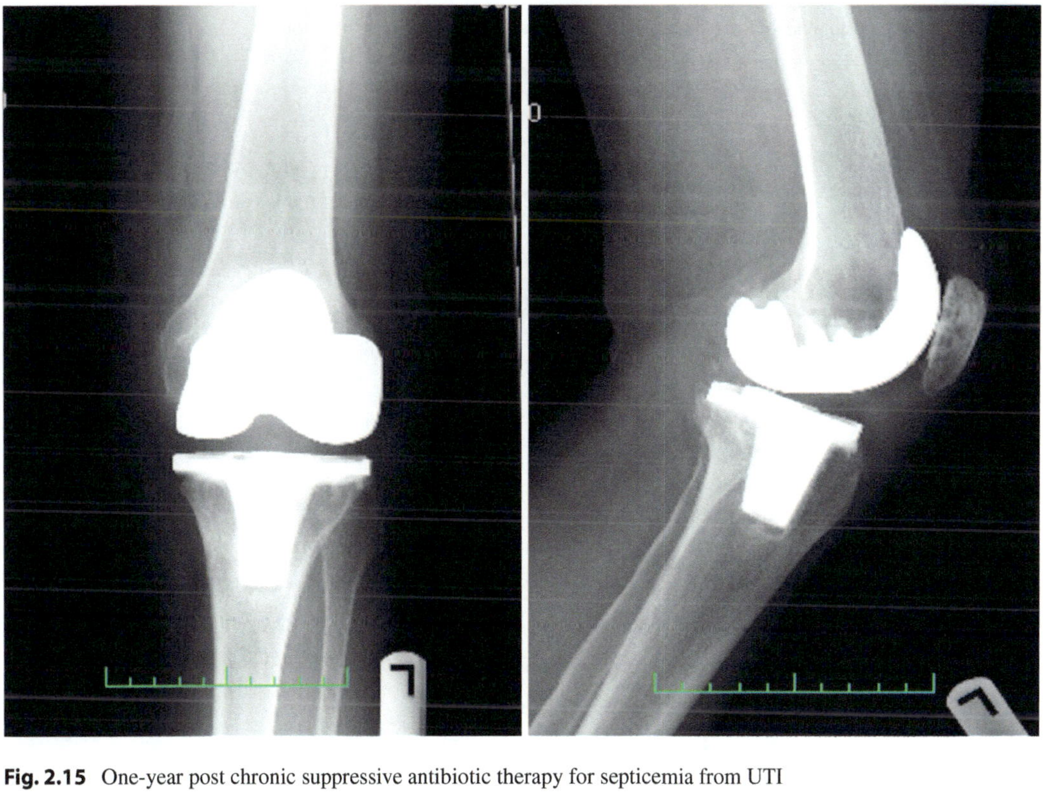

Fig. 2.15 One-year post chronic suppressive antibiotic therapy for septicemia from UTI

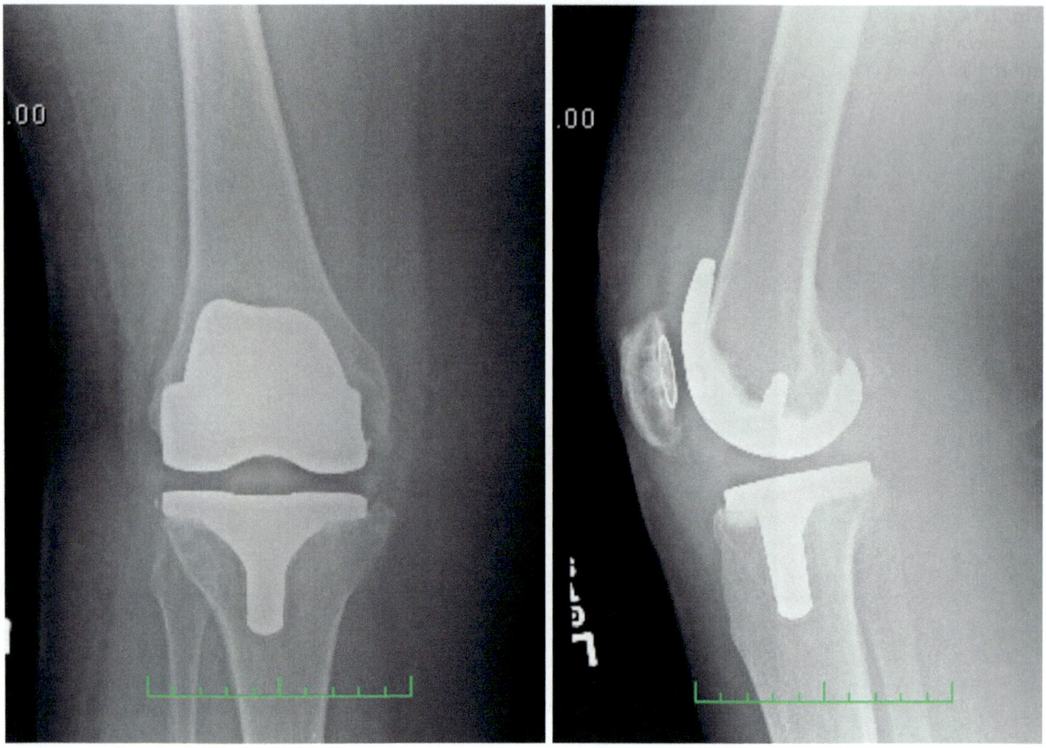

Fig. 2.16 2 years postoperative total knee arthroplasty; seen at time of acute infection

Fig. 2.17 Antibiotic prostalac

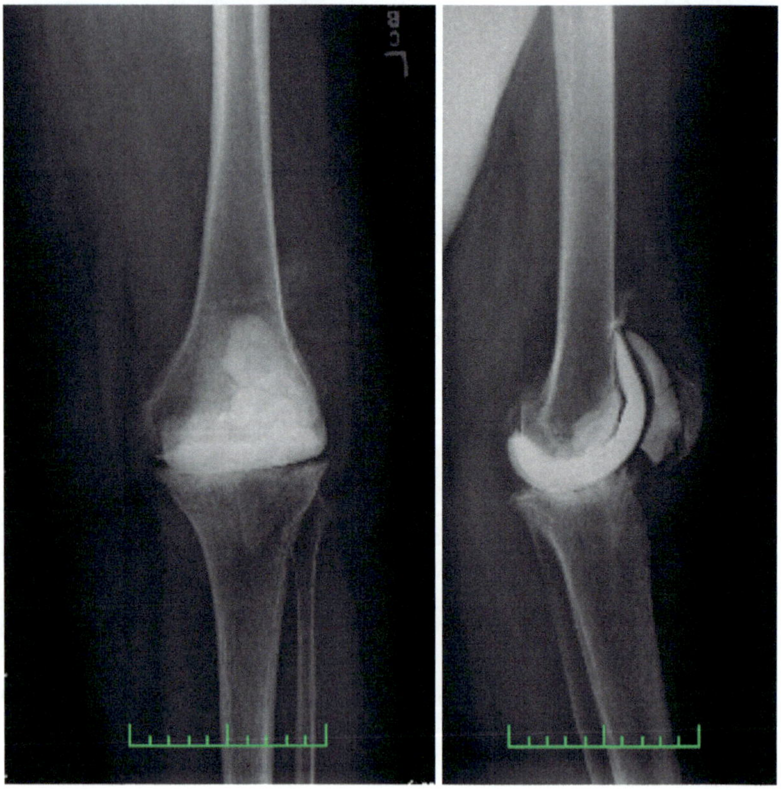

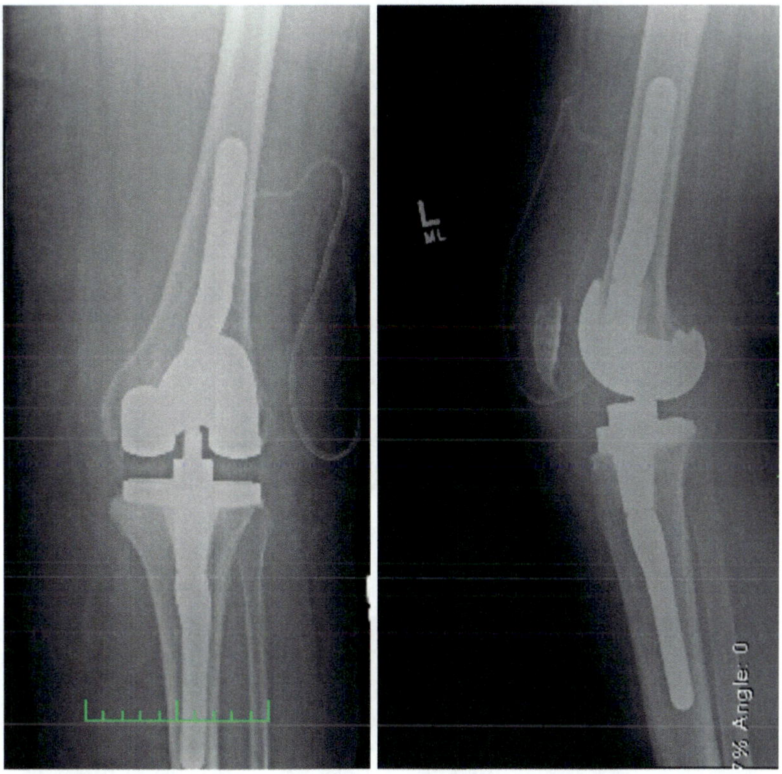

Fig. 2.18 Postoperative 2-Stage revision arthroplasty

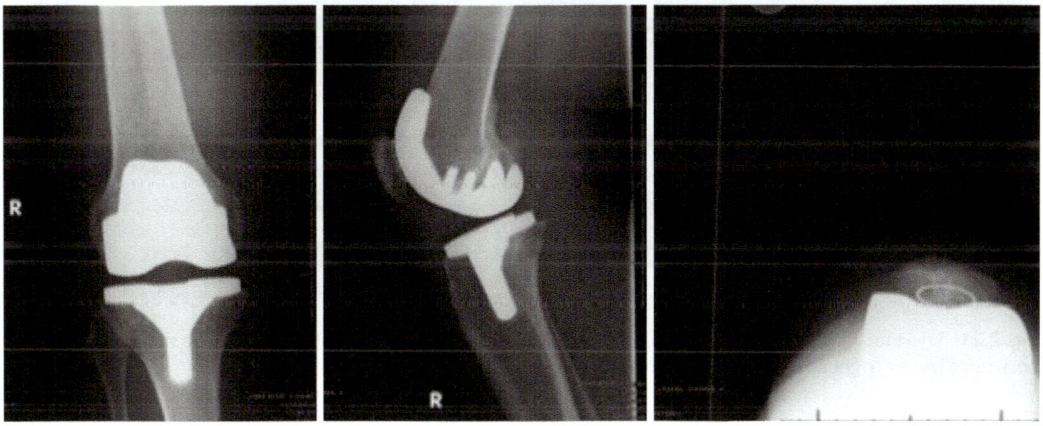

Fig. 2.19 3 months Post-op x-rays

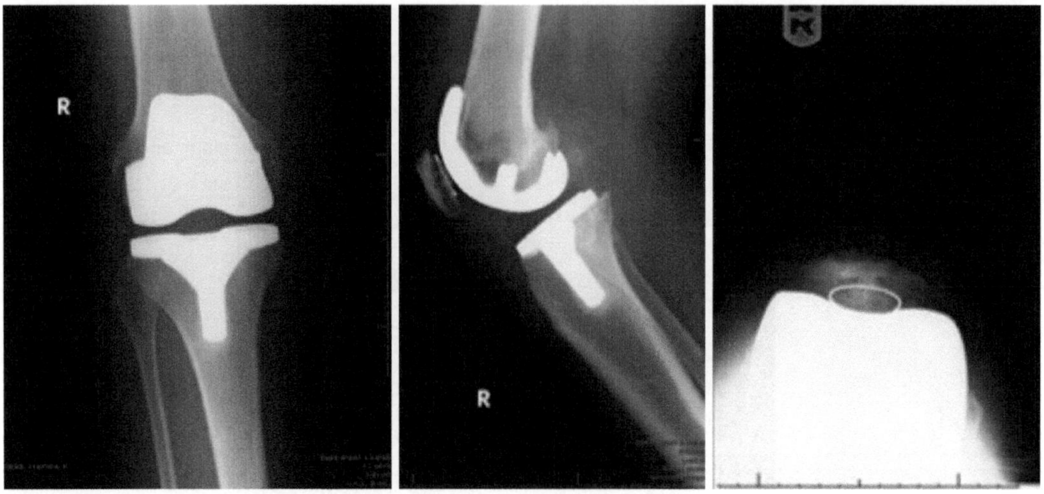

Fig. 2.20 6 months post op when patient presents with symptoms

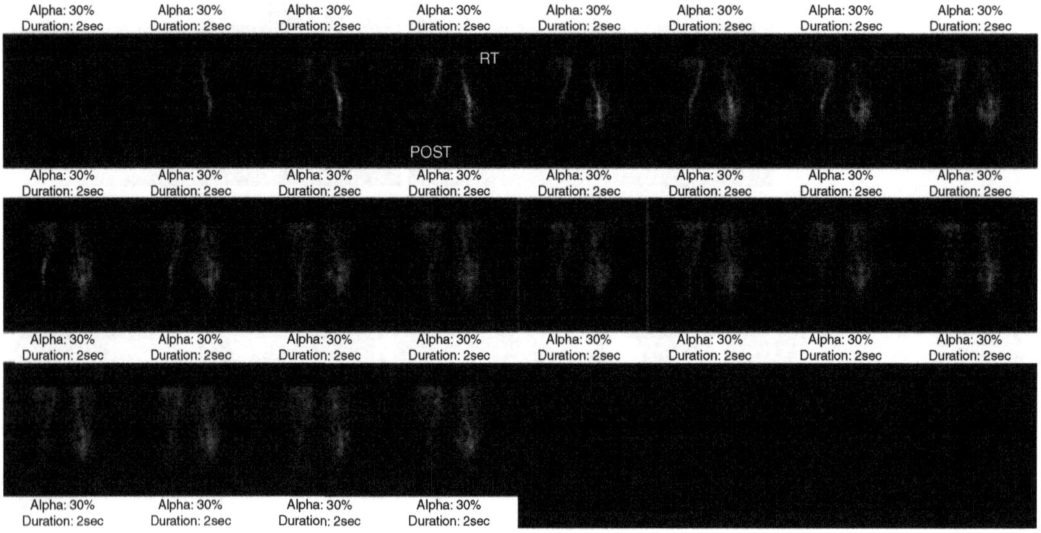

Fig. 2.21 Dynamic Flow-Phase Technetium-99 Scan is showing asymmetric flow to the prosthetic right knee (these are posterior view so “right knee” is on left); indicative of loosening or infection

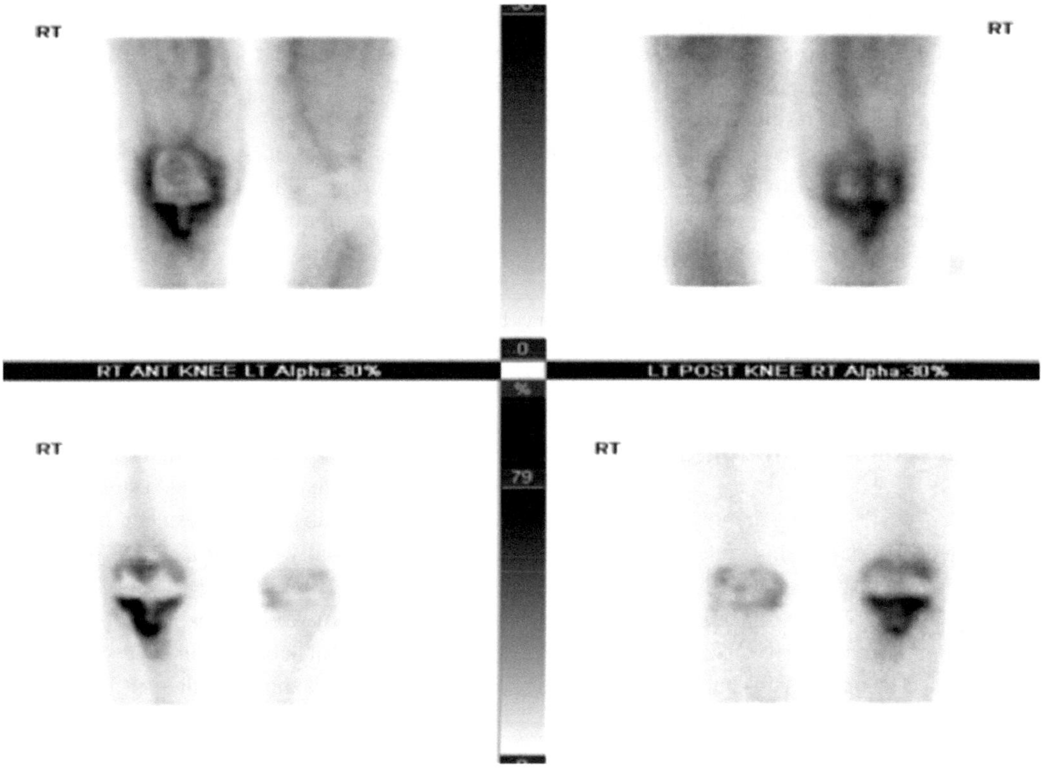

Fig. 2.22 Static Technetium-99 Scan is showing increased uptake around the tibial component

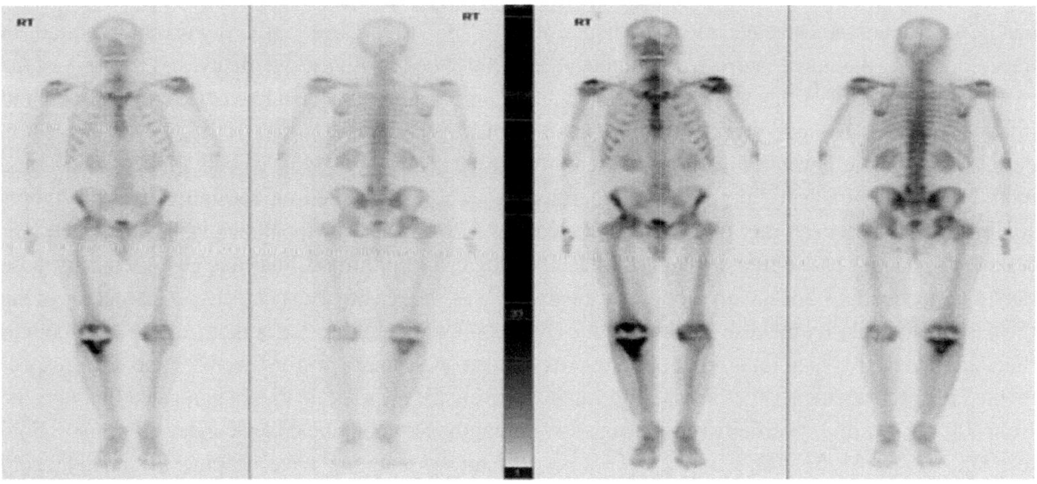

Fig. 2.23 Whole body scan

Combined Bone and Gallium-67 Imaging

In 1979, Reing evaluated 79 joint replacements with both bone and gallium scans [52]. At that time, as it is known today, Gallium-67 labeled leukocytes accumulate in areas of septic and aseptic inflammation, in bone marrow, and in areas of increased bone metabolism [51]. In that initial landmark study, technetium bone scan had 100% sensitivity, but only 15% specificity; in contrast, utilizing gallium-67 scan, the sensitivity was 95%, but the specificity improved to 100% [52]. Over the span of the past 40 years, multiple studies have reproduced these study goals, albeit with greater variability and lesser results [51]. According to Love and co-workers, combined bone/gallium imaging was 75% sensitive, 59% specific, and 66% accurate in diagnosing prosthetic joint infections. This technique has been replaced by indium-111 labeled leukocyte imaging, due to its inability to significantly differentiate infected from non-infected prosthetic joints [51].

Labeled Leukocyte Imaging

Labeled leukocyte imaging theoretically should be best suited for diagnosing infected prosthetic joints. White blood cells typically only accumulate in areas of increased bone mineral turnover related to infection. Since the early 1980s, this technique has produced in inconsistent and varying results [51]. The technique requires the patient to have their venous blood drawn and then the leukocytes isolated and labeled with indium-111 oxine or Technetium-99 hexamethyl propylene amine oxide (HMPAO) [53]. By this technique, predominantly neutrophils are labeled, as the radioactive tracer destroys the more sensitive lymphocytes [51]. Thus the utility of this test is for more acute infectious processes that are neutrophil-dependent, than the more chronic infections, which are more lymphocyte-mediated processes. Numerous studies have reported on this procedure. Labeled leukocyte imaging has a greater diagnostic accuracy than technetium bone scan alone, but, again there is great variability in these studies results. By literature review, for such imaging following prosthetic knee replacement, the sensitivity ranges from 40% to 96% and specificity ranges from 76% to 100% [48, 50, 51, 53, 54].

Indium-111 Labeled Leukocyte Imaging and Sulfur Colloid Marrow Scanning

The combination of indium-111 labeled leukocyte and sulfur colloid bone marrow imaging reflects the accumulation of radiotracer in fixed macrophages, or the reticuloendothelial cells, of bone marrow. In normal individuals, these should be spatially congruent; that is, the distribution of labeled leukocyte and marrow scanned images should be similar [51]. In the setting of prosthetic joint infection or osteomyelitis, the indium-111 labeled leukocytes will preferentially accumulate, whereas, the technetium-99 labeled sulfur colloid will be relatively absent. The resultant images are dissimilar or spatially incongruent, thus indicative of infection [55] (Figs. 2.11, 2.12, and 2.24).

Palestro and co-workers reported in 1991 that the combination of labeled leukocyte and sulfur colloid marrow scanning resulted in 95% accuracy in diagnosing prosthetic knee infection. This finding was considered superior to the accuracy of labeled leukocyte scintigraphy alone (78%), bone scintigraphy alone (74%), or combined labeled leukocyte and bone scintigraphy (75%) [50].

Similarly, Love and co-workers reported in 2004, the sensitivity, specificity, and accuracy of the combination of labeled leukocyte and sulfur colloid marrow scanning were 100%, 91%, and 95%, respectively [39]. Most recently in 2009, Love and co-workers reported on 150 failed joint prostheses with surgically, histopathologically, and microbiologically confirmed final diagnoses [51]. In these cases, the sensitivity, specificity, and accuracy of the combination of labeled leukocyte and sulfur colloid marrow scanning were 96%, 87%, and 91%, respectively [51]. Based on these aggregated findings, the combination of labeled leukocyte and sulfur colloid marrow scanning have become the relative gold

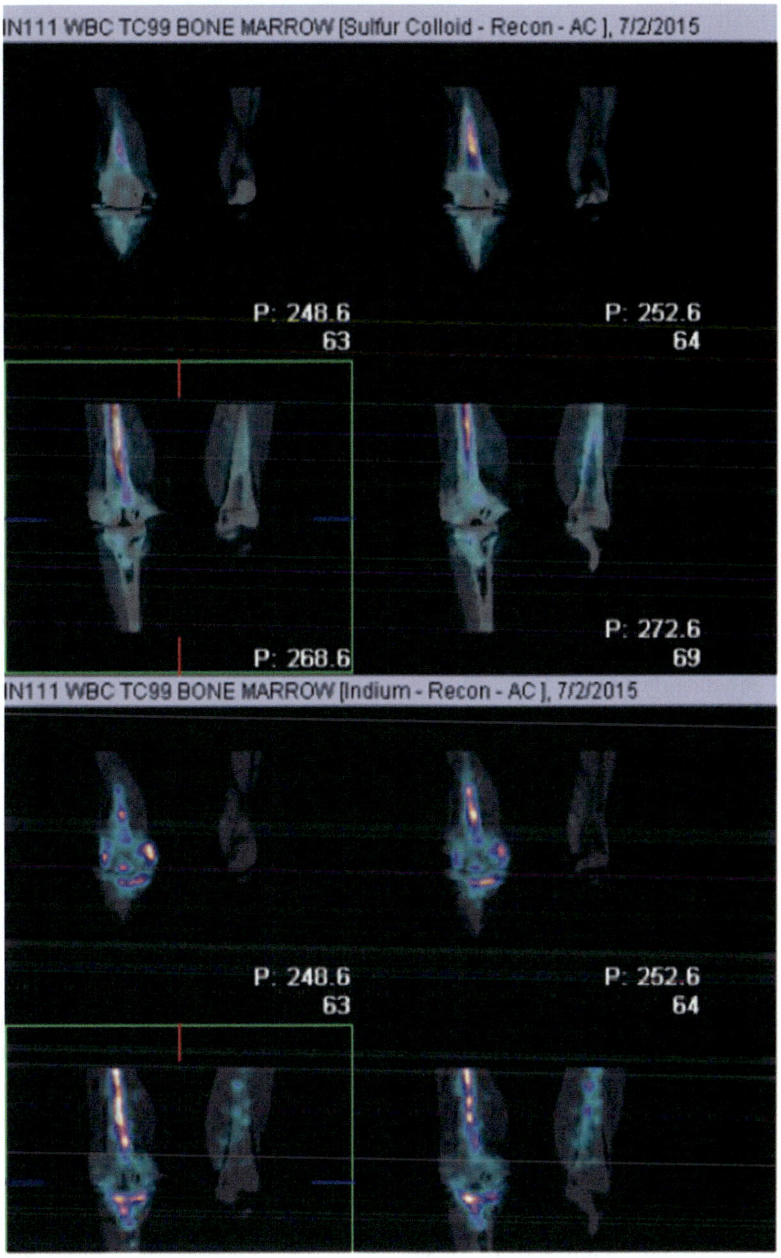

Fig. 2.24 Sulfur-Colloid & Indium-111 Scans are showing differential uptake in proximal tibia consistent with infection

standard for radionuclide imaging in the detection of prosthetic joint infections.

Molecular Techniques

As the field of molecular biology continues to progress, techniques have been developed utilizing the identification of common bacterial chromosomal regions as a means to detect the presence of bacteria. These techniques have been applied to the detection of bacteria within joints. The current standard of care in orthopedics regarding the diagnosis of prosthetic joint infections is a positive synovial joint fluid culture. Identification of an exact organism, followed by the determination of precise antimicrobial sensitivities, allow for the proper management of this condition.

The polymerase chain reaction (PCR) is a molecular technique in which complementary base-pair chains are separated (denatured) and then polymerized to increase the number of copies of that specific DNA, or RNA sample. By this process of amplification, detection of specific bacterial genetic material is possible, thus making it a highly sensitive test. Conversely, since bacteria are so widespread and present on even normal tissue, it may produce false-positive results. Secondly, the persistence of bacterial DNA after cell death or bacterial contamination in the recombinantly prepared reagents is another presumed reason for the high rate of false-positive results [56, 57].

Initial studies by multiple authors sought to identify specific bacteria in joint fluid. Lee, Poole, Liebling, and Nocton all described the use of polymerase chain reaction to identify specific organisms in joint fluid [58–61]. Following those initial studies in the 1990s, multiple investigators consequently found varied findings questioning the accuracy of PCR in the detection of prosthetic joint infections [62]. The afore-described ubiquitous nature of bacteria resulted in a measurably high false-positive rate.

What next developed was the use of what is called broad-range PCR. This method refers to a chromosomal region that is conserved among all bacterial species and is thereby targeted for amplification [63]. The 16S ribosomal RNA gene is one such gene that is universal to all bacteria and has been extensively studied. The advantage of using this gene is the ability to detect the presence of bacteria, regardless of individual species. Similarly, its disadvantage, again, is the detection of bacteria that have not caused a prosthetic joint infection but are a result of contamination and thus producing a false-positive result.

In 1999, Tunney reported the use of broad-range PCR with immunofluorescence to determine the rates of bacterial infection in total hip revisions. 120 patients were included in this study in which a strict anaerobic bacteriologic practice was utilized during the process of sonication of retrieved prostheses; this resulted in only a 22% incidence of infection [64]. When immunofluorescence microscopy with specific monoclonal antibody for Propionibacterium and polyclonal antiserum for Staphylococcus species was utilized on these sonicated samples, the incidence of bacterial detection increased to 63% [64]. Finally, bacterial DNA was detected in 72% of sonicated samples using PCR amplification for the 16S rRNA gene. The author stated that the incidence of prosthetic joint infections were grossly underestimated by current culture detection methods and that additional testing with PCR may be indicated as part of the assessment for these infections [64].

In contrast, in 2005, Panousis used, and then reported on broad-range PCR to determine the presence of bacteria in 91 consecutive patients having revision joint arthroplasty [65]. Their results found PCR to have a sensitivity of 92% and a specificity of only 74% [65]. That author did not recommend the routine use of broad-range PCR due to the apparent high false positives.

More recently, in 2011, Rampini published a prospective study in which broad-range 16S ribosomal RNA gene polymerase chain reaction was utilized on samples where routine bacterial cultures proved negative [66]. In 394 specimens, there was >90% concordance for broad-range PCR and routine bacterial culture. In 231 specimens with negative routine bacterial culture, broad-range PCR showed a 43% sensitivity, 100% specificity, 100% positive predictive value, and 80% negative predictive value [66]. These authors concluded that broad-range PCR is "particularly useful in the identification of bacterial pathogens" [66].

To further this technique, Deirmengian writes "…in an effort to counter the disadvantages of broad-range or universal PCR, several authors have introduced strategies that attempt to decrease the potential false-positive or contamination rate…" [63]. In a technique referred to as "multiplexing," multiple, bacterial species-specific PCR tests are performed simultaneously on specimens. In 2003, Tarkin et al. utilized a specific PCR technique aimed at amplification of the *mecA* gene in methicillin-resistant *Staphylococcus aureus* (MRSA) [67]. When using this technique, aimed specifically at addressing detection of MRSA, their results showed a 97% concordance with routine culture. Achermann et al. in 2010, evaluated, prospectively, 37 joint infections with culture, sonication, and multiple PCRs. Routine cultures identified 59% of the organisms, whereas multiplex PCR identified 100% [68].

In an attempt to reduce the false-positive rates utilizing DNA PCR, newer techniques using RNA have been described. Whereas bacterial DNA sequences can survive longer after bacteria death, RNA sequences have a much shorter half-life to degradation, and therefore, a lower likelihood of being detected unless active bacterial infection occurs. In this technique, reverse transcriptase polymerase chain reaction (RT-PCR) is performed amplifying RNA sequences in a fashion similar to that utilizing DNA sequences. In 2008, Birmingham elegantly demonstrated this concept by performing experimentation on synovial fluid with live and killed bacteria [69]. Bergin et al., in 2010, published results utilizing RT-PCR with universal primers to detect bacterial rRNA, with a goal to reduce false-positive results seen in traditional broad-range PCR assays [57]. Sixty-four patients with symptomatic knee effusions undergoing revision knee arthroplasty were included in the study group. The test correctly identified all six patients with confirmed infection, and all 58 patients who did not have an infection. The study demonstrated 100% sensitivity, 100% specificity, and 100% positive predictive value [57].

It the current time, DNA and RNA PCR is a potent technology in detecting prosthetic joint infections. Limitations of this technology include cost, technical considerations on methodology and equipment, for routine hospital use. These factors make it utilization more limited to use in the academic centers, rather than community hospitals. Further refinement of the technique and protocols will eventually make this more accessible, but also strengthen the body of literature supporting its use.

Intraoperative Evaluation

The long workup of the suspected peri-prosthetic joint infection preoperatively can give you a certain affirmation once you are in the operating room. However, if there is still concern for infection, and the clinical picture, serologic studies, synovial studies, and radiographic studies are not convincing, and then intraoperative evaluation is your final evidence. Several things can be evaluated intraoperatively including Gram stain, the culture of synovial fluid/tissue, and frozen sections.

Gram staining can detect the presence of neutrophils in the sample as well as the presence of organisms. How much value does this test add to the diagnosis is something that has been questioned. Studies have shown that it, in fact, does not add a significant amount of value to the workup. Ghanem et al. shows in his study that Gram staining failed to diagnose prosthetic joint infection in 47% of cases of total knee replacements and a stained organism were observed in only 30% of these cases [70].

Similarly, in the study by Spanghel et al., he found that Gram staining had a sensitivity of 19% and NPV of 89% on his prospective study of 202 cases. For these reasons, many surgeons have abandoned Gram staining for more reliable tests such as culture and frozen sections [71].

Histopathologic study of a specimen to isolate the causative bacterial species is important in treatment and prognosis. These specimens taken intraoperatively are surgeon dependent, and a few considerations should be taken. The first consideration is that multiple specimens should be taken from various locations around the knee joint. Any area of suspected biofilm formation should be debrided and sent to pathology for analysis. Specimens should not be taken from superficial locations, such as skin because the risk of contaminants due to the colonizing bacteria found at those locations. If specimens are taken from superficial sites, such as sinus tracts, it is imperative not to contaminate the rest of the specimens with this one. Therefore, it may be important to use different instrumentation to collect these specimens. The pathogens responsible for deep space joint infections are usually distinct from the colonizing flora on the skin, but it is these colonizing bacteria that most commonly infect prosthetic devices [72].

Although the MSIS criteria list a single positive culture as being minor criteria for diagnosing prosthetic joint infection, Bridget et al. concluded in their prospective study that a single culture-positive specimen was found to have little diagnostic value and recommended that three or more culture-positive samples are strongly predictive of infection [73]. This highlights the importance of multiple cultures during revision surgery to avoid false negatives and the same applies for doing frozen sections. The AAOS guidelines currently strongly recommend the use of frozen section of peri-implant tissues in revision surgery of the hip and knee when prosthetic joint infection has not been excluded. The threshold of 5 neutrophils per HPF (400×) in multiple frozen sections is a minor criterion as part of the MSIS definition of prosthetic joint infection. In a meta-analysis, Della Valle et al. determined that 10 neutrophils/HPF is a good rule in the test but that a negative result does not exclude infection. When they analyzed studies using a lower threshold (5 neutrophils/HPF) the authors found similar sensitivity but a lower specificity with a high false-positive rate [74].

More recently, in a meta-analysis of 26 studies by Tsaras et al. included over 3000 patients comparing the threshold of five cells to 10 cells/HPF. They concluded that there was no significant difference between the diagnostic accuracy of frozen section histopathology utilizing the most common thresholds of five or 10 PMNs/high-power field [75] (Fig. 2.13).

Frozen section histopathology should, therefore, be considered a valuable part of the diagnostic workup for patients undergoing revision arthroplasty, especially when the potential for infection remains after a thorough preoperative evaluation.

Case Studies

1. An 88-year-old woman, 6 years status post left total knee replacement (2004) presented to the office with the complaint of a swollen, painful, erythematous, hot knee with significantly the diminished range of motion. The patient had had no complaints related to her knee arthroplasty before this time. The patient 3 weeks prior to this event had been hospitalized for management of urosepsis. Radiographs at this visit (2010) (Fig. 2.14) did not reveal any bony changes, such as radiolucencies consistent with loosening, from prior radiographs. Knee joint fluid aspiration revealed WBC: 22,000/cc. Serum ESR and c-reactive protein were elevated. The patient was admitted for surgical management of this condition. The patient declined prosthetic removal, antibiotic prostalac placement with two-stage revision. Rather, the patient preferred management with open irrigation and debridement with polyethylene exchange, along with oral antibiotics for chronic suppressive therapy. Knee joint fluid cultures revealed *E. coli*, sensitive to ampicillin. The patient has been managed with ampicillin 500 mg BID for the past 5 years. She remains asymptomatic and has not had radiographic evidence of loosening (Figs. 2.14 and 2.15).
2. A 66-year-old woman 2 years status post bilateral knee arthroplasty in 2009 was receiving management and chemotherapy for breast cancer. The patient has surgery for placement of a PICC line in December 2011. The patient presented in January 2012 with a painful, swollen, erythematous, and hot left knee with significantly diminished range of motion. The patient had no complaints related to her knee arthroplasties before this time. Radiographs at this visit did not reveal any radiographic evidence of loosening (see Fig. 2.16). Knee joint fluid aspiration revealed WBC: 35,000/cc. The patient was admitted for surgical management of this condition.

   We recommended the patient undergo two-stage exchange arthroplasty to ensure adequate eradication of the bacterial load. The patient consented to this plan. The patient underwent initial removal of all prosthetic components with the placement of antibiotic prostalac containing 2 g of Vancomycin, 2 g of Tobramycin (see Fig. 2.17). Intraoperative cultures grew Streptococcus species that were sensitive to ceftriaxone. The patient underwent 6-week management of this infection with intravenous antibiotic. Before surgical re-implantation, knee joint fluid aspirate did not reveal any increased WBC nor bacterial growth. Serum ESR and c-reactive protein were normalized.

At 8 weeks post-prostalac implantation, the patient returned to the operating room for revision knee arthroplasty using stemmed femoral and tibial implants, along with a posterior-semi-constrained post-polyethylene (Fig. 2.18). We likewise utilized antibiotic containing 1 g of Vancomycin and 1 g of Tobramycin. The patient has had excellent knee function for the past 3 years, having stable, 0–115 degrees of flexion motion, and no recurrent pain or swelling.

3. A 62-year-old man 5 months postoperatively began to experience right knee swelling (Fig. 2.19). The patient had an unremarkable recovery and by 2 months postoperative, had returned to the gym, performing rather rigorous exercise routines. These included 30 min on a stationary bicycle, 30 min on the elliptical machine, followed by another hour of resistive strengthening exercises. He performed this routine 6 days a week. He had been advised on decreasing some of this routine due to concerns of prosthetic wear. After his presentation with knee swelling, he was advised to curtail further his activity level. The patient returned at approximately 6 months postoperatively having the complaint of continued knee swelling and pain, despite discontinuing his exercise routine (Fig. 2.20). During that interview, it was learned that at 4 months postoperatively he had required surgical incision and drainage of an infected pilonidal cyst. The patient underwent diagnostic evaluation with knee aspiration for routine cultures and sensitivities, along with triple-phase bone scan (Figs. 2.22 and 2.23), indium scan, and sulfur colloid scan (see Fig. 2.24). Serum sedimentation rate returned at 60 mm/s; serum c-reactive protein level returned significantly abnormally elevated. Knee joint cultures revealed methicillin-sensitive Staphylococcus species. The patient underwent two-stage revision arthroplasty (Fig. 2.25). An antibiotic prostalac spacer was placed (Fig. 2.26). The patient

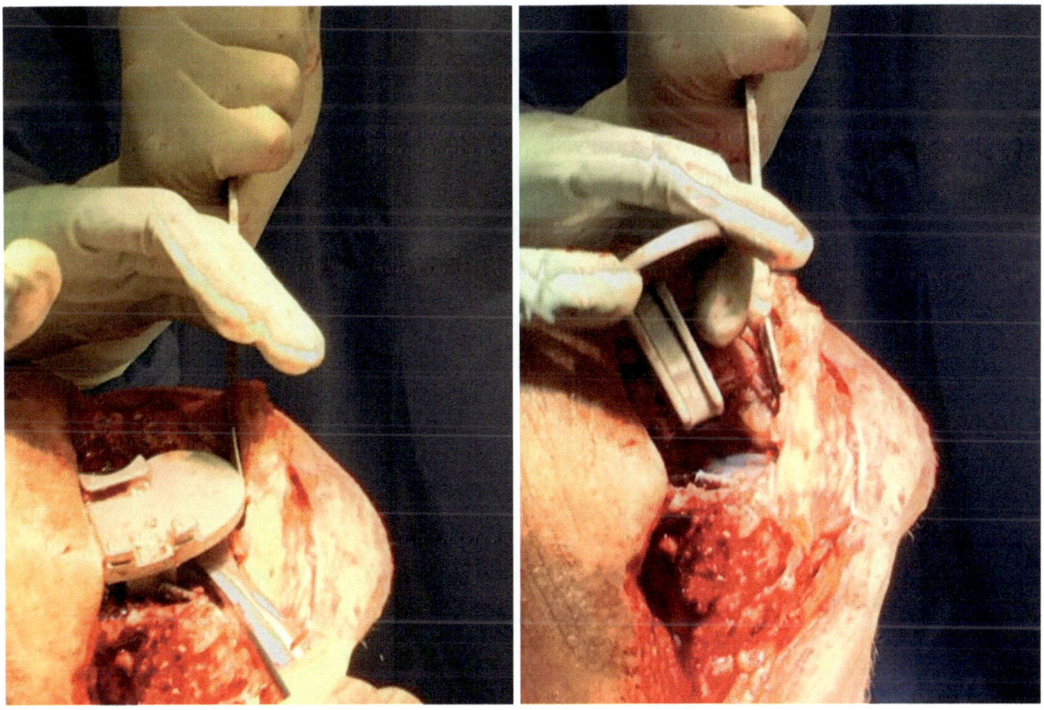

Fig. 2.25 Loose tibial component removed effortlessly by levering with a Cobb elevator

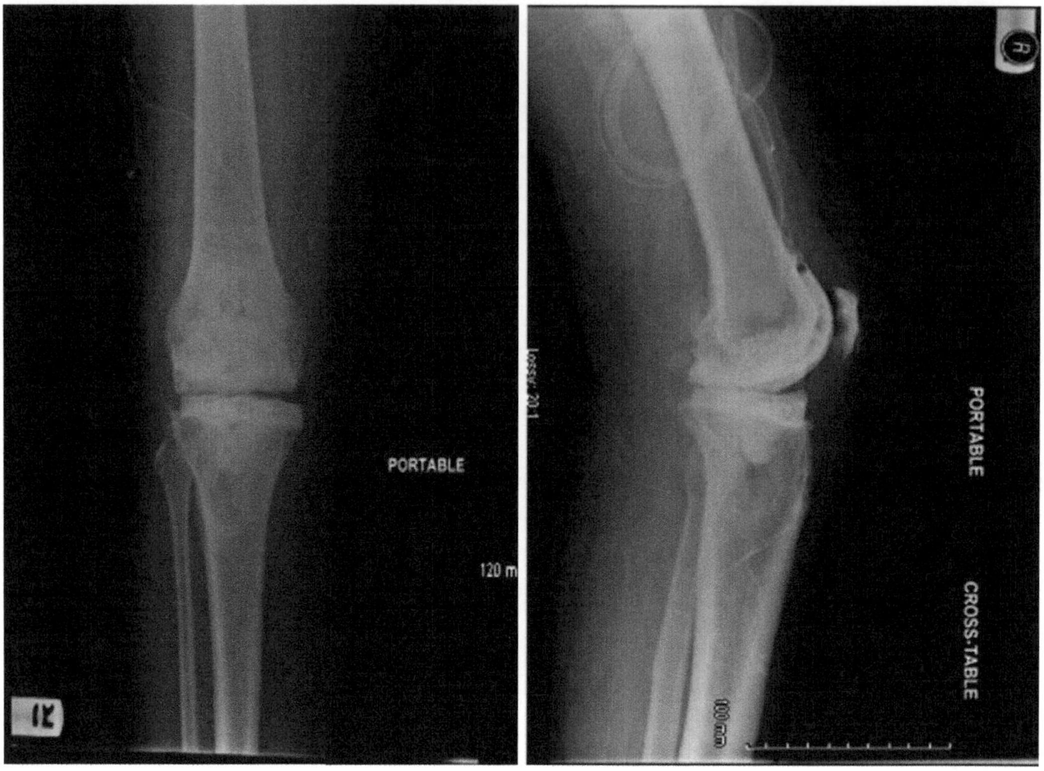

Fig. 2.26 Antibiotic prostalac

received 6 weeks of intravenous and oral antibiotic therapy. Before implantation of the revision arthroplasty, preoperative knee joint cultures did not reveal any growth. Likewise, intraoperative frozen sections were negative for elevated inflammatory cells [see intraoperative photos]. The patient has had an unremarkable revision arthroplasty with 0–115 degrees of motion and painless ambulation (Fig. 2.27).

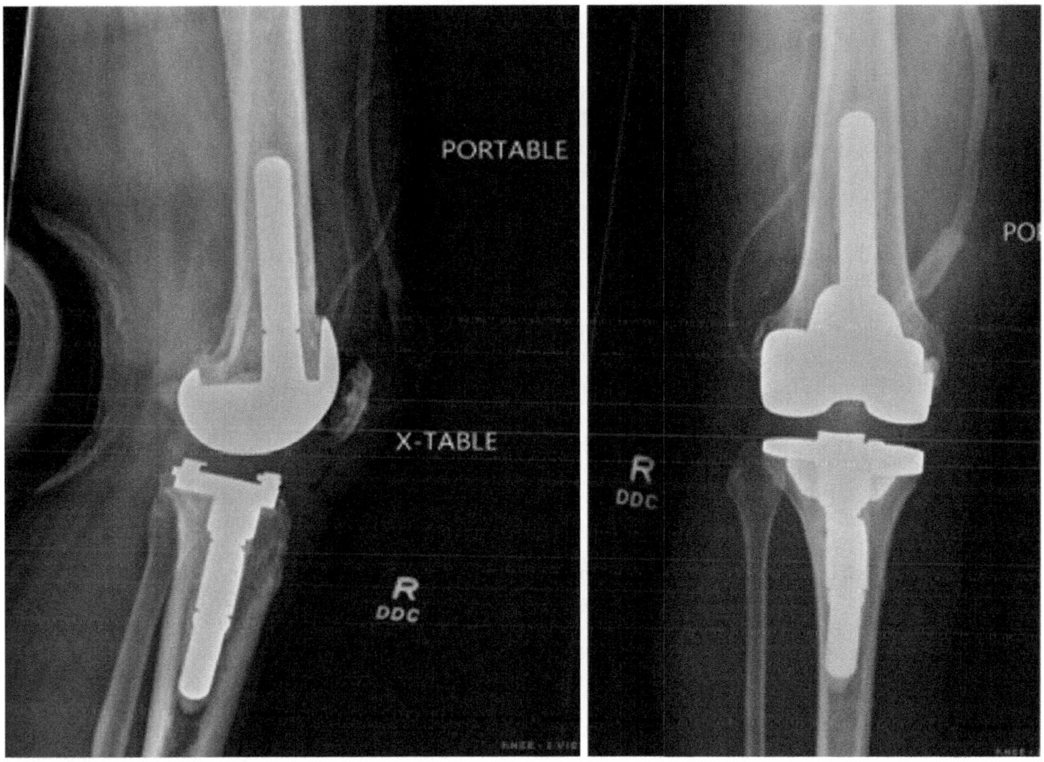

Fig. 2.27 Final revision knee radiographs

Summary

The purpose of this chapter was to aid the clinician in the diagnosis of prosthetic knee infections. The individual's goal is to utilize this information in the formation of a step-wise diagnostic process, such that the great majority of these catastrophic and debilitating conditions are accurately and expeditiously diagnosed and treated. To reiterate, the fact that there is no, one-test that accurately reveals this process and diagnoses this condition, makes the diagnosis of the infected prosthetic joint dependent upon an initial high index of suspicion when there is the onset of a painful, prosthetic joint.

References

1. Polybius. (264 B.C.) The rise of the Roman Empire. Translated by Ian Scott-Kilvert. London: Penguin; 1979.
2. Bozic KJ, Kurtz SM, Lau E, Ong K, Vail TP, Berry DJ. The epidemiology of revision total hip arthroplasty in the United States. J Bone Joint Surg Am. 2009;91(1):128–33.
3. Bozic KJ, Kurtz SM, Lau E, et al. The epidemiology of revision total knee arthroplasty in the United States. Clin Orthop. 2010;468(1):45–51. https://doi.org/10.1007/s11999-009-0945-0.
4. Parvizi J, Pawasarat IM, Azzam KA, Joshi A, Hansen EN, Bozic KJ. Periprosthetic joint infection: the economic impact of methicillin-resistant infections. J Arthroplast. 2010;25(6 Suppl):103–7. https://doi.org/10.1016/j.arth.2010.04.011.
5. Kurtz SM, Lau E, Watson H, Schmier JK, Parvizi J. Economic burden of peri-prosthetic joint infection in the United States. J Arthroplasty. 2012;27(8 Suppl):61–5.e1. https://doi.org/10.1016/j.arth.2012.02.022.
6. Mandell GL. Mandell, Douglas, and Bennett's principles and practice of infectious diseases. Karger.com. 2005. http://www.karger.com/Article/Abstract/7313.
7. Dr. Nicola Stanley-Wall. School of Life Sciences. 26 Oct 2015. http://www.lifesci.dundee.ac.uk/people/nicola-stanley-wall.
8. Parvizi J, Alijanipour P, Barberi EF, Hickok NJ, Phillips KS, Shapiro IM, Schwarz EM, Stevens MH, Wang Y, Shirtliff ME. Novel developments in the prevention, diagnosis, and treatment of periprosthetic joint infections. J Am Acad Orthop Surg. 2015;23 Suppl:S32–43.

9. Zimmerli W, Tampuz A, Ochsner PE. Prosthetic-joint infections. N Engl J Med. 2004;351(16):1645–54. https://doi.org/10.1056/NEJMra040181.
10. Shirtliff ME, Mader JT, Camper AK. Molecular interactions in biofilms. Chem Biol. 2002;9(8):859–71.
11. Costerton JW, Stewart PS, Greenberg EP. Bacterial biofilms: a common cause of persistent infections. Science. 1999;284(5418):1318–22.
12. Coventry MB. Treatment of infections occurring in total hip arthroplasty. Orthop Clin North Am. 1975;6:991–1003.
13. Spangehl M. Diagnosis of periprosthetic joint infection: serology. In: Parvizi J, editor. The knee. Reconstruction, replacement and revision, vol. 2. Brooklandville: Data Trace Publishing Company; 2013. p. 101.1–101.15.
14. Tsukayama DT, Estrada R, Gustilo RB. Infection after total hip arthroplasty. A study of the treatment of one hundred and six infections. J Bone Joint Surg Am. 1996;78:512–23.
15. Parvizi J, Zmistowski B, Berbari EF, Bauer TW, Springer BD, Della Valle CJ, et al. New definition for peri-prosthetic joint infection: from the workgroup of the musculoskeletal infection society. Clin Orthop Relat Res. 2011;469(11):2992–4. https://doi.org/10.1007/s11999-011-2102-9.
16. Zmistowski Consensus meeting 2013.
17. Husain T, Kim D. C-reactive protein and erythrocyte sedimentation rate in orthopaedics. Univ Pa Orthop J. 2002;15:13–6.
18. Alijanipour P, Adeli B, Hansen EN, Chen AF, Parvizi J. Intraoperative purulence is not reliable for diagnosing periprosthetic joint infection. J Arthroplasty. 2015;30(8):1403–6.
19. Hurley JV. Acute inflammation. Edinburgh: Churchill Livingstone; 1972.
20. Shahi A, Parvizi J. Prevention of periprosthetic joint infection. Arch Bone Joint Surg. 2015;3(2):72–81.
21. Brown NM. Serum and synovial fluid analysis for diagnosing chronic periprosthetic infection in patients with inflammatory arthritis. J Bone Joint Surg Am. 2012;94(7):594. https://doi.org/10.2106/JBJS.J.01318.
22. Della Valle C, Parvizi J, Bauer TW, Dicesare PE, Evans RP, Segreti J, et al. Diagnosis of peri-prosthetic joint infections of the hip and knee. J Am Acad Orthop Surg. 2010;18(12):760–70.
23. Elgeidi. Interleukin-6 and other inflammatory markers in the diagnosis of peri-prosthetic joint infection. Int Orthop. 2014;38(12):2591–5. https://doi.org/10.1007/s00264-014-2475-y.
24. Trampuz A, Piper KE, Jacobson MJ, et al. Sonication of removed hip and knee prostheses for diagnosis of infection. N Engl J Med. 2007;357(7):654–63.
25. Zamani B, Jamali R, Ehteram H. Synovial fluid adenosine deaminase and high-sensitivity C-reactive protein activity in differentiating monoarthritis. Rheumatol Int. 2012;32(1):183–8.
26. Parvizi J, Jacovides C, Adeli B, Jung KA, Hozack WJ. Mark B. Coventry Award: synovial C-reactive protein: a prospective evaluation of a molecular marker for peri-prosthetic knee joint infection. Clin Orthop Relat Res. 2012;470(1):54–60.
27. Bedair H, Ting N, Jacovides C, Saxena A, Moric M, Parvizi J, Della Valle CJ. The Mark Coventry Award: diagnosis of early postoperative TKA infection using synovial fluid analysis. Clin Orthop Relat Res. 2011;469(1):34–40. https://doi.org/10.1007/s11999-010-1433-2.
28. Tischler EH, Cavanaugh PK, Parvizi J. Leukocyte esterase strip test: matched for musculoskeletal infection society criteria. J Bone Joint Surg. 2014;96-A(22):1917–20.
29. Parvizi J, Jacovides C, Antoci V, Ghanem E. Diagnosis of periprosthetic joint infection: the utility of a simple yet unappreciated enzyme. J Bone Joint Surg Am. 2011;93(24):2242–8.
30. Wetters NG, Berend KR, Lombardi AV, Morris MJ, Tucker TL, Della Valle CJ. Leukocyte esterase reagent strips for the rapid diagnosis of periprosthetic joint infection. J Arthroplasty. 2012;27(8 Suppl):8–11.
31. Deirmengian C, Kardos K, Kilmartin P, Cameron A, Schiller K, Parvizi J. Combined measurement of synovial fluid α-Defensin and C-reactive protein levels: highly accurate for diagnosing periprosthetic joint infection. J Bone Joint Surg Am. 2014;96(17):1439–45.
32. Deirmengian C, Kardos K, Kilmartin P, Cameron A, Schiller K, Parvizi J. Diagnosing periprosthetic joint infection: has the era of the biomarker arrived? Clin Orthop Relat Res. 2014;472:3254–62. https://doi.org/10.1007/s11999-014-3543-8.
33. Wang CJ, Juang TW, Wang JW, et al. The often poor clinical outcome of infected total knee arthroplasty. J Arthroplasty. 2002;17:608–14.
34. Manaster BJ. Total knee arthroplasty: postoperative radiologic findings. AJR Am J Roentgenol. 1995;165(4):899–904.
35. Lyons CW, Berquist TH, Lyons JC, et al. Evaluation of radiographic findings in painful hip arthroplasties. Clin Orthop Relat Res. 1985;195:239–51.
36. Math KR, Zaidi SF, Petchparap C, et al. Imaging of total knee arthroplasty. Semin Musculoskeletal Radiol. 2006;10(1):47–63.
37. Chryssikos T, Parvizi J, Ghanem E. FDG-PET imaging can diagnose periprosthetic infection of the hip. Clin Orthop Relat Res. 2008;466:1338–42.
38. Zhuang H, Duarte PS, Pordehnad M, et al. The promising role of 18F-FDG PET in detecting infected lower limb prosthesis implants. J Nucl Med. 2001;42(1):44–8.
39. Love C, Marwin S. Diagnosis infection in the failed joint replacement: a comparison of coincidence detection 18F-FDG and 111In-labeled leukocyte-99mTc-sulfur colloid marrow imaging. J Nucl Med. 2004;45:1864–71.
40. Manthey N, Reinhard P, Moog F, et al. The use of [18F] fluorodeoxyglucose positron emission tomography to differentiate between synovitis, loosening

and infection of hip and knee prostheses. Nucl Med Commun. 2002;23(7):645–53.
41. Reinartz P. FDG-PET in patients with painful hip and knee arthroplasty: technical breakthrough or just more of the same. Q J Nucl Med Mol Imaging. 2009;53(1):41–50.
42. Peterson JJ. Postoperative infection. Radiol Clin N Am. 2006;44(3):645–8.
43. Pill S, Parvizi J, Tang P. Comparison of fluorodeoxyglucose positron emission tomography and 111Indium–white blood cell imaging in the diagnosis of periprosthetic infection of the hip. J Arthroplasty. 2006;21:91–7.
44. Sofka CM. Optimizing techniques for musculoskeletal imaging of the postoperative patient. Radiol Clin N Am. 2006;44(3):323–9.
45. Robson M, Bydder G. Clinical ultrashort echo time imaging of bone and other connective tissues. NMR Biomed. 2006;19:765–80.
46. Bancroft LW. MR imaging of infectious processes of the knee. Radiol Clin N Am. 2007;45(6):931–41.
47. Love C, Marwin S, Palestro C. Nuclear medicine and the infected joint replacement. Semin Nucl Med. 2009;39(1):77–8.
48. Murphy B, Miraude E, van Roij A, Kavanagh E. Diagnosis of periprosthetic joint infection: imaging. In: Parvizi J, editor. The knee. Reconstruction, replacement and revision, vol. 2. Brooklandville: Data Trace Publishing Company; 2013. p. 105.1–105.13.
49. Hofmann AA, Wyatt RWB, Daniels AU, et al. Bone scans after total knee arthroplasty in asymptomatic patients. Clin Orthop. 1990;251:183–8.
50. Palestro CJ, Swyer AJ, Kim CK, et al. Infected knee prostheses: diagnosis with In-111 leukocyte, Tc-99m sulfur colloid, and Tc-99m MDP imaging. Radiology. 1991;179:645–8.
51. Love C, Marwin S, Palestro C. Nuclear medicine and the infected joint replacement. Semin Nucl Med. 2009;39(1):66–78.
52. Reing CM, Richin PF, Kenmore PI. Differential bone-scanning in the evaluation of a painful total joint replacement. J Bone Joint Surg Am. 1979;61 A:933–6.
53. Pelosi E, Baiocco C, Pennone M, et al. 99mTc-HMPAO-leukocyte scintigraphy in patients with symptomatic total hip or knee arthroplasty: improved diagnostic accuracy by means of semi-quantitative evaluation. J Nucl Med. 2004;45(3):438–44.
54. Scher DM, Pak K, Lonner JH, et al. The predictive value of Indium-111 leukocyte scans in the diagnosis of infected total hip, knee and resection arthroplasties. J Arthroplast. 2000;15(3):295–300.
55. Palestro CJ, Love C, Tronco GG, et al. Combined labeled leukocyte and technetium-99m sulfur colloid marrow imaging for diagnosing musculoskeletal infection: principles, technique, interpretation, indications, and limitations. Radiographics. 2006;26:859–70.
56. Parvizi J, Erkocak O, Della VC. Current concepts review culture-negative periprosthetic joint infection. J Bone Joint Surg Am. 2014;96:430–6.
57. Bergin PF, Doppelt JD, Hamilton WG, Mirick GE, Jones AE, Sritulanondha S, Helm JM, Tuan RS. Detection of peri-prosthetic infections with use of ribosomal RNA-based polymerase chain reaction. J Bone Joint Surg Am. 2010;92(3):654–63.
58. Lee AH, Ramanujam T, Ware P, et al. Molecular diagnosis of *Ureaplasma urealyticum* septic arthritis in a patient with hypogammaglobulinemia. Arthritis Rheum. 1992;35(4):443–8.
59. Poole ES, Highton J, Wilkins RJ, et al. A search for *Chlamydia trachomatis* in synovial fluids from patients with reactive arthritis using the polymerase chain reaction and antigen detection methods. Br J Rheumatol. 1992;31(1):31–4.
60. Liebling MR, Arkfeld DG, Michelini GA, et al. Identification of *Neisseria gonorrhoeae* in synovial fluid suing the polymerase chain reaction. Arthritis Rheum. 1994;37(5):702–9.
61. Nocton JJ, Dressler F, Rutledge BJ, et al. Detection of Borrelia burgdorferi DNA by polymerase chain reaction in synovial fluid from patients with Lyme arthritis. N Engl J Med. 1994;330(4):229–34.
62. Gallo J, Raska M, Dendis M, et al. Molecular diagnosis of prosthetic joint infection. A review of evidence. Biomed Pap Med Fac Univ Palacky Olomouc Czech Repub. 2004;148(2):123–9.
63. Deirmengian C, Siemon J. Diagnosis of periprosthetic joint infection: molecular techniques. In: Parvizi J, editor. The knee. Reconstruction, replacement and revision, vol. 2. Brooklandville: Data Trace Publishing Company; 2013. p. 102.1–7.
64. Tunney MM, Patrick S, Curran MD, et al. Detection of prosthetic hip infection at revision arthroplasty by immunofluorescence microscopy and PCR amplification of the bacterial 16S rRNA gene. J Clin Microbiol. 1999;37(10):3281–90.
65. Panousis K, Grigoris P, Butcher I, et al. Poor predictive value of broad-range PCR for the detection of arthroplasty infection in 92 cases. Acta Orthop. 2005;76(3):341–6.
66. Rampini SK, Bloemberg GV, Keller PM, Buchler AC, Dollenmaier G, Speck RF, Bottger EC. Broad-range 16S rRNA gene polymerase chain reaction for diagnosis of culture-negative bacterial infections. Clin Infect Dis. 2011;53(12):1245–51.
67. Tarkin IS, Henry TJ, Fey PI, et al. PCR rapidly detects methicillin-resistant staphylococci peri-prosthetic infection. Clin Orthop Relat Res. 2003;414:89–94.
68. Achermann Y, Vogt M, Leunig M, et al. Improved diagnosis of peri-prosthetic joint infection by multiplex PCR of sonication fluid from removed implants. J Clin Microbiol. 2010;48(4):1208–14.
69. Birmingham P, Helm JM, Manner PA, Tuan RS. Simulated joint infection assessment by rapid detection of live bacteria with real-time reverse transcription polymerase chain reaction. J Bone Joint Surg Am. 2008;90(3):602–8.
70. Ghanem E, Ketonis C, Restrepo C, Joshi A, Barrack R, Parvizi J. Periprosthetic infection: where do

we stand with regard to Gram stain? Acta Orthop. 2009;80(1):37–40.
71. Spangehl MJ, Masterson E, Masri BA, O'Connell JX, Duncan CP. The role of intraoperative Gram stain in the diagnosis of infection during revision total hip arthroplasty. J Arthroplast. 1999;14(8):952–6.
72. Steckelberg JM, Osmon DR. Prosthetic joint infections. In: Bisno AL, Waldvogel FA, editors. Infections associated with indwelling medical devices. 2nd ed. Washington, DC: American Society for Microbiology; 1994. p. 259–90.
73. Atkins BL, Athanasou N. Prospective evaluation of criteria for microbiological diagnosis of prosthetic-joint infection at revision arthroplasty. The OSIRIS Collaborative Study Group. J Clin Microbiol. 1998;36(10):2932–9.
74. Della Valle CJ, Sporer SM, Jacobs JJ, Berger RA, Rosenberg AG, Paprosky WG. Preoperative testing for sepsis before revision total knee arthroplasty. J Arthroplast. 2007;22(6 Suppl 2):90–3.
75. Tsaras G, Maduka-Ezeh A, Inwards CY. Utility of intraoperative frozen section histopathology in the diagnosis of periprosthetic joint infection. JBJS. 2012;94(18):1700–11.

Pre-operative Workup and Planning for Periprosthetic Fractures of the Hip and Knee

3

Edward M. DelSole and James D. Slover

Introduction

The term "periprosthetic fracture" refers to a fracture around a joint arthroplasty. The incidence of periprosthetic fractures is 0.045–0.13%, and this is rising due to the increasing number of primary and revision hip and knee arthroplasty procedures [1]. These injuries are a substantial financial burden on the healthcare system, with revisions for fracture being more costly than revision for both aseptic loosening and deep infection due to significantly increased operative times, blood loss, and hospital stay than revision for other reasons [2].

The consequences of periprosthetic fracture are significant. Bhattacharyya et al. reported a 1-year mortality of 11% following periprosthetic fracture of the femur despite patients with fracture having similar comorbidity indices to patients undergoing primary arthroplasty [3]. This study also reported that delay of surgical intervention for longer than 48 h was associated with an increase in mortality. Therefore, expedited medical evaluation and surgical management is needed. Lindahl demonstrated that a periprosthetic fracture contributes to 1-year mortality independent of medical comorbidities, underscoring that the fracture itself may be a sentinel health event for the patient [4].

Periprosthetic fractures can occur intraoperatively (considered "early") or at any time interval after the index arthroplasty (considered "late") as a result of low- or high-energy traumatic events. The management of periprosthetic fractures is dependent upon multiple factors including the nature of injury, the fracture pattern, the stability of the implant, the quality of remaining host bone, and the patient's comorbid medical status. Prior to any operative management, all of these factors should be closely evaluated in order to appropriately plan for surgery.

The focus of this chapter is to describe the initial evaluation and management of patients who have sustained periprosthetic fractures about a total hip or total knee arthroplasty. Evaluation of medical issues and radiographic studies will be discussed. Radiographic classification systems will be presented along with their implications on pre-operative planning.

E. M. DelSole
Department of Orthopaedic Surgery, Tower Health, Keystone Spine and Pain Management, Wyomissing, PA, USA
e-mail: edelsole@kos-spine.com

J. D. Slover (✉)
Zucker School of Medicine at Hofstra/Northwell, Hempstead, NY, USA

Lenox Hill Hospital, New York, NY, USA
e-mail: jslover@northwell.edu

R. S. Yoon et al. (eds.), *Trauma and Infection Control in Revision Hip and Knee Arthroplasty*,
https://doi.org/10.1007/978-3-031-71971-4_3

Part I: Clinical Evaluation of Periprosthetic Fractures

The goals of evaluation and treatment includes early comprehensive medical evaluation and optimization, surgical fracture reduction and fixation, achievement of a stable and well-fixed prosthesis, and early post-surgical mobilization to prevent the morbidity of prolonged recumbency such as venous thromboembolic events, pneumonia, and pressure ulcers.

Like fractures of the native hip, patients who sustain late periprosthetic fractures of the hip or knee will do so either spontaneously secondary to compromised bone due to osteoporosis or osteolysis, or as the result of significant trauma. It is important to understand that these two patients are pathologically distinct and must be considered as such.

Initially, the high-energy trauma patient should be evaluated according to the Advanced Trauma Life Support (ATLS) protocol. The systematic evaluation of the airway, breathing, circulation and perfusion, neurologic disability, and full exposure of the trauma patient should be performed immediately and the patient should be stabilized emergently. Assessment of medical history, current medications, and last meal is important. Thorough orthopaedic evaluation should be performed, including a complete secondary survey. Plain films of the chest, pelvis, and any obviously injured extremity should be obtained. Surgical stabilization of the extremities should be performed after collaboration with the general surgery team to determine the optimal timing of early total care or damage control procedures.

Patients with spontaneous periprosthetic fractures or those with low energy trauma should be systematically evaluated with a complete history and physical examination. History should include the injury event and any signs of prosthesis compromise that may have precipitated it. The patient should be asked if they had pain in the injured joint or extremity prior to the fracture, which may be suggestive of prior loosening, osteolysis, or an adverse soft-tissue response to the implant or its wear particles. Careful history of trauma should be elucidated. An attempt should be made to distinguish patients who fell and subsequently felt pain in the affected extremity from those who felt acute pain in the extremity prior to falling because this latter case may have sustained a fracture prior to a fall which is concerning for prosthesis loosening, osteolysis, and osteoporosis.

The possibility of a pre-existing periprosthetic joint infection (PJI) should be explored through careful history and clinical evaluation. If there is any clinical suspicion for infection, further workup by laboratory studies, intra-operative evaluation, and potentially intra-operative frozen section should be performed. There are presently no defined algorithms for specifically ruling out a PJI in the setting of a periprosthetic fracture and ultimately the determination may need to be made intra-operatively.

Pre-operatively we do not routinely use traction stabilization for all patients. Traction by means of a transosseous pin and weighted pulley system is reasonable to perform if the fracture is sufficiently distal in the femur to cause an unstable thigh deformity. In this setting, traction may decrease deformity, pain, and blood loss [5]. Additionally, traction is an important tool if the timing of definitive fixation is unknown. In this setting, traction may be helpful to maintain the length of the femur, ultimately allowing for easier definitive reduction and fixation.

Physical Examination

A routine orthopaedic physical examination should be performed. The skin should be inspected closely for integrity of prior scars, erythema, drainage, or other local soft-tissue reactions. Palpation should be performed to assess areas of pain, deformity, joint hypermobility/laxity, or soft-tissue mass. A complete neurovascular examination should be performed with special tests performed based upon the mechanism of injury. If the history and mechanism is suspicious for knee dislocation, an ankle-brachial index should be performed to evaluate for vascular injury [6]. The surgeon should evaluate the competence of the knee extensor mechanism. Joint stability should be assessed if possible.

Pre-operative Medical Evaluation

The consequences of periprosthetic fracture are severe. Bhattacharyya et al. reported a 1-year mortality of 11% following periprosthetic fracture of the femur despite patients with fracture having similar comorbidity indices to patients undergoing primary arthroplasty [3]. This study also reported that delay of surgical intervention for longer than 48 h was associated with an increase in mortality. Thus expedited medical evaluation and surgical management is encouraged.

Initial management should include pre-operative bloodwork including complete blood count, metabolic panel, coagulation studies, and blood type and screening. The authors recommend placement of a Foley catheter for fluid management and to minimize the need for painful bed mobilization prior to surgery. Perioperative thromboembolism prophylaxis should be initiated if not medically contraindicated.

Radiographic Evaluation

The radiographic evaluation of a periprosthetic fracture should include orthogonal plain X-rays of the affected extremity. Periprosthetic fractures at the hip or knee necessitate full-length orthogonal films of the femur and tibia in order to plan for possible placement of plates or stems. Regardless of anatomic location, the radiographs should be evaluated with careful attention to fracture pattern, location, comminution, bone quality, and implant loosening. A well-fixed implant demonstrates contact between the bone-implant or bone-cement interfaces without separation [7]. Classification of the fracture should be made to help guide treatment.

Although not routinely used, computed tomography (CT) and magnetic resonance (MR) imaging studies can be considered when fracture is suspected but not evident on X-rays [7–9]. Similarly, these imaging modalities may be used to better delineate the extent of periprosthetic osteolysis and pelvic discontinuity. While plain films in general are the standard for diagnosing periprosthetic osteolysis, these have been shown to have relatively poor sensitivity, especially for lesions in the ischium and acetabular rim for which there is a sensitivity of <15% [10]. Computed tomography (CT) though not routinely used in the pre-operative evaluation of periprosthetic fractures may provide additional information related to osteolytic bone losses. CT has been shown to identify up to 75% of osteolytic lesions in the hip although lesions in the pubis are more difficult to detect [11]. Better still is MR, which has been shown to detect up to 95% of osteolytic lesions regardless of lesion location. Both modalities are highly effective at determining the volume of the lesion [11, 12].

Additionally, if prior operative reports are unavailable, an attempt should be made to determine the type of implant involved in the fracture from plain radiography. The system used for the index procedure may influence the necessary tools needed for successful revision surgery. Existing bearing surfaces should be evaluated to anticipate potential intra-operative issues. For example, metal-on-metal articulations may corrode and cause significant local metallosis, which leads to adverse soft-tissue reactions, necrosis of soft tissue, and ultimately a complicated surgical approach and closure [13].

Part II: Periprosthetic Fracture Radiographic Evaluation and Classification Systems

The surgical tactic for a periprosthetic fracture is dependent upon fracture pattern and location, the fixation of the component, remaining host bone stock, and the quality of that bone. These principles inform most modern periprosthetic fracture classification systems and guide the surgical management of these injuries.

Periprosthetic fractures around the acetabulum may occur both intra-operatively during press-fitting of the cup or at a later time after surgery [14, 15]. The most widely cited classification of periprosthetic acetabular fractures is that of Paprosky (Table 3.1) [16]. In his classification system, type I and II fractures are those which

Table 3.1 The Paprosky classification of periprosthetic acetabulum fractures [16]

Type I	Intra-operative fractures caused by acetabular component insertion
Type II	Intra-operative fracture caused by acetabular component removal
Type III	Traumatic fracture
Type IV	Spontaneous fractures
Type V	Pelvic discontinuity

occur during surgical implantation of the cup or removal of a cup, respectively. Depending upon the fracture pattern, type I fractures are treated with either component retention if stable, exchange for a component with supplemental screw fixation, or removal of the implant followed by anatomic fracture reduction and rigid internal fixation followed by line-to-line acetabular component placement with screw fixation. Treatment of type II fractures is dependent upon the residual host bone stock and involves placing a porous coated acetabular component with supplemental screw fixation with or without bone graft. For type II fractures with extensive bone loss (<50% remaining host bone) reconstruction usually involves placement of a cage construct to span the defect, obtaining fixation in the ilium and ischium. Type III fractures are acute fractures that result from trauma. For type III injuries with a stable acetabular component, non-surgical treatment is recommended with a period of protected weight bearing. For type III fractures with unstable component, surgical treatment with component removal, fracture reduction and internal fixation, and placement of a line-to-line type acetabular component is typically recommended. Type IV fractures occur spontaneously without trauma. Similar to type II fractures, type IV can be reconstructed using porous-coated hemispherical components with screw fixation. However, those with extensive bone loss may require reconstruction cages. Type V fractures involve a pelvic discontinuity and are treated with reconstruction cages, periacetabular augments, and structural allografts. When these fractures occur, anteroposterior pelvis and Judet oblique radiographs should be performed to appropriately classify the fracture [17–19].

Table 3.2 The Vancouver classification of periprosthetic femur fractures [20]

Type A	Fracture of the greater or lesser trochanter
Type B1	Fracture about a well-fixed stem
Type B2	Fracture about a loose stem with good remaining bone stock
Type B3	Fracture about a loose stem with poor remaining bone stock
Type C	Fracture well distal to the implant stem

Periprosthetic fractures of the proximal femur are most commonly classified according to the Vancouver Classification, which describes a fracture's position, implant stability, and quality of remaining bone stock (Table 3.2) [20]. A Vancouver type A fracture involves the greater or lesser trochanter and typically represents an avulsion fracture of an osteolytic segment in the setting of a low energy mechanism (Fig. 3.1) [21]. These are typically treated non-operatively with weight bearing to tolerance or, if displaced and occurring intra-operatively, with fracture reduction and fixation with a clawed trochanteric plate [22]. Vancouver A fractures of the lesser trochanter are similarly treated with weight bearing to tolerance or, if involving substantial medical cortex, are treated surgically with cerclage wiring and revision if the stem has destabilized. Vancouver B fractures occur around the femoral stem. This type is subdivided into types B1, B2, and B3, which further describe the fracture based upon its location, the stability of the femoral stem, and the quality of surrounding bone stock. B1 fractures occur around a well-fixed femoral stem (Fig. 3.2) and are treated typically with open reduction and internal fixation using plates, screws, cables, or cortical onlay allografts. B2 fractures occur around a loose femoral stem with good regional bone stock (Figs. 3.3 and 3.4). B3 fractures occur around a loose femoral stem with poor regional bone stock. For B2 and B3 fractures, revision with a fully coated stem with distal fixation is performed in conjunction with fracture fixation. In B3 fractures, bone replacing techniques such as impaction grafting or use of an allograft prosthesis or proximal femoral replacement may be indicated. Vancouver type C frac-

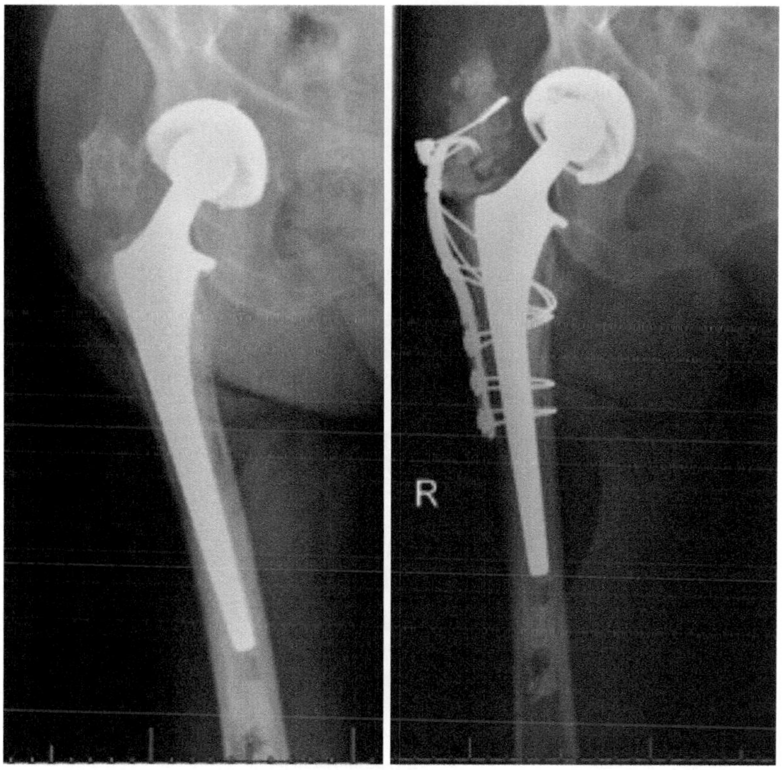

Fig. 3.1 This is an 87-year-old female who sustained a Vancouver type A fracture of the greater trochanter with resultant hip instability and recurrent dislocation. Her fracture was treated with ORIF using a greater trochanter plate and cable system. The acetabular component was concomitantly revised to a revision cup with a constrained polyethylene liner in response to her instability

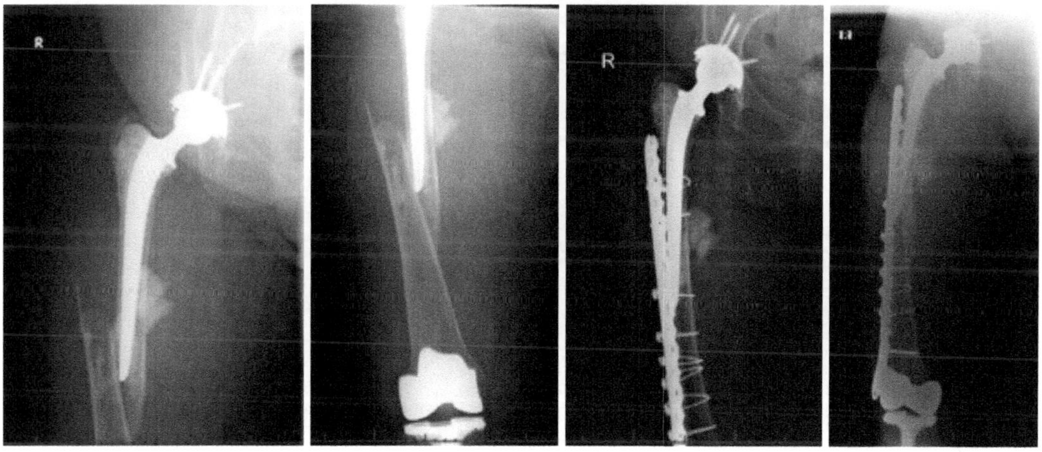

Fig. 3.2 A 79-year-old female sustained a Vancouver Type B1 fracture near the distal aspect of a well-fixed cemented stem. Careful inspection of these radiographs demonstrates an intact cement mantle without evidence of delamination from the proximal bone or the implant itself. This fracture was treated with ORIF using a lateral periarticular locking plate and cabling system

tures occur distal to a well-fixed femoral stem and are typically treated with open reduction and a long laterally applied plate and screw construct.

The classification systems of periprosthetic supracondylar distal femur fractures about a total knee arthroplasty are multiple and often determine the need for surgery or non-surgical management. The Su classification system is one useful system for determining surgical options for patients who require operative intervention

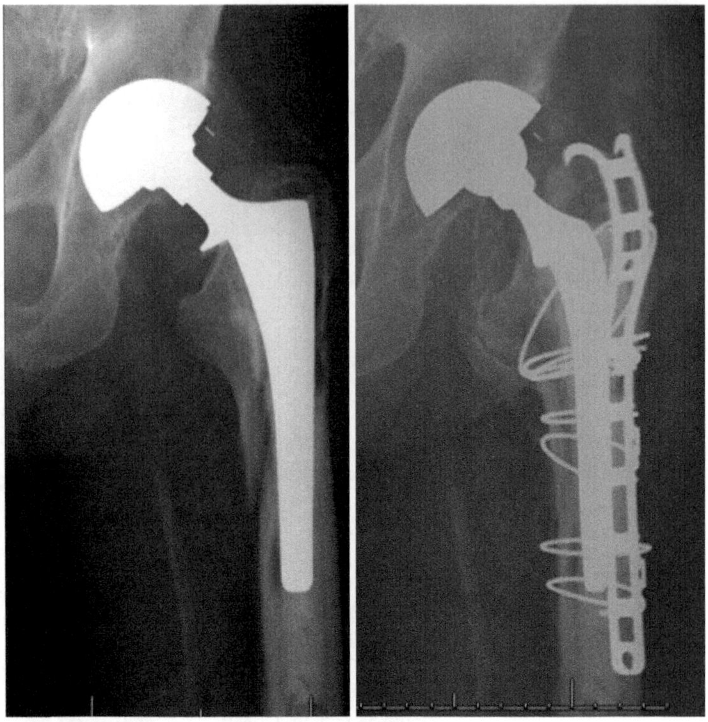

Fig. 3.3 A 97-year-old male who sustained a Vancouver B2 fracture about a loose cemented femoral stem. Inspection of the injury radiograph demonstrates loosening, evidenced by radiolucency between the cement mantle and bone in Gruen's zones 1 and 2. This was treated with revision cemented THA and ORIF of the fracture using a greater trochanter plate and Dall-Miles cable system

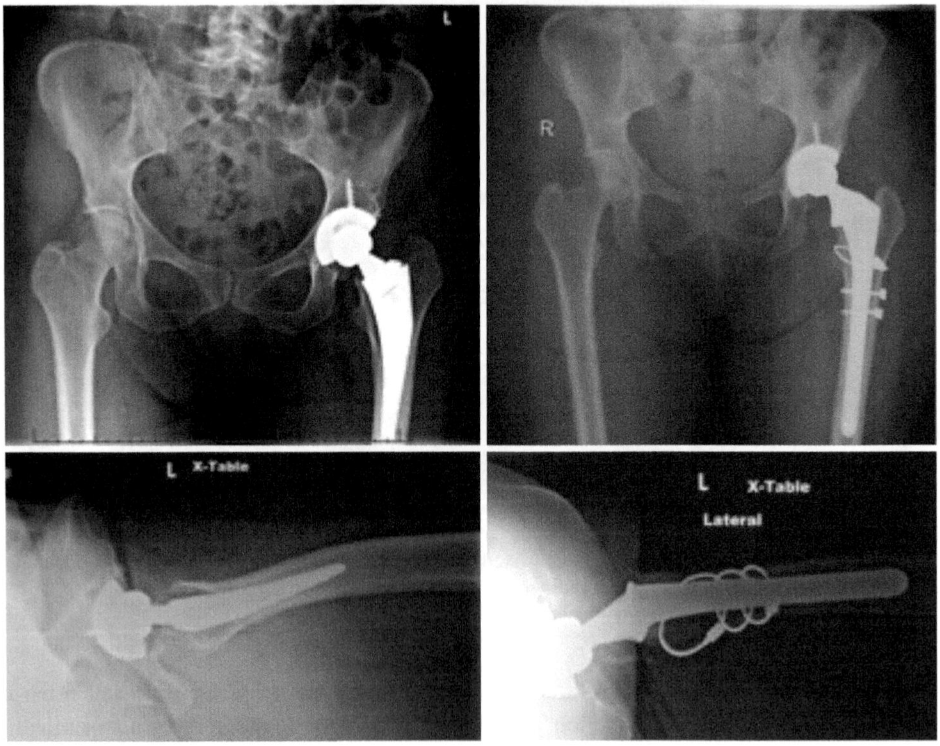

Fig. 3.4 A 76-year-old female sustained a Vancouver B2 fracture. The loose stem is evidenced by subsidence, and loosening was confirmed intra-operatively. This injury was managed with revision to a long diaphyseal fitting component and cables

(Table 3.3) [23]. In this system, type I fractures are those occurring well proximal to the femoral component. These fractures are typically treated with intramedullary nails. Type II fractures are those occurring at the proximal aspect of the prosthesis and extend proximally. These fractures typically require fixation with a fixed-angle device or retrograde nail if the prosthesis has an open box. Type III fractures are those with any fracture line extending distal to the femoral component's anterior flange (Fig. 3.5). These may be amenable to fixation with a fixed-angle device though some will require revision to a long-stemmed distal femoral replacement. The fixation of the component should be evaluated intra-operatively for each of these fracture types, as revision would be necessary in all cases if the femoral component were loose.

Periprosthetic fractures of the tibia are also classified based upon the location of the fracture, fixation status of the tibial component, remaining proximal tibial bone stock, and whether or not they occur intra-operatively [24]. In the Felix classification system, type I fractures are tibial plateau fractures around a well-fixed stem (Table 3.4). Type IA fractures, which are those with stable implants are treated with open reduction and internal fixation. Type IB fractures, which are those with unstable implants are most

Table 3.3 The Su classification of periprosthetic distal femur fractures [23]

Type 1	Fracture proximal to the femoral knee component
Type 2	Fracture which originates at the proximal aspect of femoral component and migrates proximally
Type 3	Fracture line extends distal to the anterior flange of the femoral component

Table 3.4 The Felix classification of periprosthetic proximal tibia fractures [24]

Type I	Tibial plateau fracture about a well-fixed tibial component
Type II	Tibial plateau fracture around the prosthetic stem with associated osteolysis
Type III	Tibial fractures which occur distal to the stem and do not cause prosthetic loosening
Type IV	Tibial fracture which involves the tibial tubercle

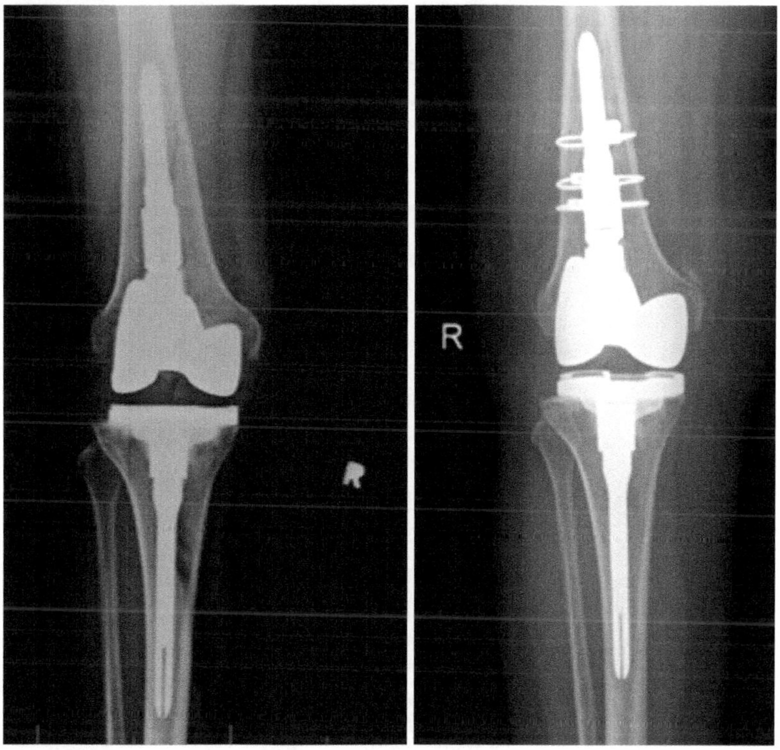

Fig. 3.5 A 56-year-old female sustained a Su Type 3 periprosthetic fracture of the distal femur. The fracture line extends distal to the anterior flange of the femoral component; however, the fracture is non-displaced and the implant was found to be stable. The fracture was treated with open reduction and circumferential cable fixation

commonly treated with revision. Type IC fractures, which occur intra-operatively, are treated with reduction and fragment-specific fixation as well as conversion to a long-stemmed tibial component with post-operative protected weight bearing. Type II fractures are those that occur around the prosthetic stem and are frequently associated with periprosthetic osteolysis. Type IIA fractures can be treated with casting and non-weight bearing. Type IIB fractures typically occur around a long-stemmed prosthesis with osteolysis and can be treated with revision arthroplasty. Type IIC fractures should be treated however necessary to achieve anatomic reduction and stable tibial component fixation prior to surgical closure. Type III fractures are those which occur distal to the component and do not cause prosthetic loosening (Fig. 3.6). Type IIIA fractures have been treated non-operatively with casting and restricted weight bearing. Type IIIB fractures have been treated with initial casting and staged tibial component revision after fracture healing has occurred. Type IIIC fractures can be treated with cast immobilization or revision to a long-stemmed tibial component during the index procedure. Type IV fractures are those which involve the tibial tubercle. These fractures can be treated with extension casting or open reduction and internal fixation depending upon the degree of displacement.

Periprosthetic fractures of the patella are most commonly classified in the manner published by Ortiguera and Berry (Table 3.5) [25]. This classification is guided by the integrity of the extensor mechanism, fixation status of the patellar

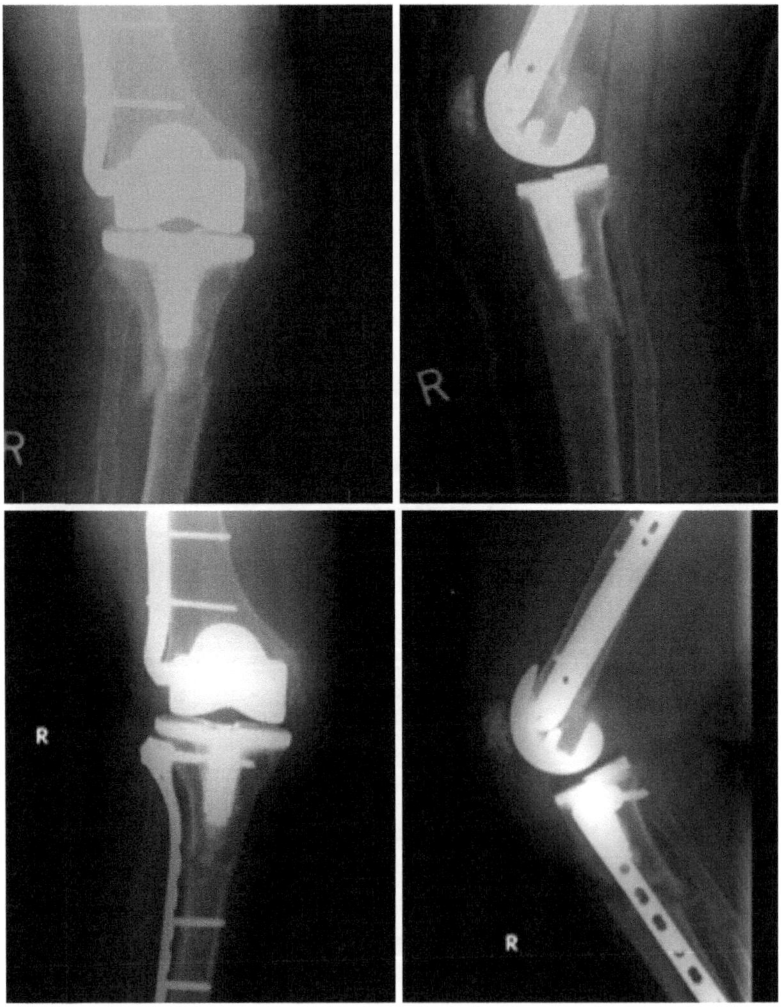

Fig. 3.6 A 68-year-old female with a right TKA sustained a Felix type 3 fracture about the tibial component. The fracture was minimally displaced and did not extend into the periprosthetic metaphyseal bone. The implant itself was stable. This fracture was treated by ORIF using a lateral periarticular locking plate

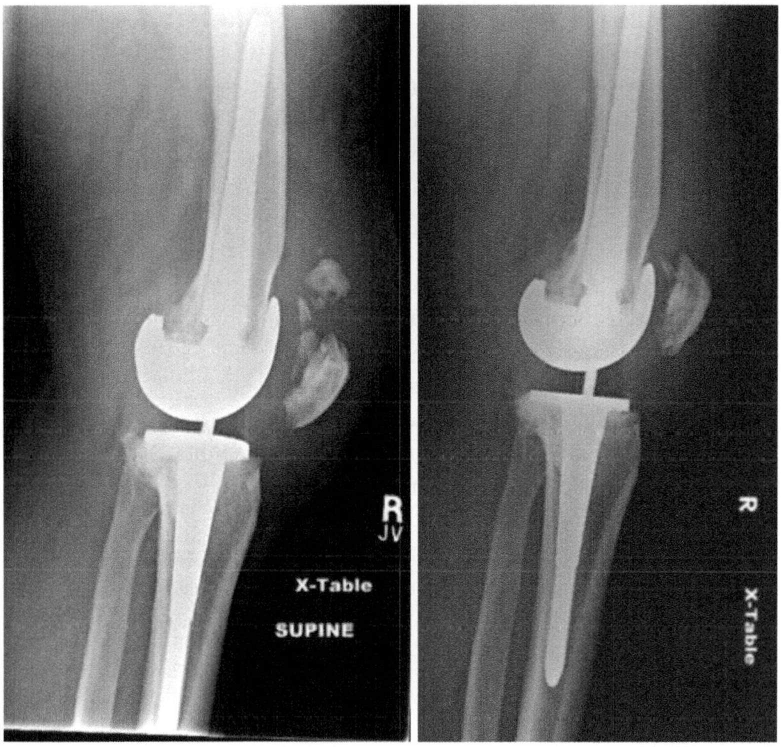

Fig. 3.7 A 71-year-old male sustained an Ortiguera Type 2 fracture with a stable prosthesis and a disrupted quadriceps tendon. The patient was treated with partial patellectomy of the proximal comminution and quadriceps tendon advancement and fixation using non-absorbable suture

Table 3.5 Ortiguera and Berry classification of periprosthetic patella fractures [25]

Type I	Fracture around a patellar implant with an intact extensor mechanism
Type II	Fracture around a patellar implant with a disrupted extensor mechanism
Type III	Fracture around a patellar implant with an intact extensor mechanism and a loose component

implant, and the quality of the host bone. Type I fractures are around a stable implant with an intact extensor mechanism and can be treated with observation or immobilization. Type II fractures involve a disrupted extensor mechanism (Fig. 3.7). These difficult injuries can be treated with prolonged immobilization in extension or with surgical fixation or partial patellectomy and advancement of the extensor mechanism. Type III fractures occur with an intact extensor mechanism with a loose component. These can be treated with observation alone or by resection arthroplasty, internal fixation, and concomitant or staged revision patellar resurfacing. With poor remaining patellar bone stock, resection arthroplasty can be performed with subsequent patelloplasty or complete patellectomy.

Conclusion

Periprosthetic fractures are complex injuries that present unique surgical challenges. To avoid pitfalls while caring for these patients, we recommend a careful and standardized pre-operative plan which includes a thorough history and physical exam, expeditious pre-operative medical workup and optimization, and timely surgical intervention within 48 h if possible. Radiographic classification is essential in order to plan the surgical tactic. Early post-operative mobilization is essential and may help to prevent the early complications of prolonged recumbence.

Author's Preferred Method/Take Home Points

- Periprosthetic fractures are major sentinel health events and require careful pre-surgical planning.
- A careful physical examination and an expeditious pre-operative medical workup are essential.
- Radiographic evaluation should focus on the location and pattern of the fracture, as well as the fixation status of the implant and the quality of the remaining host bone surrounding the implant. Radiographic classification directly guides surgical management.
- An attempt should be made to understand the nature of the existing implants within the patient in order to anticipate complications during approach, fracture care, and wound closure.

Glossary

Arthroplasty A surgical procedure which involves exposure of a joint, excision of bone and soft tissue, and reconstruction of the joint with articulating implants of variable material which allow for extremity motion.

Fracture The event in which bone, when under an applied stress, reaches its Newtonian yield point and subsequently breaks.

Hip The human joint composed of the articulation of the acetabulum of the pelvis and the femoral head.

Knee The human joint composed of the articulations of the distal femur, proximal tibia, and patella.

Osteolysis Pathologic demineralization of bone, which occurs around an orthopaedic implant and can be visualized on plain radiograph, typically in response to microscopic wear particles from arthroplasty.

Periprosthetic fracture A fracture of bone occurring at or around an orthopaedic implant.

Revision A surgical procedure which involves removal of an orthopaedic implant and replacement of a new implant typically due to some prior mechanical failure of the original implant.

References

1. Lindahl H, Malchau H, Herberts P, Garellick G. Periprosthetic femoral fractures classification and demographics of 1049 periprosthetic femoral fractures from the Swedish National Hip Arthroplasty Register. J Arthroplasty. 2005;20(7):857–65. https://doi.org/10.1016/j.arth.2005.02.001.
2. Vanhegan IS, Malik AK, Jayakumar P. A financial analysis of revision hip arthroplasty: the economic burden in relation to the national tariff. J Bone Joint Surg Br. 2012;94-B(5):619–23. https://doi.org/10.1302/0301-620X.94B5.
3. Bhattacharyya T, Chang D, Meigs JB, Estok DM, Malchau H. Mortality after periprosthetic fracture of the femur. J Bone Joint Surg Am. 2007;89(12):2658–62. https://doi.org/10.2106/JBJS.F.01538.
4. Lindahl H, Oden A, Garellick G, Malchau H. The excess mortality due to periprosthetic femur fracture. A study from the Swedish national hip arthroplasty register. Bone. 2007;40(5):1294–8. https://doi.org/10.1016/j.bone.2007.01.003.
5. Winant EM. The use of skeletal traction in the treatment of fractures of the femur. J Bone Joint Surg. 1949;31A(1):87–93.
6. Fanelli GC, Stannard JP, Stuart MJ, MacDonald PB, Marx RG, Whelan DB, et al. Management of complex knee ligament injuries. J Bone Joint Surg Am. 2010;92(12):2235–46. https://doi.org/10.1016/S0021-9355(10)71511-3.
7. Fritz J, Lurie B, Miller TT. Imaging of hip arthroplasty. Semin Musculoskelet Radiol. 2013;17(3):316–27. https://doi.org/10.1055/s-0033-1348098.
8. Cook SM, Pellicci PM, Potter HG. Use of magnetic resonance imaging in the diagnosis of an occult fracture of the femoral component after total hip arthroplasty. J Bone Joint Surg. 2004;os-86(1):149–53. https://doi.org/10.1007/s002640050119.
9. Fritz J, Lurie B, Potter HG. MR imaging of knee arthroplasty implants. Radiographics. 2015;35(5):1–19. https://doi.org/10.1148/rg.2015140216.
10. Claus AM, Engh CA, Sychterz CJ, Xenos JS, Orishimo KF, Engh CA. Radiographic definition of pelvic osteolysis following total hip arthroplasty. J Bone Joint Surg. 2003;85-A(8):1519–26. https://doi.org/10.1097/00003086-200112000-00007.
11. Walde TA, Weiland DE, Leung SB, Kitamura N, Sychterz CJ, Engh CA Jr, et al. Comparison of CT, MRI, and radiographs in assessing pelvic osteolysis. Clin Orthop Relat Res. 2005;437:138–44. https://doi.org/10.1097/01.blo.0000164028.14504.46.
12. Weiland DE, Walde TA, Leung SB, Sychterz CJ, Ho S, Engh CA, Potter HG. Magnetic resonance imaging in the evaluation of periprosthetic acetabular osteolysis: a cadaveric study. J Orthop Res. 2006;23(4):713–9. https://doi.org/10.1016/j.orthres.2005.02.007.

13. Fehring KA, Fehring TK. Modes of failure in metal-on-metal total hip arthroplasty. Orthop Clin North Am. 2015;46(2):185–92. https://doi.org/10.1016/j.ocl.2014.11.001.
14. Chitre A, Wynn Jones H, Shah N, Clayson A. Complications of total hip arthroplasty: periprosthetic fractures of the acetabulum. Curr Rev Musculoskelet Med. 2013;6(4):357–63. https://doi.org/10.1007/s12178-013-9188-5.
15. Sharkey PF, Hozack WJ, Callaghan JJ, Kim YS. Acetabular fracture associated with cementless acetabular component insertion: a report of 13 cases. J Arthroplasty. 1999;14(4):426–31. https://doi.org/10.1016/S0883-5403(99)90097-9.
16. DellaValle CJ, Momberger NG, Paprosky WG. Periprosthetic fractures of the acetabulum associated with a total hip arthroplasty. Instr Course Lect. 2003;52:281–90.
17. Callaghan JJ. Periprosthetic fractures of the acetabulum during and following total hip arthroplasty. J Bone Joint Surg. 1997;79(9):1416–21.
18. Judet R, Judet J, Letournel E. Fractures of the acetabulum: classification and surgical approaches for open reduction. Preliminary report. J Bone Joint Surg Am. 1964;46:1615–46.
19. Letournel E. Acetabulum fractures: classification and management. Clin Orthop Relat Res. 1980;151:81–106.
20. Masri BA, Meek R, Duncan CP. Periprosthetic fractures evaluation and treatment. Clin Orthop Relat Res. 2004;420:80–95. https://doi.org/10.1097/01.blo.0000122241.70546.eb.
21. Haidukewych GJ, Langford JR, Liporace FA. Revision for periprosthetic fractures of the hip and knee. Instr Course Lect. 2013;62:333–40.
22. Ricci WM. Periprosthetic femur fractures. J Orthop Trauma. 2015;29(3):130–7. https://doi.org/10.1097/BOT.0000000000000282.
23. Su ET, DeWal H, Di Cesare PE. Periprosthetic femoral fractures above total knee replacements. J Am Acad Orthop Surg. 2004;12(1):12–20.
24. Felix NA, Stuart MJ, Hanssen AD. Periprosthetic fractures of the tibia associated with total knee arthroplasty. Clin Orthop Relat Res. 1997;345:113–24.
25. Ortiguera CJ, Berry DJ. Patellar fracture after total knee arthroplasty. J Bone Joint Surg. 2002;84-A(4):532–40.

4 Addressing the Femoral Side: From Minimal to Severe Bone Loss

Brian M. Culp, Robert A. Sershon, and Brett R. Levine

Introduction

Longer patient life expectancies, as well as the ever-increasing numbers of primary THA being performed annually, will result in a greater incidence of revision THA in years to come [1]. This increased demand will require a large number of surgeons capable of addressing the burden. A variety of pathologic processes lead to femoral-sided failure, including aseptic loosening, stress shielding, periprosthetic fracture, infection, corrosion, implant failure, and technical errors from the index surgery. While the etiology responsible for THA revision can vary, a fairly consistent set of problems are encountered when revising a malfunctioning femoral component. These issues include altered proximal femoral anatomy/remodeling, loss of femoral bone stock, management of a pedestal or retained cement/hardware, and deficient abductor muscle tension. These anatomical dilemmas may be exacerbated intra-operatively during removal of the failed endoprosthesis or cement mantle, or when performing a debridement in the setting of infection. The surgeon must deal with these challenges while achieving the goals of the revision, namely adequate fixation, restoration of anatomy, and maintenance of hip kinematics.

B. M. Culp · R. A. Sershon · B. R. Levine (✉)
Department of Orthopedic Surgery, Rush University Medical Center, Chicago, IL, USA

In this chapter, the authors will explore common problems a surgeon may encounter during femoral component revision and break each of these down into several manageable challenges. The remainder of this chapter will provide case-based examples of challenges one may encounter during revision of the femoral component. It is our goal to provide the reader with preoperative, intraoperative, and postoperative guidance for the clinical decisions that needs to occur on a patient-by-patient basis. We hope to provide a systematic approach to reviewing the preoperative radiographs, recommend the appropriate tools and implants necessary to solve anticipated problems, and develop an understanding of the various prostheses and pearls to utilize them for specific situations.

Background

The concerns of femoral bone loss, abnormal proximal femoral morphology, management of a pedestal or retained cement, and soft tissue deficiency are present in varying degrees in all cases of revision THA. It can be helpful to mentally separate each of these problems into individual categories, compartmentalizing the necessary tools available to solve each of them. Arguably, the most challenging to address is bone loss, as this will ultimately dictate which prosthetic option the surgeon should use. The implant chosen must

R. S. Yoon et al. (eds.), *Trauma and Infection Control in Revision Hip and Knee Arthroplasty*,
https://doi.org/10.1007/978-3-031-71971-4_4

achieve sufficient fixation to prevent subsidence or rotation, allow for early weight bearing, restore the local anatomy to provide adequate hip stability, and have a good long-term track record. This task becomes more challenging as the quantity and quality of the bone decreases. While preoperative radiographs provide information regarding the anticipated amount of bone loss the surgeon will encounter, it is important to remember that films typically underestimates the actual bone loss found intraoperatively. A critical evaluation of preoperative radiographs allows for enhanced preoperative planning of the desired design and intrinsic properties of the femoral implant required to provide sufficient stability and fixation. However, it is important to create a backup plan during the planning process.

Preoperative radiographs are classically assessed using three main systems for femoral bone loss. These include the American Academy of Orthopaedic Surgeons (AAOS), the Mallory classification, and the Paprosky classification systems [2–4]. Tables 4.1, 4.2, and 4.3 highlight each classification system. While each classification system provides some utility, the Paprosky classification system provides a good framework for guiding prosthesis selection, and is the preferred system at our institution.

Altered proximal femoral anatomy most frequently manifests itself in femoral retroversion and varus angulation, likely due to the deforming forces crossing the hip joint in the setting of failing fixation. When preparing a preoperative plan, one must utilize implant options that do not rely on normal proximal femoral anatomy for support. For example, the surgeon must be able to put the components in the correct anteversion, regardless of the location of available bone. This may be solved with modular prostheses or cylindrical, distally fixed monoblock stems that allow the surgeon to correct for this abnormal morphology. Modularity has the benefit of being able to change the length and diameter of the proximal segment, which may be more versatile in managing leg lengths and bone defects. Furthermore, modular stems provide the ability to restore the appropriate leg length and offset independent from the location of ultimate stem fixation. While modular components provide such benefits, there are certain drawbacks associated with their use. Additional interfaces have increased opportunity for component corrosion or wear. Furthermore, junctional sites of certain modular components have had problems with mechanically assisted crevice corrosion and, ultimately, fatigue fractures of the implants. It is imperative when planning surgery to consider when and where to use modular implants, as it is often contraindicated to utilize these prostheses in the setting of minimal proximal and junctional bony support. While many of these problems have been resolved with improved component manufacturing, the surgeon must still consider them when choosing to use this option.

Proximal femoral varus remodeling raises other issues regarding component implantation. Excess varus angulation, when present, may pre-

Table 4.1 Mallory bone loss classification

Type 1	Intact metaphyseal and diaphyseal bone
Type 2	Metaphyseal bone destruction with an intact cortical tube
Type 3	Metaphyseal bone destruction with cortical damage
3A	Cortical destruction in the region of the lesser trochanter
3B	Cortical destruction extends to the region from the lesser trochanter to the isthmus
3C	Cortical destruction of the isthmus and further distally

Table 4.2 AAOS classification

Type 1	Segmental defect
Type 2	Cavitary defect
Type 3	Combined segmental and cavitary defects
Type 4	Rotation or angular deformity
Type 5	Femoral stenosis
Type 6	Femoral discontinuity

Table 4.3 Paprosky femoral bone loss classification

Type 1	Minimal metaphyseal bone loss with intact diaphysis
Type 2	Extensive metaphyseal bone loss with intact diaphysis
Type 3A	Metaphyseal bone is nonsupportive and greater than 4 cm of intact diaphysis
Type 3B	Metaphyseal bone is nonsupportive and less than 4 cm of intact diaphysis
Type 4	Extensive metaphyseal and diaphyseal bone loss with a widened canal. Nonsupportive isthmus

vent adequate preparation of the femoral canal with straight reamers. Additionally, the chosen prosthesis may not seat properly within the angulated bone. Early three-point stem fixation, rather than full seating of the implant, can result in undersizing of the component and failure to maximize host bone-implant contact. This increases the risk of both varus alignment and early implant failure. In this circumstance, an extended trochanteric osteotomy (ETO) may be required to allow straight reaming of the canal or to accommodate the proximal aspect of the prosthesis. The use of an ETO also provides excellent exposure to manage a distal pedestal or retained cement when present. This technique can be utilized during revision THA for component removal, improved exposure, or to facilitate replanting the revision components and has an excellent history with osteotomy site union rates of 98% after 2.6 years [5]. An ETO also minimizes the possible complication of canal perforation during reaming and can permit advancement of the trochanter to aid in tension of the abductors. Further description of the procedure and indications will be discussed later in this chapter.

The integrity of the soft tissues around the hip is yet another area of concern when planning for revision THA. This topic encompasses a broad area of consideration, which includes the presence, or absence of abductor muscles to tension the hip, the blood supply to the femoral bone, the existence of heterotopic bone, and the avoidance of complications secondary to neurovascular injury. Special attention should be paid to preoperative abductor function. This can be assessed on preoperative clinical examination and radiographs, with a particular focus on the region of the greater trochanter. If the integrity of the abductor complex is in question, the surgeon should be prepared to utilize a system that can accommodate constraint, or consider dual-mobility technology, which has recently demonstrated the ability to compensate for abductor deficiency. Intraoperatively, careful technique should be utilized with dissection around the femur, gluteus maximus tendon and abductors to prevent damage to local neurovascular structures. It is also advisable to consider the sciatic nerve and local vascular structures when attempting to restore leg length in chronically shortened lower extremities, as over-lengthening (>2–3 cm) may result in undue tension on the sciatic nerve, difficulty reducing an osteotomy, and an overall increase in postoperative complications.

In general, we favor using the Paprosky classification of femoral bone loss in an algorithmic fashion to anticipate surgical needs [3]. Type 1 defects possess fairly normal host bone, allowing multiple types of prostheses to result in a successful outcome. Type 1 defects can be treated with cemented or cementless fixation. When cementless fixation is used, one should consider a prosthesis that engages either the metaphyseal-diaphyseal junction or the diaphysis. In many instances, a primary stem may suffice, or otherwise a short, full-coated stem may be all that is required to get sufficient bone contact to gain stability. For Paprosky type 2 defects, where metaphyseal bone loss will not allow proximal fixation, fixation into an intact diaphysis is highly recommended. Once again, a standard length extensively coated, distal-fixed stem works nicely for this scenario. For type 3a bone loss, which has greater than 4 cm of intact femoral diaphysis, the use of long, fully coated, cylindrical prostheses have been shown to perform well with low rates of subsidence or loosening. Large stems greater than 19 mm may have less reliability with a fully coated, monoblock cylindrical stem. In this circumstance, as well as in the setting of type 3b bone loss where less than 4 cm of intact isthmus remains, a splined, tapered stem can achieve excellent fixation. For bone loss that leaves a patulous canal with essentially no cortical bone for adequate fixation, options include impaction bone grafting, cemented stems, composite allograft fixation, or a megaprosthesis.

Preoperative Planning and Radiographs

The breadth of challenges that present during revision THA can be better dealt with when one possesses the appropriate tools and equipment, highlighting the importance of thorough preoperative planning. This starts with radiographic assessment. The patient should have adequate radiographs, which include an X-ray AP pelvis, AP hip, frog leg lateral, and full-length femoral X-rays. It is important to scrutinize the implant-bone interface or bone-cement interface for radiolucencies (particularly if progressive from prior radiographs). Assessment of the greater trochanter and the shoulder of bone above the existing prosthesis can give the treating surgeon information in regard to the degree of difficulty that will be encountered during stem extraction. If a significant amount of trochanteric overhang is seen, safe extraction of a stem can become quite difficult. Furthermore, proximal stress shielding and/or osteolysis can leave the greater trochanter in a fragile state, making component removal even more problematic. Osteotomy planning should occur in these situations to help with exposure or component removal. Attention should also be paid to the calcar in order to determine if there is adequate host bone present to support a prosthesis or if a calcar-replacing body may be needed. Proximal metaphyseal bone stock is frequently deficient, imiting the number of appropriate implant choices.

Moving distally, the isthmus of the femur should be carefully evaluated. The length of the isthmus is measured from the top of the apparent intact femoral canal to the level at which the diaphysis begins to flare out. The measured length of intact isthmus available will assist in planning the appropriate level at which fixation the new femoral implant will occur. The presence or absence of a distal pedestal is also important to recognize preoperatively. Never underestimate a pedestal, as they can be stout enough to require an ETO in order to safely traverse the area of dense, sclerotic bone. Finally, distal femoral views provide information regarding potential blocks for distal femoral implant placement, such as an ipsilateral total knee prosthesis, distal deformity, or prior hardware.

Preoperative templating is a valuable exercise that can help ensure a good outcome at the time of the revision surgery. Templating can give the surgeon a visual perspective of how their planned implant will fit at the time of surgery and help with formulating a backup plan in event that X-rays are misleading or an intraoperative adjustment needs to be made. Templating of the affected leg can be performed, or alternatively, the contralateral leg can be used as a guide to restoring normal anatomy. Limb length discrepancy can be estimated from the preoperative radiographs and an appropriate plan should be made to help restore this difference. The planned implant can be templated for the canal size, for length (i.e., to assure the anchor point is distal to a planned osteotomy), and for fit in the setting of femoral bow or deformity. Plans for an ETO should be made at this time and the distance from the tip of the greater trochanter to the desired level of the osteotomy should be measured (this determination is based on the length of the residing stem, femoral deformity, and osseointegration status of the implant).

Paprosky Type I Femur

Paprosky Type I femoral defects are described as having minimal proximal bone loss with supportive cancellous metaphyseal bone and a normal diaphysis. Type I defects are commonly seen in failed hip resurfacing procedures or when revising a cementless femoral component that has failed to demonstrate osteointegration. Preoperative planning for type I femurs should predominately focus on radiographic signs of implant loosening, implant design, proximal femoral bone stock, femoral canal diameter, and evidence of femoral remodeling. Cross table lateral radiographs may give evidence of remodeling, which typically is retroversion. If the current imp nt is cemented, the bone-cement interface should also be assessed to see how difficult it might be to remove cement.

Relatively normal host bone typically present in type I femurs permits the use of a variety of femoral implants that can use either cemented or uncemented fixation. In most cases of type 1 bone loss, primary arthroplasty implants can be utilized in a reliable fashion. Cemented prostheses are possible in this setting due to the relative proximal bone preservation, which allows for adequate cement interdigitation. If removing a cemented prosthesis, it is important to scrutinize the cement mantle on the preoperative radiographs. Adjacent to the prior mantle, there may be a neocortex that must be debrided to ensure contact with the remaining cancellous bone. If the surgeon chooses to revise using a cemented component, a standard or oversized cement restrictor should be utilized, and third-generation cementing techniques are recommended to ensure maximal interdigitation with the remaining bone. Alternatively, if the existing cement mantle is pristine and can accommodate it, a cement-into-cement technique can be used.

If choosing non-cemented fixation, either a proximally engaging or a distally engaging femoral stem can be used. Proximal porous coating provides the advantage of proximal bone loading to prevent stress shielding, as well as offering the option of modularity for cases of abnormal version or proximal/distal mismatch. Stem-in-sleeve designs also perform well for this task. There have been reports of good outcomes for these prostheses in the revision setting for type I or II femurs with upwards of 96% of component ingrowth and over 95% component survival at 4 years [6]. Alternatively, proximally porous-coated stems with a diaphyseal engaging component can also achieve excellent fixation. Yet another available option is a cylindrical, diaphyseal engaging stem, which permit fixation regardless of proximal remodeling and have demonstrated an excellent track record for ingrowth. Ultimately, surgeons can employ nearly any primary prosthesis available in the setting of a type I femoral defect and are advised to utilize the component they are most comfortable implanting.

Case 1

The patient is a 68-year-old female 3 years status post a primary left hip resurfacing performed at an outside institution that presented with left hip pain. Her index resurfacing was uncomplicated. The patient reported having a painless, well-functioning joint for 2.5 years, until recently developing symptoms. Her left hip pain radiated down the thigh to the knee and was activity related. Radiographic imaging obtained at the initial visit demonstrated evidence acetabular component loosening and significant femoral neck narrowing (Figs. 4.1 and 4.2). Preoperative infectious work-up showed normal values for the erythrocyte sedimentation rate (ESR) and C reactive protein (CRP). Preoperative films show a resurfacing arthroplasty with maintained proximal femoral bone stock and radiographic evidence of acetabular loosening. The lateral radiographs show normal femoral version.

Operation

The prior posterior approach was utilized. This incision was extended proximally and distally for enhanced visualization and identification of normal tissue plains. Using electrocaudery, the dissection was taken down to the level of the deep fascia. The fascial layer, which is often scarred down in the revision setting, was elevated and carefully developed. The hip was then aspirated and sent for intraoperative cell count. The short external rotators and capsule were taken down in a single sleeve and retracted posteriorly to protect the sciatic nerve. Deep cultures were taken and capsular biopsy for was sent for frozen section, which was negative for inflammatory cells. Cell count returned as negative for infection.

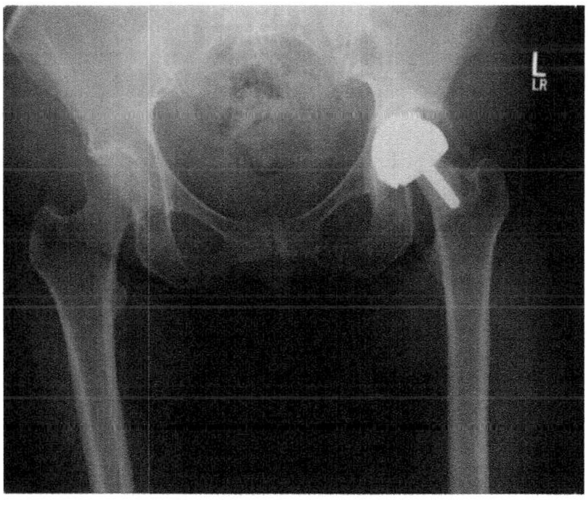

Fig. 4.1 AP pelvis radiograph with a grossly loose monoblock, cobalt-chromium acetabular component, and narrowing of the femoral neck around the resurfacing implant. The femoral defect would be considered a Paprosky Type 1 defect

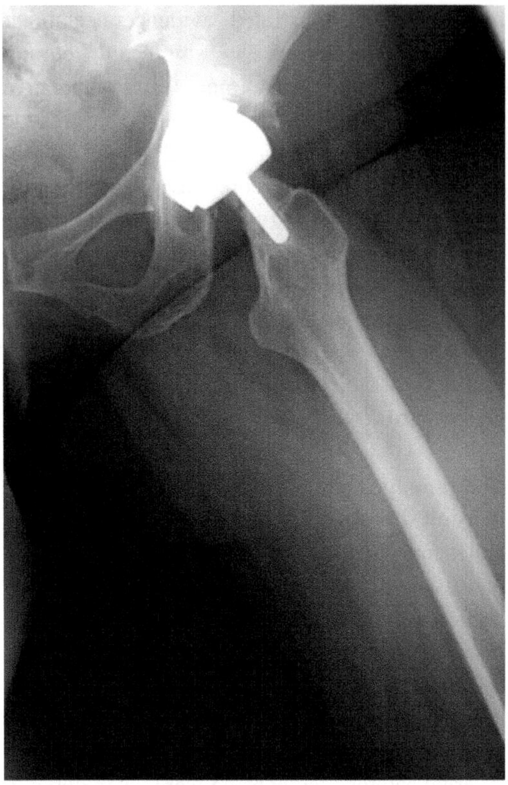

Fig. 4.2 Frog lateral radiograph of the left hip with a grossly loose acetabular component and narrowing of the femoral neck around the resurfacing implant

Significant metallosis was visualized throughout the joint, but the abductors and adjacent soft tissues were fairly normal. The neck osteotomy site was cut at this time to improve visualization. The neck was severely sclerotic, which is not an uncommon finding in the setting of hip resurfacing implants. The acetabular component was found to be loose and easily removed. The acetabulum was debrided, prepared, and the acetabular revision was performed.

The femur was lifted from the wound using a femoral elevator. This stage is done with caution to prevent excess levering on the proximal femur, which often has poor quality bone in the revision setting. The femur was prepared with straight reamers by hand for the planned cylindrical, distal-fixed femoral stem. We then successfully reamed using hand power up to a size 15.5 for a size 16 trial stem Excellent fit was achieved with good rotational and axial stability. Hand powered reaming may have an added advantage of tactile feedback for the surgeon, especially when he does not frequently perform this technique. The hip was trialed and the definitive stem was inserted in the desired anteversion. The head was implanted and the hip was reduced and found to be stable in multiple positions of stress. This stage should be done with particular attention, as instability is the most frequent complication of revision hip replacement. Leg lengths are assessed both clinically and using bony landmarks planned during templating. Closure of the short external rotators and capsular sleeve can be performed through bone tunnels, or with soft tissue advancement to the local structures. Drains are placed deep and the fascia, fat, and dermal layers are closed with particular attention paid to closing down dead space.

Postoperative Course

Due to the relatively pristine anatomy and bone quality the patient was made weight bearing as tolerated and physical therapy was initiated during the first postoperative week with special focus placed on abductor strengthening. Posterior hip precautions were maintained for 6 weeks after surgery. The patient ultimately progressed well and has returned to full function and is now 3 years from surgery with stable radiographs and has subsequently had her contralateral hip replaced (Figs. 4.3 and 4.4).

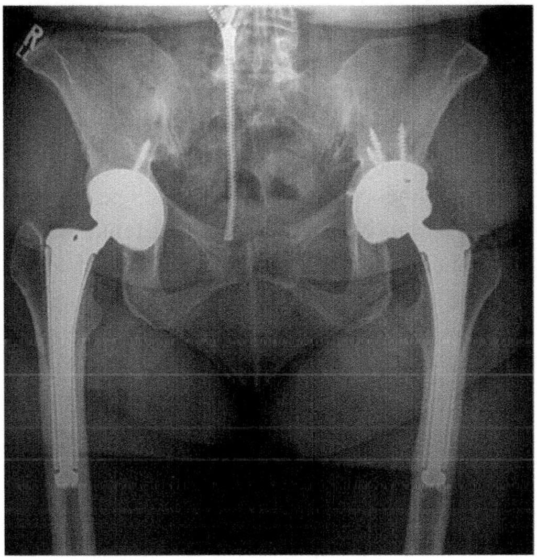

Fig. 4.3 AP pelvis radiograph 3 years after revision left THA for a failed hip resurfacing. The Type 1 defect was managed with a composite distally fixed femoral component. Her right hip underwent an uncomplicated interval THA as well

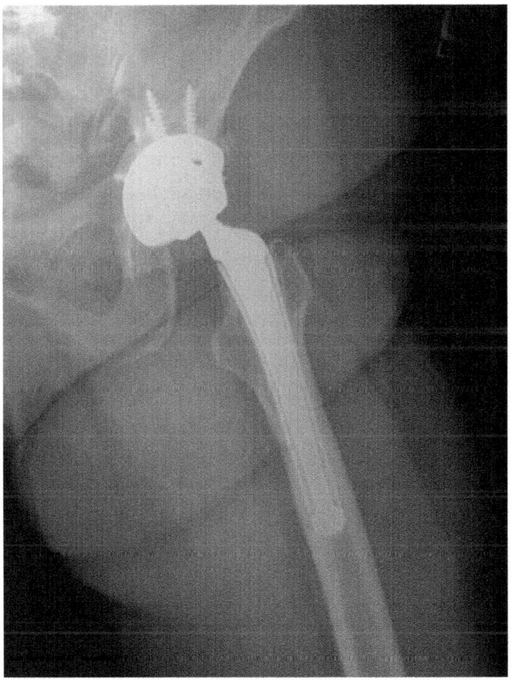

Fig. 4.4 Frog lateral radiograph of the left hip 3 years after revision THA for a failed hip resurfacing. The Type 1 defect was managed with a composite distally fixed femoral component

Paprosky Type 2 Femur

Type 2 Paprosky femoral defects are noted to have deficient metaphyseal bone with an intact and supportive diaphysis. This can occur in the setting of loose proximal-fitting components, which have led to significant bone loss in the metaphyseal region, either due to the removal process or due to the implant itself. It can also occur in the setting prosthetic infection or with short-cemented stems in conjunction with a limited cement mantle. Without proximal cancellous bone and support, the implant must rely at least in part on diaphyseal fixation for stability. The diaphysis is typically intact for its entire length, so a variety of stems that bypass the weakened metaphysis can be chosen. Cemented components can be used, but have historically poor results [7]. The lack of cancellous bone for interdigitation of the cement may lead to early loosening or cement mantle failure; regardless, cemented stems are still useful tools to have in one's armamentarium. This is especially true for patients with a history of radiation to the region, or in the circumstance when bone ingrowth is unlikely. Care should be taken not to ream or broach too vigorously upon preparation to ensure any viable host bone is left intact to permit a good cement mantle. Once again, third-generation cement techniques, including cement restrictors, canal preparation, vacuum mixing, and pressurization will have a better outcome if this form of fixation is utilized.

Uncemented prostheses have more predicable outcomes and are the preferred prostheses in this setting. There are a number of good options available to create a stable construct. These include a proximally porous-coated revision stem or a stem-in-sleeve design. Alternatively, standard length cylindrical implants or short tapered stems are good options. These components may incorporate a calcar-replacing geometry to augment their axial stability and aid in proximal loading. Furthermore, there is a higher frequency of bone remodeling in the setting of type II bone loss, requiring some level of modularity to accommodate the abnormal anatomy. Splined, tapered, cylindrical, distally fixed stems are also reasonable options. These stems have recently gained popularity due to surgeon familiarity with tapered implants and the materials properties of titanium alloy versus cobalt-chromium implants.

Case 2

A 54-year-old patient was referred in for evaluation of a painful metal on metal THA. Preoperative inflammatory markers were normal, and a hip aspiration was negative for infection. Serum metal levels were above expected ranges, and radiographs showed a progressive radiolucent line at the superior lateral aspect of the acetabular shell (Fig. 4.5). A bone scan was obtained confirming the suspicion of a loose acetabular component. There was uptake around the proximal femur as well. An RI with metal suppression protocol was performed showing no adverse local soft tissue reaction with intact abductors. The decision was made to revise the components.

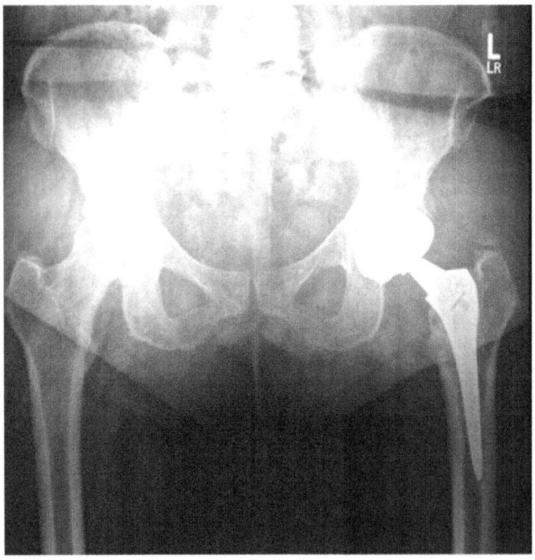

Fig. 4.5 AP pelvis radiograph with a flat-wedge, modular tapered stem in place. The acetabular component appears to show signs of loosening and metal levels were increased. The patient was indicated for a left revision THA

Operation

A posterior approach was utilized, rather than the anterior approach from the index surgery. The fascia was split and the posterior sleeve was elevated in one continuous fashion. The femoral head was removed and the modular femoral neck component was found to be cold welded to the femoral stem. When neck removal was attempted, the femoral body was found to be grossly loose and was pulled out by hand. The acetabular component was then easily explanted with minimal bone loss. The acetabulum was debrided and reamed, and a hemispherical shell was impacted in place with good fixation and support. The femur was then debrided with a reverse crochet hook and curettes. The metaphyseal region was found to be nonsupportive consistent with Paprosky Type II bone loss. A stem with diaphyseal fixation was therefore chosen for replantation. The femur was reamed using flexible reamers, followed by straight reamers by hand to a size 12.5 mm. The definitive size 13 cylindrical stem was implanted and found to have good scratch fit. The proximal bone was inspected and found to be supportive of the stem. Proximal bony support is especially important when implanting cylindrical stems below a size 13.5 mm, as these have a higher reported incidence of implant fracture [8]. High offset necks or heavier patients also increase this fracture risk, as these situations result in higher cantilever bending forces on the component. For this reason, proximal bony support is highly recommended when implanting a small diameter stem with distal fixation. Furthermore, allograft augmentation can be considered if proximal bone support is lacking or if an ETO is utilized.

Postoperative Course

The patient was progressed to weight bearing as tolerated over the first 6 weeks after surgery. Posterior hip precautions were maintained for a similar length of time. The patient went onto an uneventful postoperative course return to a normal level of function (Fig. 4.6).

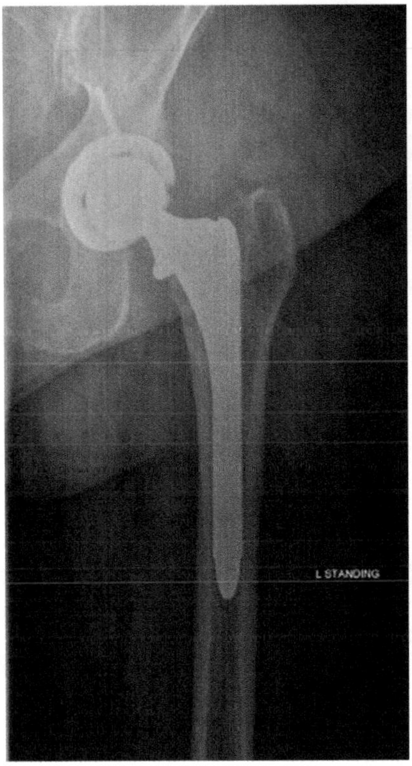

Fig. 4.6 AP radiograph of the left hip shows a well-fixed cylindrical stem with distal fixation. After removal of the flat wedge taper for corrosion and aseptic loosening, this stem design was utilized to treat the remaining Type 2 Paprosky femoral defect

Paprosky Type 3A Femur

Paprosky type IIIA femoral defects exhibit extensive metaphyseal bone loss and are defined as having more than 4 cm of intact diaphysis available for distal fixation in the femoral isthmus. The lack of proximal metaphyseal bone requires all type III femurs to rely upon distal fixation for stem stability. Scratch fit provided by extensively coated femoral stems, both monoblock and modular, allows reliable distal fixation in the presence of 4 cm or more of intact diaphysis as seen in type IIIA. Excellent long-term outcomes have been reported utilizing extensively porous-coated femoral stems [9–11]. These stems have the ability to get good fixation irrespective of the presence of proximal bone support in a majority of cases. Cylindrical, cobalt chrome stems, however, do have the previously mentioned risk of prosthesis fracture in the setting of implants smaller than 13 mm in diameter. Furthermore, they have been shown have a higher failure rate in stems with diameters larger than 18 mm [12]. In these circumstances, it is preferable to use a tapered stem with splines. Tapered stems with splines, both modular and non-modular, were developed to achieve high initial stability in cases of proximal bone deficiency. These prostheses rely on reaming the femoral diaphysis into a conical shape that provides axial stability to the tapered stem. Splines provide rotational stability and help secure the stem in the desired position. Modular, tapered, splined titanium implants have regained popularity in recent years as better manufacturing techniques have decreased failure concerns at modular junctions. However, proximal osseous support at the modular junction is recommended in these implants as corrosion and fatigue fracture have been reported in the literature [13, 14].

Whether tapered or cylindrical, diaphyseal engaging designs rely on straight reaming of the femur to create the appropriate geometry. An ETO is an invaluable tool in this setting to permit appropriate reaming as well as to prevent complications such as canal perforation. It is often a good technique to begin with flexible reamers before switching to straight reamers to ensure the canal path is followed. When the cortical bone is weak or deficient, the surgeon can consider reaming under fluoroscopic guidance, especially when becoming familiar with this technique.

Case 3

The patient is a 58-year-old male who is 2 years status post a primary right THA at an outside institution presenting with right hip pain. The index arthroplasty was complicated by an intraoperative calcar split fracture, which was addressed with a single, proximal cable and component retention. His initial postoperative course was uneventful. The patient reported having a painless, well-functioning THA for 1.5 years, until developing symptoms just prior to his presentation in the office. His pain was activity

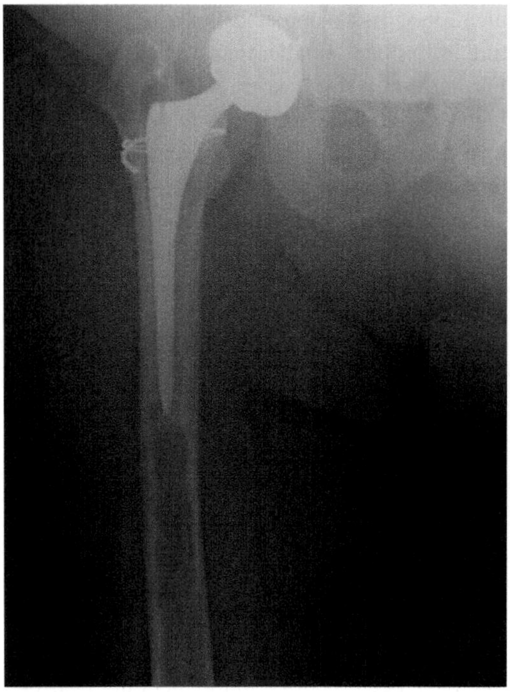

Fig. 4.7 AP of the right hip with what appears to subsidence of the femoral component with some bone loss through the metaphyseal region and proximal third of the femur. The defect is a Paprosky Type 3A defect

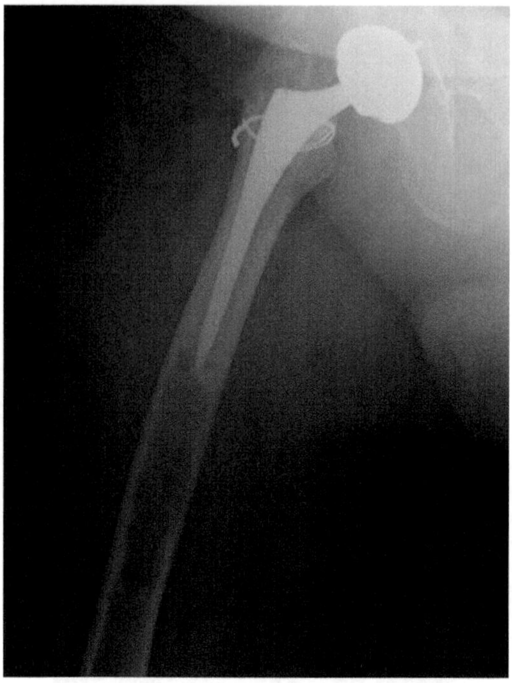

Fig. 4.8 Frog lateral of the right hip showing subsidence of the femoral stem with distal osteolysis noted and evidence the formation of a pedestal

related and there were no reported symptoms concerning for infection other than pain. Radiographic imaging obtained at the initial visit (Figs. 4.7, 4.8, and 4.9) demonstrated evidence of femoral component loosening. Standard preoperative work-up, including ESR and CRP, were performed and were negative for infection. The original surgeon performed a core biopsy below the prosthesis to evaluate the distal area for osteolysis.

Preoperative planning for type IIIa femurs should focus on radiographic signs of implant loosening, current implant design, proximal and distal bone stock, canal diameter, and femoral remodeling to allow the surgeon to appropriately prepare for difficult intraoperative situations. In our patient, preoperative films show a proximally coated tapered stem with radiographic evidence of loosening. This is best demonstrated by the formation of an intramedullary weight bearing pedestal at the distal tip of the stem, extensive radiolucent lines throughout the proximal stem-bone interface, and implant subsidence. In this scenario, it is less likely an ETO will be utilized for stem removal. However, the surgeon should be prepared to perform an ETO in the event the stem proves to be well-fixed and difficult to remove. Evidence of a deficient proximal metaphysis with a robust proximal diaphyseal cortex in our patient alerts the surgeon that distal stem fixation is necessary. Preserved femoral anteversion without evidence of substantial proximal femoral remodeling on the lateral radiograph suggests that either a fully coated monoblock or a modular stem are acceptable implants. Femoral remodeling into retroversion occurs most commonly secondary to a stem that has been loose for longer periods of time and may make appropriate version of a monoblock stem more difficult to achieve [15]. In cases where femoral retroversion is detected preoperatively, a modular titanium fluted stem may be a more appropriate option, as this allows the surgeon to more easily align the stem to their desired anteversion.

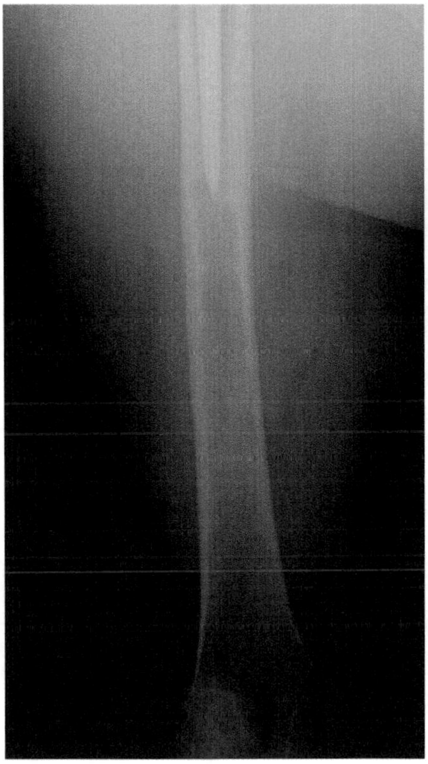

Fig. 4.9 AP of the right femur showing the distal extent and of the area of osteolysis below the femoral stem. You can see elements of sclerosis and osteolysis at the distal tip of the stem confirming the loosening of the implant in this Type 3A defect

Operation

The prior posterior surgical scar was utilized and extended proximally and distally for enhanced visualization and identification of normal tissue plains. Fluid was aspirated from the hip capsule and sent for cell count, and culture as the exposure was continued. Deep cultures and capsule for frozen section were also sent for further infection work-up, all of which came back negative for infection.

Following exposure, the hip was dislocated and the femoral head was addressed first. During attempted removal of the femoral head, it was noted that the femoral stem was grossly loose and moving quite easily within the canal. The head was removed and the stem was immediately addressed. A small shoulder of bone and fibrous tissue near the base of the greater trochanter that could potentially block stem removal and contribute to additional iatrogenic bone loss or trochanter fracture was noted. A high-speed pencil-tipped burr was utilized to clear the shoulder of the prosthesis. An implant-specific explant tool was then introduced, and an uncomplicated stem removal resulted.

Following stem removal, we sequentially used a series of flexible reamers to prepare the medullary canal, sending off tissue for frozen section and cultures. Reaming was performed to a size 18, which was appropriate for a 18 × 265 mm stem. Attention was then directed to the cup, and the liner was removed. The cup was found to be well-fixed and in acceptable position, requiring no further interventions to the acetabular side. A highly cross-linked polyethylene was impacted, and our attention was again turned toward the femur. A trial size 18 × 265 modular Wagner-SL taper (Zimmer, Warsaw, IN) with trial size 36 mm, −3.5 head were inserted and the hip was reduced. Excellent alignment, leg length, rotational stability, and range of motion were noted. The hip was dislocated, extensive pulsatile irrigation was performed, and the final size 18 × 265 mm Wagner SL-taper revision stem with 36 mm, −3.5 cobalt chrome head were impacted. Again, noting appropriate clinical alignment and stability. We then closed our deep capsule and rotators, followed by fascial, subcutaneous, and skin closure in layers.

Failure secondary to aseptic femoral loosening is a rare occurrence in these long, fully coated revision stems. It should be noted that a monoblock or modular stem would have been appropriate in this patient given the lack of proximal femoral remodeling and canal diameter of 18 mm. However, as previously addressed, femoral construct failure secondary to aseptic loosening in monoblock, fully porous-coated stems have been reported in cases where the canal diameter is greater than 18 mm. In this scenario, a modular titanium fluted stem is preferred for distal fixation [16–19].

Postoperative Course

The patient's postoperative course was uncomplicated. He maintained touch down weight bearing for 6 weeks to allow bony ingrowth and to pre-

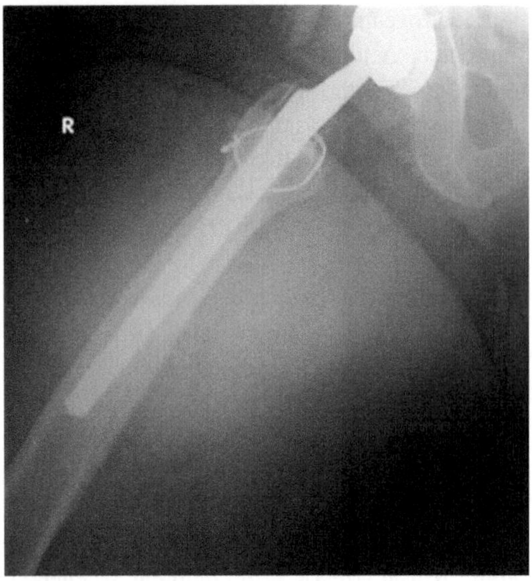

Fig. 4.10 Frog lateral of the right hip status post a revision of the femoral component for loosening. A long cylindrical, splined-tapered stem was utilized to fill the defect. A monoblock implant was utilized to manage this revision THA

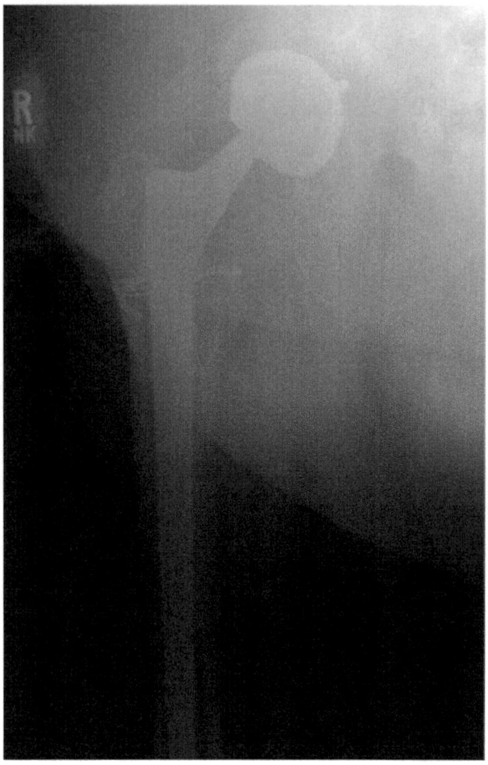

Fig. 4.11 AP radiograph of the right hip shows a well-placed revision THA with an 18 mm × 265 mm splined, tapered femoral stem in place. This bypasses the prior pedestal and fills the femur and the preoperative Type 3A defect

vent stem subsidence. Postoperative radiographs demonstrated stable implants without evidence of stem subsidence at 2 and 6 weeks. Weight bearing was progressed to 30% at 6 weeks, 60% at 8 weeks, and 100% with assist device at 10 weeks. Radiographs at 3 months again demonstrated a stable implant and all weight bearing and posterior hip precautions were discontinued at this time (Figs. 4.10, 4.11, and 4.12). Physical therapy was initiated during the first postoperative week with special focus placed on abductor strengthening. Gradual increases in strengthening and stretching exercises were implemented through 3 months. He has ultimately done well and has moved onto have his contralateral hip and bilateral knees replaced in the future.

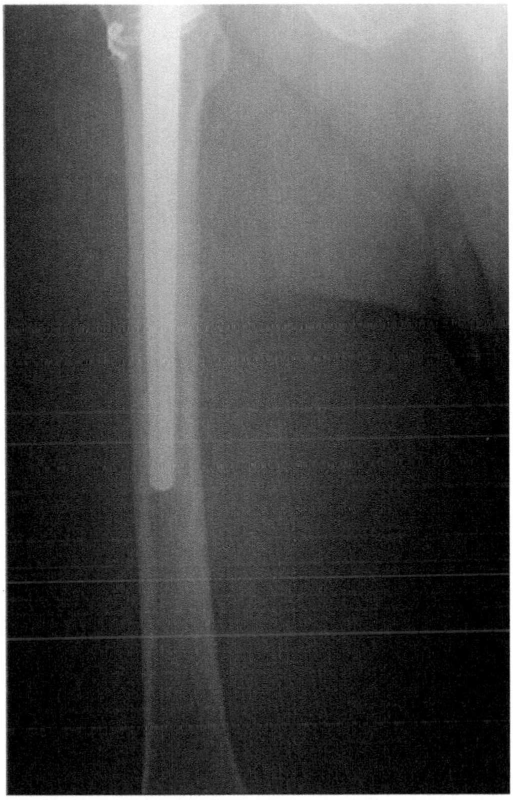

Fig. 4.12 AP radiograph of the right femur shows a well-fixed THA femoral stem. The stem bypasses the prior bony defect to gain good fixation into the femur and prevent any areas that could serve as a future stress-riser

Paprosky Type 3B Femur

Type IIIB femoral defects are classified as having a less than 4 cm of the femoral isthmus available for distal fixation. Long-term fixation can be reliably achieved using a modular or non-modular fluted, tapered stem in this setting [17, 19–23]. Unlike type 3A defects, where cylindrical monoblock stems under 18 mm in diameter have historically done well, the ability to achieve reliable long-term diaphyseal fixation with the use of an extensively porous-coated cylindrical stem may be exceeded in the case of 3B femoral defects [16–19]. A splined, tapered stem allows the femoral component to effectively wedge into the remaining isthmus, with the flutes providing added rotational stability. However, even with a wedge fit, subsidence still occurs. Gaining satisfactory distal fixation with a large enough implant must be balanced with the risk of intraoperative femur fracture during stem insertion [24].

Impaction grafting is another technique available in type 3B femurs. Impaction grafting requires removal of the old stem, femoral canal debridement, placement of a distal plug, and aggressive packing of morselized cancellous allograft surrounding a guide rod or broach. This technique allows cementation of a new prosthesis into the reconstituted femur [25, 26]. Impaction grafting requires an intact or reconstructed femoral cortex to contain the impacted graft and pressurized cement and has reported acceptable mid- to long-term survivorship [27–29]. However, periprosthetic fracture and stem subsidence during the postoperative period are reported as common complications associated with this technique [27–29].

Case 4

This is a case of a 60-year-old female who presented with 1 year of progressively worsening of left groin pain. She had undergone a previously uncomplicated left THA 2 years prior. Symptoms predominantly occurred with activity. Preoperative radiographs revealed acetabular component loosening with associated bone resorption (Figs. 4.13 and 4.14). Infection labs were drawn and demonstrated elevated ESR and CRP. The left hip was subsequently aspirated, with cell count and culture confirming a periprosthetic joint infection. The index THA was explanted through a posterior approach, utilizing an ETO to remove the extensively porous-coated stem. An articulating antibiotic spacer was inserted and the patient was consequently treated with 6 weeks of intravenous antibiotics (Figs. 4.15 and 4.16). Replantation was planned 8 weeks later, following completing of antibiotics and resolution of inflammatory labs.

When implant removal is not straightforward from above, extra equipment may be required. In cases of well-fixed cemented or cementless femoral components, we recommend having the following instruments accessible: implant-specific

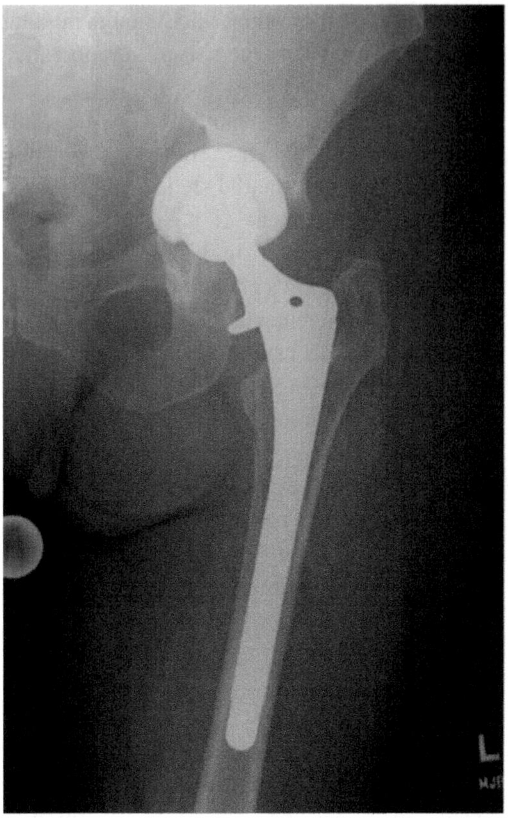

Fig. 4.13 AP radiograph of the left hip shows a well-fixed cylindrical, distally fixed femoral component and a grossly loose acetabulum with a protrusion into the pelvis. The patient was diagnosed with a PJI and indicated for a two-stage exchange procedure

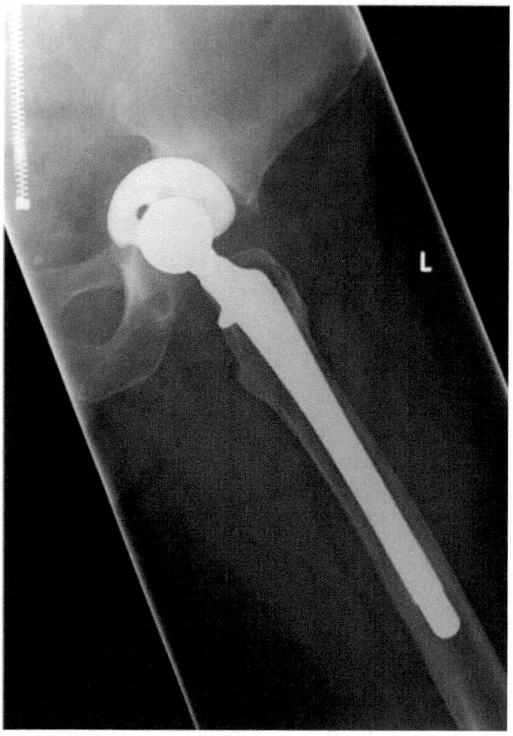

Fig. 4.14 Frog-lateral radiograph of the left hip shows a well-fixed cylindrical, distally fixed femoral component and a grossly loose acetabulum with a protrusion into the pelvis. The patient was diagnosed with a PJI and indicated for a two-stage exchange procedure

explant tools, flexible osteotomes, high-speed burrs (pencil tip, carbide tip, metal cutting), trephines, ultrasonic cement removal tools, and universal extraction tool sets. Utilizing an ETO is particularly useful in the setting of well-fixed cementless stems, distal cement extraction, varus remodeling, and larger femoral prostheses [30]. Furthermore, an ETO is helpful when replanting a long stem that requires preparation of the diaphysis more distally. Possible disadvantages of utilizing an ETO include nonunion, greater trochanteric fracture, neurovascular injury, and implant subsidence in the event of fracture remodeling.

The modern extended trochanteric osteotomy, or extended proximal femoral osteotomy, was originally described by Younger et al. [31]. The ETO is traditionally performed through a posterior approach, extending as far distal as necessary to complete to osteotomy. The osteotomy may be performed prior to or following dislocation and prior to or after removal of the femoral stem. ETO is more easily performed following dislocation; however, dislocation may not always be possible. Once the proximal femur has been adequately exposed, the femur should be positioned in internal rotation so that the posterior boarder is facing up toward the ceiling. The vastus lateralis origin is maintained; however, the bulk of its proximal extent is elevated along its posterior border and retracted posteriorly to facility further proximal femoral exposure. The osteotomy is then marked out along the exposed posterior femur.

The osteotomy is marked just anterolateral to the linea aspera and extends proximally from the quadrate tubercle (at the base of the greater trochanter) to a predetermined point on the femoral shaft distally. The distal extent of the osteotomy

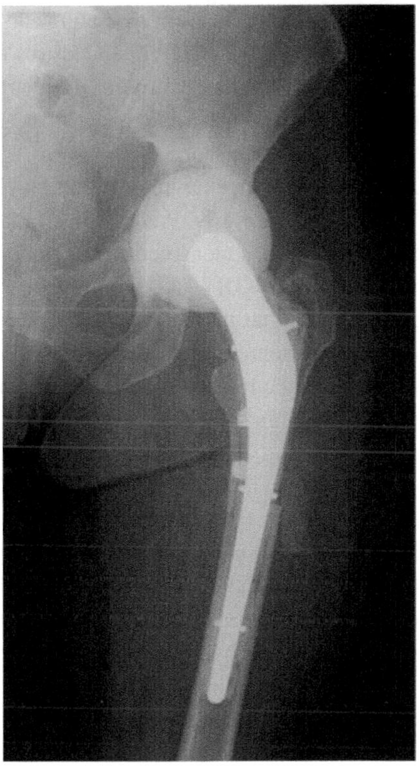

Fig. 4.15 AP radiograph of the left hip shows implant removal with placement of a dynamic spacer as part of the two-stage procedure. The prior stem was cut in half and trephines were used to extract it distally, leaving a Type 3B femoral defect

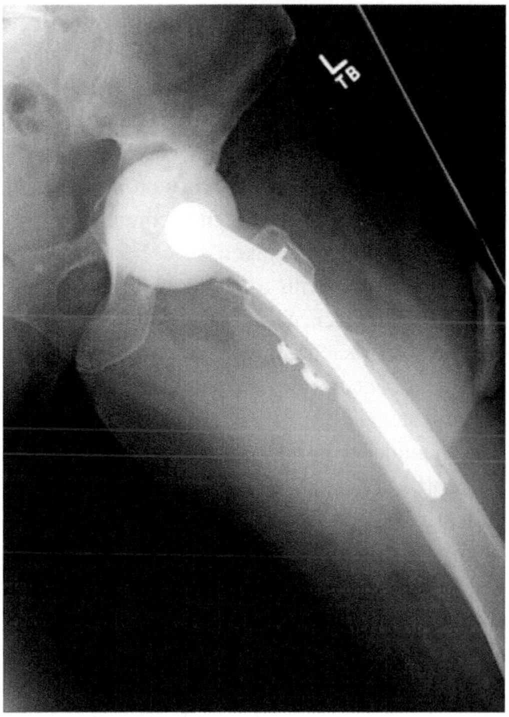

Fig. 4.16 Lateral radiograph of the left hip shows implant removal with placement of a dynamic spacer as part of the two-stage procedure. The prior stem was cut in half and rephines were used to extract it distally, leaving a Type 3B femoral defect

should ensure adequate exposure of the distal cement or bone-stem interface. A prophylactic cerclage wire is placed 2 cm distal to the osteotomy to prevent fracture propagation. Using a high-speed pencil burr, multiple holes spaced approximately 10 mm apart are created along the desired posterior osteotomy line. The burr should reach bi-cortically, extending through the femur to the anterolateral cortex. In the presence of a femoral stem, the burr will skid past the edge of the prosthesis. This should result in a segment of bone approximately one-third the circumference of the femur, involving the posterolateral one-third of the proximal femur. Connecting the burr holes posteriorly and cutting the cortex laterally at the distal extent completes the posterior osteotomy. It should be noted that it is common for the burr to lack the length to pass from posterior to anterior in the proximal femur. If this occurs, an oscillating saw is usually required to complete the proximal extent of the osteotomy in the anterolateral cortex. Wide osteotomes are subsequently utilized across the osteotomy, from posterior to anterior, to crack open the previously perforated anterior cortex and lever the osteotomy anteriorly. This creates a controlled fracture through the anterolateral perforations, and leaving anterior soft tissue connections undisturbed. The gluteus medius and minimus and vastus lateralis remain attached to the greater trochanter on the reflected segment of bone.

With the proximal segment of femur reflected, the lateral surface of stem will be completely exposed. Direct access to the anterior and posterior surfaces is now available, and the process of stem removal may begin. We continue with the high-speed pencil or metal-cutting burr, as it has proven useful in disrupting the bone-cement or bone-prosthesis interface without substantial iatrogenic bone loss. In cemented stems, the distal cement is removed from proximal to distal by drilling the cement column with progressively larger drills, followed by chipping and removal with osteotomes. In situations where the cement mantle extends beyond the osteotomy, cement taps can be used to engage the cement after progressive drilling has taken place, followed by cement removal with a slaphammer or cement hook. This sequence is repeated until adequate cement is extracted, allowing for at least 4 cm of endosteal contact prior to insertion of a revision femoral stem.

Sequential reaming of the canal ensues until appropriate distal canal fill is achieved. The revision prosthesis is inserted, and the proximal osteotomy fragment is then addressed to assure excellent contact with the cementless stem once the osteotomy fixation is secured. This is performed by using a high-speed barrel burr for cement removal and to modify the fragment to fit over the lateral shoulder of the prosthesis. Multiple cables are employed to secure the osteotomy size fragment of bone. Appropriate abductor tensioning can be achieved by removing a distal portion of the osteotomy, thus advancing the trochanter distally. Bone-graft is placed along the osteotomy site and cortical strut grafts may be used to supplement weak areas of host bone.

Operation

The prior posterior surgical incision was utilized. Hip capsule and deep aspirate were sent for frozen section, cell count, and culture. Dissection continued, followed by hip dislocation with resultant presentation of the spacer and ETO site. It was noted at this time that the previous ETO was not fully healed, as the ETO could be opened quite easily upon removal of the cables. We then removed our cement spacer and performed a thorough debridement from the skin down to the level of the bone. The acetabulum was prepared, reamed, and a revision trabecular metal shell was placed with screw augmentation. The femur was first addressed by placing a cable distal to the osteotomy site as a prophylactic measure to prevent fracture propagation during trialing and final stem implantation. It is recommended to wait to fully tighten this cable until the trial is partially seated. This will prevent damage to a possibly fragile shell of cortical bone.

This scenario is an example of proximal bone loss with intact diaphysis. Preoperative planning of intact isthmus was measured to be under 4 cm in length (Paprosky 3B). This highlights several planning factors that the surgeon must consider. First, it is pertinent to consider your definitive revision plan at the time of the initial component removal. This begins by planning the length of the ETO. Leaving a longer segment of intact diaphyseal bone will allow for better available bone stock during replantation. The ETO should be no longer than is necessary to remove the initial component. In the setting of extensive distal ingrowth, as seen here, this may require leaving a short segment of diaphysis. Additionally, recording the size of the reamer that was used to debride the canal from the initial infection can give the surgeon the ability to anticipate the size of the canal during replantation.

At times, with sufficient time between an osteotomy and a replantation, the ETO site may go onto complete healing. This cannot be relied upon for proximal fixation, however, and a stem that gains diaphyseal fixation is recommended in the setting of an ETO. It should also be noted that the proximal femur had normal morphology at the time of the placement of the dynamic spacer. In this case, proximal femoral anatomy was maintained until definitive fixation, potentially allowing the utilization of a monoblock stem. This may not always be the case, and therefore it is advisable to always have modular prosthesis options available to accommodate any changes in geometry and version.

At the time of spacer placement, the canal was reamed to 17.5 mm and a 17 mm spacer was inserted. This gave advanced consideration to the possibility that the canal may be slightly larger when the replantation was performed. Ultimately, a 19 mm canal was identified upon preparation. Because a canal diameter of greater than 18 mm was present, a modular, fluted-tapered, titanium stem was chosen given the amount of diaphyseal bone available for fixation, and overall ease of use.

With the femur elevated from the wound, flexible reamers were used to ream the canal. Straight, tapered reamers were then used up to a size 19 mm distally. The definitive splined, tapered stem was impacted until good axial fit was achieved. The head was placed, and he hip was reduced. Subsequently, two additional cables were passed around the previous osteotomy site, which closed the area down appropriately through sequential tightening. Two fiber wires were also passed around the greater trochanter from the shoulder of the stem for additional fixation. A deep drain was placed, and wound closure then proceeded.

An alternative method for revising femoral components with poor bone stock is through the use of impaction grafting. Femoral impaction bone grafting is a form of biological reconstruction that is capable of reconstituting deficient femoral bone stock for cemented revision implants. Acceptable mid- to long-term survivorship has been reported with this technique [27–29, 32].

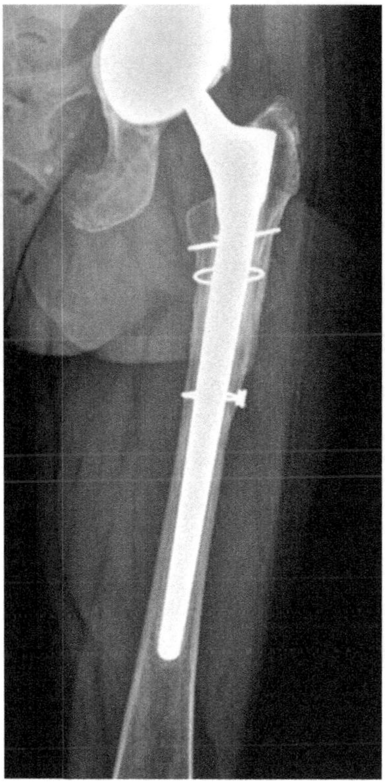

Fig. 4.17 Long-term follow-up—AP radiograph of the left femur shows reimplantation of a long splined, tapered stem to anchor in the distal bone past the prior osteotomy. A strut allograft was cabled proximally to restore the proximal femoral bonestock

Postoperative Period

The patient had an uncomplicated hospital course. Postoperatively, the patient was made touchdown weight bearing and given restricted abduction precautions. Weight bearing was progressed to 30% at 6 weeks with initiation of active abduction exercises, 60% at 8 weeks, and 100% with assist device at 10 weeks. Restricted abduction exercises were not initiated until 12 weeks. Assist device and posterior precautions were discontinued at 3 months post-op (Figs. 4.17, 4.18, and 4.19). Antibiotics were continued until cultures returned as negative.

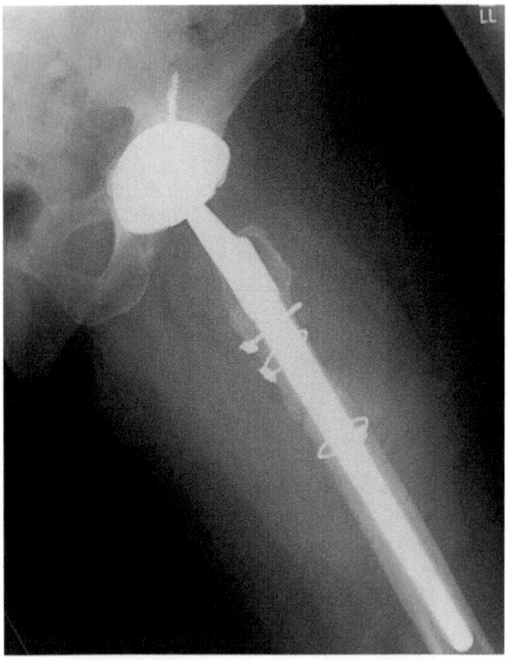

Fig. 4.18 Long-term follow-up—Frog lateral radiograph of the left femur shows reimplantation of a long splined, tapered stem to anchor in the distal bone past the prior osteotomy. A strut allograft was cabled proximally to restore the proximal femoral bonestock

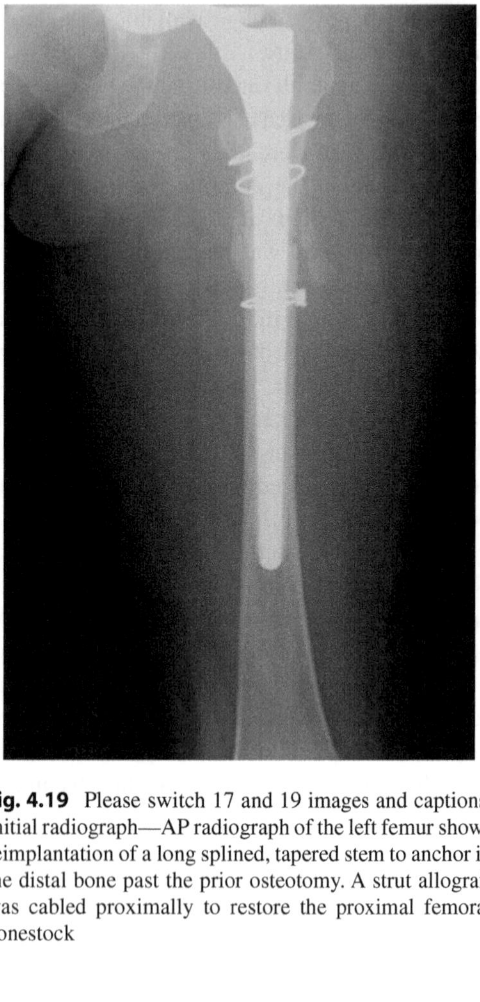

Fig. 4.19 Please switch 17 and 19 images and captions. Initial radiograph—AP radiograph of the left femur shows reimplantation of a long splined, tapered stem to anchor in the distal bone past the prior osteotomy. A strut allograft was cabled proximally to restore the proximal femoral bonestock

Paprosky Type 4 Femur

In the setting of severe bone loss, such as that seen in a Paprosky type 4 femur, the clinical decision-making must now include several other factors and goals. This type of bone loss can occur in the face of multiple revisions, extreme remodeling from chronically loose components, fracture, or infection. In these cases, there is often canal ectasia, segmental deficiency, and inadequate diaphyseal bone in which to gain fixation by any of the previously described prostheses. In these circumstances, the options available include impaction bone grafting with cemented long prosthesis, allograft prosthetic composite(APC), or a megaprosthesis.

Case 5

The patient is a 59-year-old female who had previously undergone a THA for idiopathic avascular necrosis of the hip. This subsequently became infected and failed an irrigation and liner exchange with prolonged antibiotic treatment. After a prolonged course, she was eventually explanted with placement of an articulating antibiotic impregnated cement spacer. After appropriate antibiotic treatment and work-up indicating clearance of the infection, she subsequently underwent replantation. She had multiple episodes of dislocations in the post revision period and had a periprosthetic fracture with a trochanteric fracture with escape. This was subsequently fixed using cables. This failed to provide adequate stability, and she was revised to a constrained liner (Figs. 4.20 and 4.21). This construct again became infected at a later date. Her components were removed again and a non-articulating antibiotic cement spacer was replanted, as there was not sufficient bone stock to replant an articu-

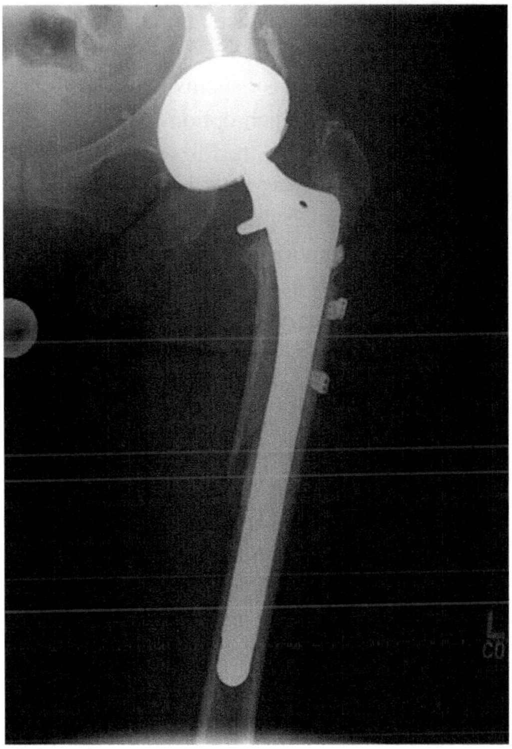

Fig. 4.20 AP radiograph of the left femur shows a Vancouver B1 fracture with a long cylindrical stem in place

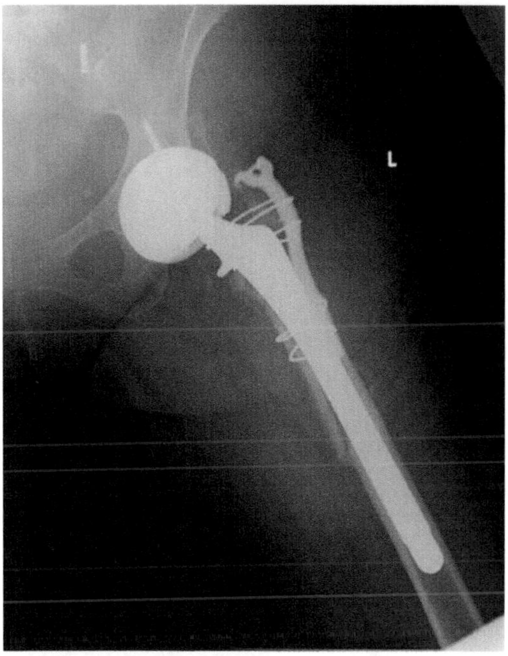

Fig. 4.21 A frog lateral radiograph is pictured with a cable plate being used to fix the proximal femur to the stem and the distal fragment. Note during this revision a constr ned liner was placed

lating spacer (Fig. 4.22). Finally, she was clinically cleared of her infection and ready for her definitive replantation.

Operation

The prior posterior surgical scar was utilized which was from the level of the lateral thigh as proximal as the posterior superior iliac spine to the distal thigh at the level of the condylar flare. Upon incising the deep fascia in line with the incision, fluid was aspirated from the site of the hip joint for intraoperative cell count. Exposure was continued, reflecting the short external rotators and capsule in one sleeve posteriorly to protect the sciatic nerve. The remaining proximal trochanteric bone was assessed and found to be in continuity with the abductors. The cement spacer was immediately visualized and removed without difficulty. The hip capsule was biopsied and sent for frozen section. Both the cell counts and frozen section proved to be negative for infection based on our institutions' standards.

The hip and acetabulum were now visualized easily. The remaining trochanter was protected for later reattachment. The acetabulum was addressed with a trabecular metal shell (Zimmer, Warsaw, IN) with multiple screws and trial liner. When addressing the femur, the sleeve of tissue around the static spacer stem was carefully dissected in a continuous fashion for later closure. The distal bone was all that remained. The transverse cut was used to freshen the proximal edge of bone stock and the canal was debrided and reamed. The trial megaprosthesis was built on the back table, estimating the desired length based off of preoperative radiographs. Once introduced, soft tissue tension and leg length were assess and found to be appropriate. The hip was reduced and checked for soft tissue tension. The final component was then implanted in a stepwise fashion, first cementing the distal segment into the remaining canal and allowing complete curing of the cement. The

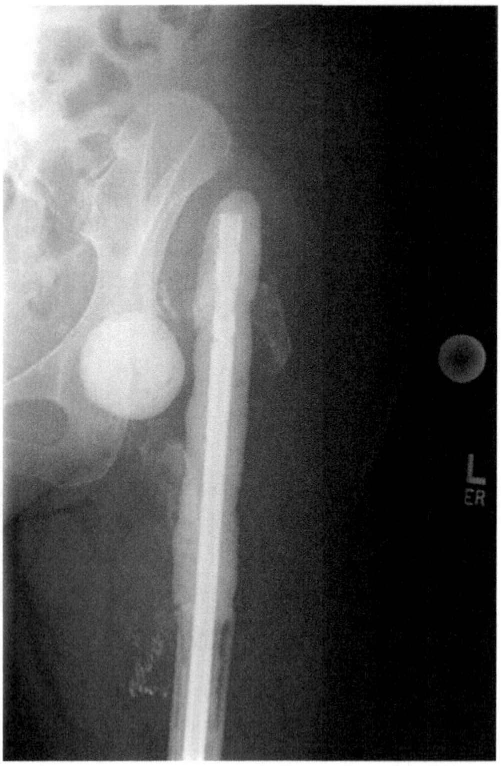

Fig. 4.22 After several dislocations and multiple surgeries, the patient ultimately developed an infection. The femoral stem was removed via an ETO. The proximal femoral bone was nonviable and fragmented and removed as part of the static spacer placement

modular segments were subsequently assembled to the well-fixed distal component. The desired length and tension were achieved. Femoral anteversion was set based off of the position of the rotated distal leg as well as the linea aspera, and the modular components were secured according to manufacturer specifications. The hip was then reduced. The remaining trochanteric bone was bolted to the side of the porous-coated proximal body, utilizing the built in fixation features of the prosthesis. The soft tissue sleeve was closed around the femoral implant and then the deep tissue planes were closed in layers.

A proximal femoral replacement was chosen for this patient for several reasons. The patient's lack of proximal canal rendered impaction grafting impossible. Although an allograft composite implant is an option, the patient's prior infection history and prolonged operative times associated with APC insertion renders introduction of an allograft prosthesis a less appealing option. Each of these techniques has benefits and down sides. When considering which option is best, the first consideration should be the life expectancy of the patient. Young patients may not gain sufficient longevity from a megaprosthesis and so an option that allows restoration of bone stock, such as impaction grafting, may be considered. Impaction grafting requires an intact femoral "tube" to allow tight packing of the morselized allograft bone [25, 27, 28, 32]. In the settings of small segmental deficiencies, mesh or strut allografts have been used to close holes in the diaphysis to allow graft impaction [28]. Morselized fresh-frozen allograft is the most frequently chosen type of graft given its availability and the amount of graft usually needed. This technique requires meticulous graft impaction using graft of moderate to small size. This size is typically larger than that produced in a bone mill, and so graft preparation is usually slow. The commonly used technique follows that as outlined in previous reports by Gie et al. [33, 34]. The bone-graft is prepared utilizing several fresh-frozen, non-irradiated femoral heads. These can be fashioned by an assistant with a saw and Rongeur instruments into coarse croutons. Meanwhile, the femoral canal is thoroughly debrided of old cement, neocortex, or fibrous debris. The femur is exposed and cerclage wires are placed around weak areas of bone, and mesh is placed to create a closed tube in any areas where defects are noted. A cement restrictor is inserted distal to the anticipated region of the new stem with the use of a guide wire. The starting packer tamp is advanced over the wire to ensure adequate length is achieved, and the bone is marked. With the distal plug secure in place, the allograft is initially introduced in small amounts using the cannulated packing tamp. Once a reasonable distal mantle of allograft has been created, the coring device is used to remove the central region of graft. The desired femoral tamps are used to push small amounts of the allograft into the remaining canal. If these fail to seat, the corer is used again to reconstitute the canal, and impaction is continued until the entire tamp is lined with allograft up to the level of the proximal marking. The proximal femur can be further reconstituted with allograft and mesh if this region is thinned or deficient. Take caution to secure any trochanteric osteotomy prior to impaction proximally. The graft is tamped tightly enough to provide rotational and axial stability for provisional trialing. After trialing is completed, a small amount of additional graft is tamped to ensure the mantle is well packed. The canal is gently lavaged and suctioned distally. Using third-generation cementing techniques, a gun is used to gently inject cement distally slowly withdrawing. Subsequently, a collarless, smooth, double-tapered prosthesis with a centralizer without wings is cemented into this newly created bone mantle with the goal of creating a high grade cement mantle interdigitation with the graft, and ultimate biologic incorporation of the graft into the remaining host bone. The top of this stem can be sealed with cement over the shoulder to prevent allograft from falling out. This is allowed to dry completely before reduction is attempted. The outcomes of this technique are fairly good when excellent technique is utilized in the appropriately selected patient [27, 28, 32]. This process is often time consuming, and therefore may not be advisable for older patients with more medical comorbidities. Additionally, the postoperative period typically requires a period of limited weight bearing to prevent subsidence and allow bony reconstitution. This postoperative requirement carries a high concern for complications for the elderly or infirmed. Furthermore, the durability of modern megaprostheses and their relative ease of use make them a more common choice for older patients.

With regard to the megaprosthesis, the technique is fairly straightforward with a few exceptions. First, the stem is often cemented into the remaining canal upon final fixation. A cement restrictor may be difficult to use due to the fact that this may be implanted near the patulous metaphyseal bone. Furthermore, the cement mantle is extremely close to the knee joint. The surgeon should probe the distal femur to ensure there are no defects, and in the event of a defect, the surgeon must use extreme caution to ensure that no cement is forced into the intraarticular space of the knee joint, as this may cause foreign body wear. It is also advisable to establish good contact between the distal porous-coated body and the diaphysis upon which it rests. This can permit ingrowth at the implant-bone interface and can better offload stresses to the cement mantle. Several techniques have been described to protect this region, including wrapping this prosthetic-bone junction with gel foam or plastic during the time of cementation. The body segment itself is fairly easy to assemble, but length is often difficult to gauge due to the lack of host bone and, often times, an implant on the contralateral leg. In these circumstances, soft tissue tension is the most frequently used guide for choosing the length of the assembled body. The surgeon should take caution not to lengthen the leg, s this may cause excess stress on the neurovascular structures, including the sciatic nerve. A drop kick test may be utilized to assess quadriceps tension as a surrogate measure for length. If the trochanter is absent, the abductor musculature may be difficult to reattach to the prosthesis. It may prove difficult even with present greater trochanteric bone, as the abductors may prove to be non-viable. In this case, the soft tissue should be attached as securely as possible to the designated location on proximal aspect of the body. Non-absorbable suture can be passed through holes in the proximal body or wrapped around the prosthesis to augment the repair. In either case, the stability of the hip may be in question. We prefer to attempt a non-constrained option when possible if the acetabular components were revised. This will allow integration of the cup without undue stress on the interface from a constrained component. "Tri-polar" technology has been emerging as a possibility for this circumstance. Should the hip prove unstable in either case, the liner can be revised to a constrained implant at a later procedure once the acetabular component has obtained ingrowth.

Postoperative Course

The patient was maintained toe touch weight bearing with hip precautions. The decision was made to use a non-constrained head based on the

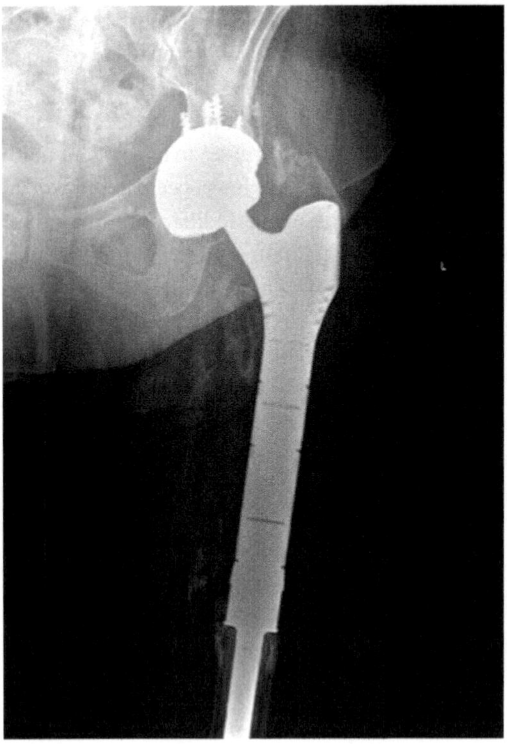

Fig. 4.23 AP radiograph of the left hip shows reimplantation of a proximal femoral replacement to treat this Type 4 femoral defect

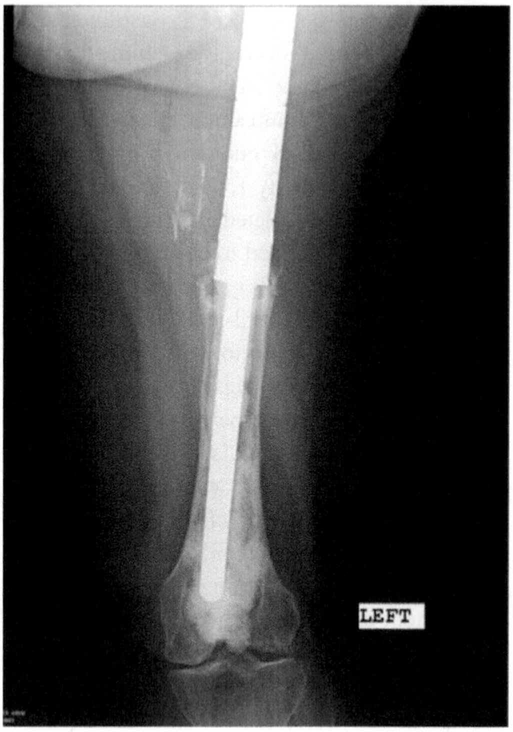

Fig. 4.24 AP radiograph of the left femur (distal) shows reimplantation of a proximal femoral replacement to treat this Type 4 femoral defect. The stem was cemented into the dis l femur as there was not enough room for a cement restrictor

relative initial stability. The consideration was also that we did not want undue stress to be placed on the new acetabular component until it had gotten ingrowth. Were it to prove unstable, we could then exchange for a constrained liner. We advanced the patient to 30% weight bearing at 6 weeks, and then 60% at 8 weeks with full weight bearing restricted until a full 3 months postoperatively (Figs. 4.23 and 4.24). We also advised the patient to use a supportive walking device for the rest of their life to protect this implant from excess stresses.

Authors' Take-Home Points

- Having the necessary tools is essential to achieving a successful surgical outcome in the revision setting. Most hospitals do not maintain a full complement of revision components and equipment in their inventory. This highlights the absolute necessity of planning for these cases. While the surgeon can use any method or classification scheme to assess the radiographs, he/she should develop a consistent and methodic approach to this exercise. In this fashion, he can plan in advance the equipment needed to perform the above techniques. We recommend that the surgeon plan not only for what is seen on the preoperative radiographs, but also for the potential to encounter more severe problems intraoperatively.
- Furthermore, the surgeon should also consider that the bone might not prove as supportive as it does at first appearance. If the surgeon cannot ensure, for example, the supportiveness of the metaphyseal region, or of the remaining diaphyseal bone, it is wise to switch to a construct with a more stable fixation approach. This can be true, for example, in a suspected Paprosky type 2 femur where the surgeon elects to utilize a cylindrical

porous-coated stem, or in a Paprosky 3a femur where the surgeon places a cylindrical, fluted stem. In general, good planning, a wide complement of tools, and a working knowledge of available options will enable the surgeon to navigate tricky situations and provide their patient with better long-term results.

Final Tips

- Spend time during preoperative planning to assess bone stock and request extra equipment for unforeseen possibilities.
- Minimize further bone loss when possible upon component removal/debridement.
- Utilize an osteotomy in circumstances that distal fixation will be required to ensure the canal is reamed straight.
- Plan your osteotomy length to preserve host diaphyseal bone when possible.
- Set patient expectations for the postoperative time period to plan for prolonged protected weight bearing. This will give the components a higher likelihood of ingrowth and prevent subsidence.
- Utilize extensile approaches.

References

1. Kurtz S, Ong K, Lau E, Mowat F, Halpern M. Projections of primary and revision hip and knee arthroplasty in the United States from 2005 to 2030. J Bone Joint Surg Am. 2007;89(4):780–5. https://doi.org/10.2106/JBJS.F.00222.
2. D'Antonio J, McCarthy JC, Bargar WL, Borden LS, Cappelo WN, Collis DK, et al. Classification of femoral abnormalities in total hip arthroplasty. Clin Orthop Relat Res. 1993;296:133–9.
3. Della Valle CJ, Paprosky WG. Classification and an algorithmic approach to the reconstruction of femoral deficiency in revision total hip arthroplasty. J Bone Joint Surg Am. 2003;85-A(Suppl 4):1–6.
4. Mallory TH. Preparation of the proximal femur in cementless total hip revision. Clin Orthop Relat Res. 1988;235:47–60.
5. Paprosky WG, Sporer SM. Controlled femoral fracture: easy in. J Arthroplast. 2003;18(3 Suppl 1):91–3. https://doi.org/10.1054/arth.2003.50074.
6. Bolognesi MP, Pietrobon R, Clifford PE, Vail TP. Comparison of a hydroxyapatite-coated sleeve and a porous-coated sleeve with a modular revision hip stem. A prospective, randomized study. J Bone Joint Surg Am. 2004;86-A(12):2720–5.
7. Haydon CM, Mehin R, Burnett S, Rorabeck CH, Bourne RB, McCalden RW, MacDonald SJ. Revision total hip arthroplasty with use of a cemented femoral component. Results at a mean of 10 years. J Bone Joint Surg Am. 2004;86-A(6):1179–85.
8. Busch CA, Charles MN, Haydon CM, Bourne RB, Rorabeck CH, Macdonald SJ, McCalden RW. Fractures of distally-fixed femoral stems after revision arthroplasty. J Bone Joint Surg Br. 2005;87(10):1333–6. https://doi.org/10.1302/0301-620X.87B10.16528.
9. Lachiewicz PF, Soileau ES. What is the survivorship of fully coated femoral components in revision hip arthroplasty? Clin Orthop Relat Res. 2015;473(2):549–54. https://doi.org/10.1007/s11999-014-3689-4.
10. Tetreault MW, Shukla SK, Yi PH, Sporer SM, Della Valle CJ. Are short fully coated stems adequate for "simple" femoral revisions? Clin Orthop Relat Res. 2014;472(2):577–83. https://doi.org/10.1007/s11999-013-3167-4.
11. Weeden SH, Paprosky WG. Minimal 11-year follow-up of extensively porous-coated stems in femoral revision total hip arthroplasty. J Arthroplasty. 2002;17(4 Suppl 1):134–7.
12. Sporer SM, Paprosky WG. Revision total hip arthroplasty: the limits of fully coated stems. Clin Orthop Relat Res. 2003;417:203–9. https://doi.org/10.1097/01.blo.0000096803.78689.0c.
13. Buttaro MA, Mayor MB, Van Citters D, Piccaluga F. Fatigue fracture of a proximally modular, distally tapered fluted implant with diaphyseal fixation. J Arthroplasty. 2007;22(5):780–3. https://doi.org/10.1016/j.arth.2006.07.007.
14. Lakstein D, Eliaz N, Levi O, Backstein D, Kosashvili Y, Safir O, Gross AE. Fracture of cementless femoral stems at the mid-stem junction in modular revision hip arthroplasty systems. J Bone Joint Surg Am. 2011;93(1):57–65. https://doi.org/10.2106/jbjs.i.01589.
15. Foran JR, Brown NM, Della Valle CJ, Levine BR, Sporer SM, Paprosky WG. Prevalence, risk factors, and management of proximal femoral remodeling in revision hip arthroplasty. J Arthroplasty. 2013;28(5):877–81. https://doi.org/10.1016/j.arth.2012.10.001.
16. Baktir A, Karaaslan F, Gencer K, Karaoglu S. Femoral revision using the Wagner SL revision stem: a single-surgeon experience featuring 11–19 years of follow-up. J Arthroplasty. 2015;30(5):827–34. https://doi.org/10.1016/j.arth.2014.12.024.
17. Konan S, Garbuz DS, Masri BA, Duncan CP. Non-modular tapered fluted titanium stems in hip revision surgery: gaining attention. Bone Joint J. 2014;96-B(11 Suppl A):56–9. https://doi.org/10.1302/0301-620x.96b11.34302.
18. Regis D, Sandri A, Bonetti I, Braggion M, Bartolozzi P. Femoral revision with the Wagner tapered

stem: a ten- to 15-year follow-up study. J Bone Joint Surg Br. 2011;93(10):1320–6. https://doi.org/10.1302/0301-620x.93b10.25927.
19. Rodriguez JA, Deshmukh AJ, Robinson J, Cornell CN, Rasquinha VJ, Ranawat AS, Ranawat CS. Reproducible fixation with a tapered, fluted, modular, titanium stem in revision hip arthroplasty at 8–15 years follow-up. J Arthroplasty. 2014;29(9 Suppl):214–8. https://doi.org/10.1016/j.arth.2013.12.035.
20. Amanatullah DF, Howard JL, Siman H, Trousdale RT, Mabry TM, Berry DJ. Revision total hip arthroplasty in patients with extensive proximal femoral bone loss using a fluted tapered modular femoral component. Bone Joint J. 2015;97-b(3):312–7. https://doi.org/10.1302/0301-620x.97b3.34684.
21. Brown NM, Tetreault M, Cipriano CA, Della Valle CJ, Paprosky W, Sporer S. Modular tapered implants for severe femoral bone loss in THA: reliable osseointegration but frequent complications. Clin Orthop Relat Res. 2015;473(2):555–60. https://doi.org/10.1007/s11999-014-3811-7.
22. Cross MB, Paprosky WG. Managing femoral bone loss in revision total hip replacement: fluted tapered modular stems. Bone Joint J. 2013;95-B(11 Suppl A):95–7. https://doi.org/10.1302/0301-620X.95B11.32763.
23. Revision Total Hip Arthroplasty Study Group. A comparison of modular tapered versus modular cylindrical stems for complex femoral revisions. J Arthroplasty. 2013;28(8 Suppl):71–3. https://doi.org/10.1016/j.arth.2013.04.052.
24. Tangsataporn S, Safir OA, Vincent AD, Abdelbary H, Gross AE, Kuzyk PR. Risk factors for subsidence of a modular tapered femoral stem used for revision total hip arthroplasty. J Arthroplasty. 2015;30(6):1030–4. https://doi.org/10.1016/j.arth.2015.01.009.
25. Schreurs BW, Arts JJ, Verdonschot N, Buma P, Slooff TJ, Gardeniers JW. Femoral component revision with use of impaction bone-grafting and a cemented polished stem. Surgical technique. J Bone Joint Surg Am. 2006;88(Suppl 1 Pt 2):259–74. https://doi.org/10.2106/jbjs.f.00340.
26. Sheth NP, Nelson CL, Paprosky WG. Femoral bone loss in revision total hip arthroplasty: evaluation and management. J Am Acad Orthop Surg. 2013;21(10):601–12. https://doi.org/10.5435/JAAOS-21-10-601.
27. Schreurs BW, Arts JJ, Verdonschot N, Buma P, Slooff TJ, Gardeniers JW. Femoral component revision with use of impaction bone-grafting and a cemented polished stem. J Bone Joint Surg Am. 2005;87(11):2499–507. https://doi.org/10.2106/jbjs.d.02547.
28. Sierra RJ, Charity J, Tsiridis E, Timperley JA, Gie GA. The use of long cemented stems for femoral impaction grafting in revision total hip arthroplasty. J Bone Joint Surg (Am Vol). 2008;90(6):1330–6. https://doi.org/10.2106/jbjs.g.00055.
29. Te Stroet MA, Rijnen WH, Gardeniers JW, van Kampen A, Schreurs BW. Satisfying outcomes scores and survivorship achieved with impaction grafting for revision THA in young patients. Clin Orthop Relat Res. 2015;473:3867–75. https://doi.org/10.1007/s11999-015-4293-y.
30. Miner TM, Momberger NG, Chong D, Paprosky WL. The extended trochanteric osteotomy in revision hip arthroplasty: a critical review of 166 cases at mean 3-year, 9-month follow-up. J Arthroplasty. 2001;16(8 Suppl 1):188–94.
31. Younger TI, Bradford MS, Magnus RE, Paprosky WG. Extended proximal femoral osteotomy. A new technique for femoral revision arthroplasty. J Arthroplasty. 1995;10(3):329–38.
32. Halliday BR, English HW, Timperley AJ, Gie GA, Ling RS. Femoral impaction grafting with cement in revision total hip replacement. Evolution of the technique and results. J Bone Joint Surg Br. 2003;85(6):809–17.
33. Gie GA, Linder L, Ling RS, Simon JP, Slooff TJ, Timperley AJ. Contained morselized allograft in revision total hip arthroplasty. Surgical technique. Orthop Clin North Am. 1993a;24(4):717–25.
34. Gie GA, Linder L, Ling RS, Simon JP, Slooff TJ, Timperley AJ. Impacted cancellous allografts and cement for revision total hip arthroplasty. J Bone Joint Surg Br. 1993c;75(1):14–21.

5 Addressing the Periprosthetic Fracture About the Acetabulum

Richard S. Yoon, Li Sun, and Frank A. Liporace

Introduction

As the number of the total hip arthroplasty rising over the last decade and projected number to be near 600,000 cases by the year 2030 [1], the expected number of periprosthetic fractures of acetabulum will also reach the all-time high. Although the periprosthetic fractures of the acetabulum are relatively uncommon after total hip arthroplasty, the presence of the fractures has been a major issue during the perioperative period, and it can lead to devastating effects to patients. The increasing complexity of surgeries directly correlates with columnar integrity and acetabular component stability. The management outcomes have been poor according to older studies regardless of the treatments. Miller [2] was the first author to describe ischiopubic fractures in patients who had total hip arthroplasty. Five hips had a ring component without cement and four hips with cement after insertion of a McKee component. The fractures failed to unite with nonoperative treatment and all patients received resection arthroplasty. McElfresh and Coventry [3] documented only one periprosthetic acetabular fracture among 5400 cemented total hip arthroplasties at the Mayo Clinic (prevalence of <0.02); however, as a result of the lack of attention to intraoperative acetabular fractures in the literature, this may have been underestimated. Sharkey et al. [4] described that 13 intraoperative acetabular fractures occurred during the insertion of cementless components; nine were diagnosed intraoperatively and four were seen in postoperative films. Haidukewych et al. [5] reviewed a series of 7121 primary total hip arthroplasties and reported the intraoperative acetabular fracture during 21 (0.4%) of 5359 performed with a cementless acetabular component. No acetabular fractures seen during any of the 1762 procedures done with cemented implant. As the cementless acetabular component becoming industrial standard, the incidence of periprosthetic acetabular fractures should not be taken lightly. More revision surgeries are performed annually which could be another potential reason that an increasing number of periprosthetic acetabular fractures are seen during component removal. As the longevity of THAs increases, more severe and complex periprosthetic acetabular fractures are being treated due to extensive osteolysis associated with polyethylene wear. Improved surgical approaches along with availability of innovative implants have significantly increased management options and improved surgical outcomes. Even with the advancement of surgical techniques and modern implant designs, materials, periprosthetic acetabular fractures remains to be one of the most difficult complications to manage

R. S. Yoon (✉) · L. Sun · F. A. Liporace
Division of Orthopaedic Trauma and Complex Adult Reconstruction, Department of Orthopaedic Surgery, Cooperman Barnabas/Jersey City Medical Center - RWJBH, Livingston/Jersey City, NJ, USA

R. S. Yoon et al. (eds.), *Trauma and Infection Control in Revision Hip and Knee Arthroplasty*,
https://doi.org/10.1007/978-3-031-71971-4_5

with many controversies. This chapter is intended to provide modern arthroplasty surgeons with general guidelines on periprosthetic acetabular fracture management based on clinical evidences. The fractures are categorized into intraoperative and postoperative fractures. Postoperative fractures have received the greatest attention in the literature. Acetabular bone loss has to be taken into consideration in this particular scenario. Management strategies of intraoperative and postoperative fractures are discussed separately.

Background

Nonunion and component loosening are common sequelae of periprosthetic acetabular fractures which could lead to dysfunction of the prosthetic hip, debilitating pain and subsequent deteriorating functional level of the patients. To achieve the best possible outcomes, it is required for modern arthroplasty surgeons to understand the diagnosis, risk factors, classification, treatments, as well as possible complications of periprosthetic acetabular fractures.

Periprosthetic acetabular fractures can occur either intraoperatively or postoperatively. Surgeons should have high index of suspicion for intraoperative acetabular fractures as they can be difficult to identify. This is crucial for making correct diagnosis and optimizing the outcomes. When a concern arises regarding a possible fracture (audible noise that suggests fractures, sudden loss of stability, etc.), a full clinical and radiographic assessment of the affected area is a must. This includes careful evaluation of component stability with use of intraoperative stress tests of the pelvis and acetabular component and often times it may require removal of the implant for a thorough examination of columns and walls of the acetabulum. Intraoperative live fluoroscopy can be helpful to determine component stability and confirm fracture patterns. The importance of recognition of intraoperative acetabular fractures cannot be overemphasized. As early identification of fracture is the key to obtain fracture stability and prevent component failure. Sharkey et al. [4] reported two of four fractures not identified intraoperatively required subsequent revision. Diagnosis of an intraoperative acetabular fracture is not always an easy task. Kim et al. [6] had 18 fractures identified on a cadaveric study, 10 were visible on initial radiographs, and 5 were visible only on oblique radiographs obtained specifically to detect such events. And 3 were not recognized until the component had been removed and the acetabulum was visually inspected.

For postoperative fractures, a thorough history and physical examination are imperative. History taking should focus on suspected episodes of injury or trauma, changing of postoperative pain pattern and other related clinical symptoms. Standard radiographs should be used for initial diagnosis, including pelvis and Judet radiographs. Advanced imaging studies are also helpful for diagnosis as well as for preoperative planning purpose. CT and MRI with metal suppression sequence becomes increasingly popular due to its ability to present more accurate detail of peri-implant structures, particularly in assessing periprosthetic fractures and implant loosening.

Surgeons should be able to recognize the risk factors for periprosthetic acetabular fractures (Table 5.1) [7], so that preventative measure can be used during perioperative period. Unlike cementless acetabular component, cemented acetabular component has not shown to be associated with periprosthetic fractures [5]. Cementless cup has been the industry standard for total hip arthroplasty and as the cementless acetabular cups becoming more popular, the prevalence of the intraoperative periprosthetic acetabular fractures is anticipated to increase. Monoblock elliptical cups have also shown to increase rate of periprosthetic acetabular fractures comparing to

Table 5.1 Risk factors for acetabular periprosthetic fracture

Surgeon-related	Underreaming; forced up fitting
Implant-related	Monoblock elliptical cups, uncemented cups
Patient-related	Age, female, sex, traumatic injury, osteolysis, rheumatoid arthritis, peptic ulcer disease, heart disease, paget disease

hemispherical cups [5]. The acetabulum was prepared with hemispheric reamer when monoblock elliptical cups were inserted. The monoblock elliptical cups significantly increase the rate of periprosthetic acetabular fractures (3.5%) comparing to hemispherical modular cups (0.09%). Majority of the fracture (76%) occurred during cup insertion. The tremendous hoop stress created by impaction could have caused significant point loading which could potentially lead to fracture of the acetabulum.

Underreaming the acetabulum with forceful insertion is also a well-established cause of intraoperative fractures [4, 8, 9]. Underreading of the acetabulum with insertion of a larger press-fit component has gained popularity to avoid screw fixation with the attendant risks of vessel perforation, screw fretting, back wear, and channeling of polyethylene debris along screw tracks. Excessive reaming coupled with increased impaction forces due to underreaming may cause pelvic dissociation [10]. Certain patient-related factors have been identified as risk factors. As the population age and the life expectancy continues to increase, so are the number of elderly patients. The older postmenopausal women with osteoporosis are particularly at risk. When this is combined with deep acetabular and cementless component insertion, it could potentially lead to higher incidence of periprosthetic fractures. Significant osteolysis has also been reported [11] to be a cause of periprosthetic acetabular fracture. The fracture was initially missed but a sudden increase in pain with loose implant prompted the suspicion of fracture. Previous generations of polyethylene prior to modern production and preservation techniques has significant impact on accelerated polyethylene wear which eventually contribute to osteolytic lesions. Minimal invasive approaches have also been associated with intraoperative acetabular fractures. Any revision surgeries, particularly revision surgeries involving removal of previous acetabular implants significantly increase the chance of periprosthetic acetabular fractures. Meticulous techniques and proper instrumentations are required.

To date, there is no consensus on the best classification system for periprosthetic acetabular fractures. As the fractures attract more attention, there is an urgent need of complete classification scheme which can provide universal guideline for surgeons.

According to an earlier study of small series of cases from Peterson and Lewallen [12], a total of 11 cases were included in the study. The periprosthetic acetabular fractures can be classified into two types based on component stability. Type I which is classified as radiographic sign of stable acetabular component: no change in position of the component comparing with the radiographs from pre-fracture state and a gentle range of motion of the hip causes little to no pain. Type II is classified as obvious displacement and radiographic sign of loosening of the acetabular component. There is notable pain of the hip associated with motion. Author did not recommend any specific treatment guideline from the study due to inherent low power, but stable Type I fracture with minimal displacement can be treated nonoperatively without compromising the function of the component. An acute revision arthroplasty should be done for Type II fractures along with supplemental plate-screw fixation and bone grafting.

Callaghan et al. [13] have categorized the periprosthetic acetabular fractures on the basis of in vitro investigation. They found a fracture occurred in 4 of 30 acetabula that had been underreamed by 2 mm and in 14 of 26 that had been underreamed by 4 mm. They identified four types of fractures based on anatomical location: anterior wall, transverse, inferior lip, and posterior wall. They also classified acetabular fractures by the time of presentation, either intraoperative or postoperative. The stability of the acetabular component is crucial, either loose or fixed which dictates the management strategy. Fractures occurred 6 to 12 months after surgery are considered as late postoperative fractures which are somewhat related to insufficiency fractures due to increased activity after THA. The best timing to treat these fractures is as early as they are recognized. Intraoperative acetabular fracture around the periphery should be thoroughly explored to make sure no transverse fractures exist. Della Valle et al. [14] classified acetabular fractures, including both intraoperative and postoperative types (Table 5.2). Type I fractures occur intraoperatively at the time of insertion of the acetabular implant and are subclassified as type A if they are diagnosed intraoperatively, are nondisplaced and are associated with a stable component; as type B if they are diagnosed intraoperatively but are associated with a displaced fracture and columnar or component instability exists; and as type C if they are not recognized intraoperatively. It can be challenging to determine between displaced and nondisplaced fractures intraoperatively. Surgeons should consider both clinical signs and intraoperative radiographic findings. The obturator and iliac oblique radiographs are particularly helpful to determine fracture displacement. Type II fractures occur at the time of component removal and are further classified as type A if there is less than 50% loss of acetabular bone stock and as type B if there is greater than 50% loss of acetabular bone stock. These occur typically in revision total hip arthroplasties when removing a well-fixed implant with significant osteolysis. The amount of remaining bone stock dictates the management choices. Type III fractures are the same as Peterson and Lewallen [12] originally described which is based on the stability of the acetabular component into type A, associated with stable implant and type B, associated with an unstable acetabular component. Type IV fractures occur without a history of trauma in association with osteolysis and are subclassified based on remaining bone stock; as type A if more than 50% of the native acetabular bone available for reconstruction; as type B if associated with more than 50% loss of host bone. It may be difficult to estimate the amount of bone loss associated with osteolysis preoperative because plain radiographs often underestimate the amount of bone loss [15]. Pelvic discontinuity is classified as Type V due to its unique clinical entity. Type V A as more than 50% host bone remained; V B as less than 50% host bone; and V C as pelvic discontinuity associated with prior pelvic irradiation.

Helfet and Ali [16] described a treatment algorithm (Fig. 5.1) for periprosthetic fractures of the acetabulum along with classification though this is currently not wildly accepted nor proven in recent literatures in terms of its usefulness.

Davidson et al. [17] proposed another classification scheme that is in addition to Vancouver classification system of periprosthetic fractures. They attempt to simply the classification by focusing on fracture stability, presence of pelvic discontinuity, failure of acetabular prosthesis, and presence of osteolysis. This applies to the acetabulum intraoperatively: type I is a nondisplaced fracture that does not compromise the stability of the component; type II is a nondisplaced fracture that potentially compromises the stability of the reconstruction, such as a transverse fracture of the acetabulum (pelvic dissociation or discontinuity) or an oblique fracture that causes separation of anterior column and dome from posterior column; type III is a displaced fracture, assuming the displacement causes instability of the acetabular component. Berry et al. [18] reported a 0.9% prevalence of periacetabular fracture with pelvic discontinuity at acetabular

Table 5.2 Classification of periprosthetic fractures of the acetabular associated with THA

Type I Intraop fractures secondary to component insertion	(A) Recognized intraop. Fracture nondisplaced and component stable	(B) Recognized intraop. Displaced fracture and unstable column or component	(C) Fractures not recognized intraop
Type II Intraop fractures secondary to component removal	(A) Loss of <50% of acetabular bone stock	(B) Loss of >50% of acetabular bone stock	
Type III Traumatic fractures	(A) Component stable	(B) Component unstable	
Type IV Spontaneous fractures	(A) Loss of <50% of acetabular bone stock	(B) Loss of >50% of acetabular bone stock	
Type V Pelvic discontinuity	(A) Loss of <50% of acetabular bone stock	(B) Loss off >50% of acetabular bone stock	(C) Prior pelvic irradiation

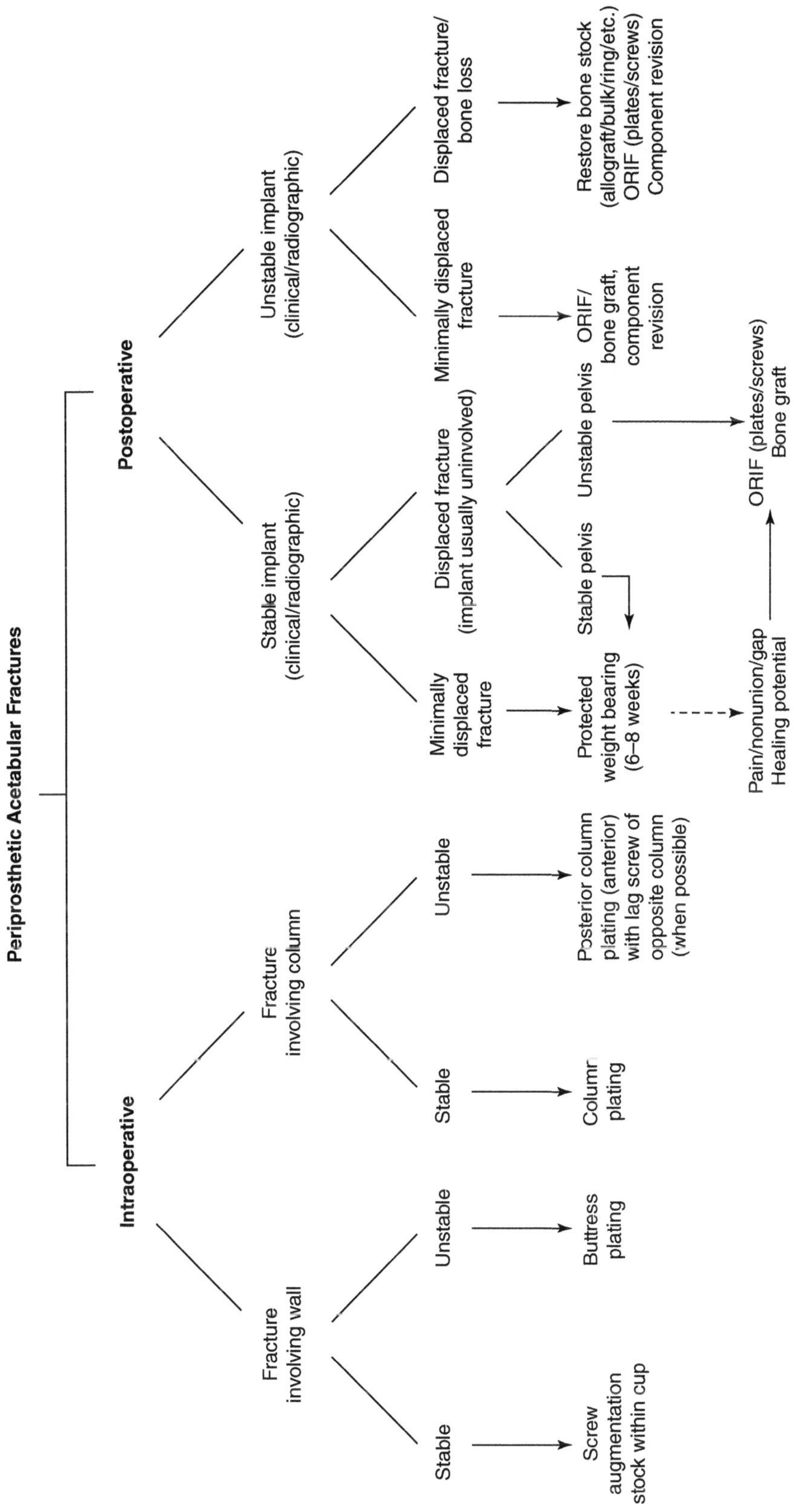

Fig. 5.1 Treatment algorithm for periprosthetic fractures of acetabulum

revision (31 of 3505). The review also described the diagnostic features of pelvic discontinuity. There include any visible fractures on the AP radiographs, with rotation or translation of the inferior portion of the pelvic relative to the superior portion. In certain cases, it is difficult to appreciate a fracture line because of obscuring hardware or metallic signal. Judet views could be helpful which may show fractures lines across the anterior and posterior columns.

Acetabular bone loss plays a significant role in managing periprosthetic fractures, particularly in revision total hip arthroplasty surgeries and late postoperative acetabular fractures. Surgeons should be familiar with classification systems and management recommendations. Many classification systems have been described over the years. The American Academy of Orthopaedic Surgeons (AAOS) introduced the classification scheme based on the presence of segmental, cavitary, or combined defects [19] (Table 5.3). Because of its lack of quantitative measure, the use of the classification is limited in clinical scenarios. There is also several other classifications described over the years. The most widely used is the Paprosky classification of acetabular bone loss ([20]) (Table 5.4). The system is based on the location of the hip center of rotation in reference to the superior obturator line, degree of teardrop destruction, amount of ischial osteolysis, and integrity of the ilioischial line. There four variables allow for objective assessment of bone loss involving the posterior column, superior weight-bearing dome, and the medial acetabular wall. It is divided into three types. In type I defects, the hemisphere of the acetabulum is globally maintained. There is no hip center change; teardrop and ilioischial line remain intact. There is no disruption of anterior and posterior columns which significantly improve the potential of achieving adequate biological fixation with stable components. In type II defects, the acetabulum is distorted but anterior and posterior column remain intact. There is less than 3 cm of superior hip center migration. Type II is subdivided into types A, B, and C. In IIA defects, the bone loss mainly occurs in anterior and superior fashion. In IIB defects, there is superior dome defect with superior and lateral hip center migration. In IIIC, the medial wall has been compromised and ilioischial line has been violated. Type III represents the most complex bone loss of acetabulum with possible association with pelvic discontinuity. There is more than 3 cm of hip center migration. Most importantly, the anterior and posterior columns are no longer supportive. Type IIIA is typically referred to as "up and out" and type IIIB as "up and in."

In general, management of periprosthetic acetabular fracture is based on fracture pattern, component stability, and location. The goal of treatment is to maximize hip function. The principle of treatment includes fracture stabilization, prevention of propagation of the fracture, mainte-

Table 5.3 American Academy of Orthopaedic Surgeons Classification of acetabular deficiencies

Type	Description
I	Segmental defect
II	Cavitary defect
III	Combined segmental and cavitary defect
IV	Pelvic discontinuity
A	Discontinuity with mild segmental or cavitary loss
B	Discontinuity with moderate to severe segmental or cavitary loss
C	Discontinuity with prior pelvic irradiation
V	Hip arthrodesis

Table 5.4 Paprosky Classification of acetabular bone loss

Type	Femoral head center migration	Kohler's line	Teardrop	Ischial osteolysis
I	None	Intact	Intact	None
II A	Mild (<3 cm)	Intact	Intact	None
II B	Moderate (<3 cm)	Intact	Intact	Mild
II C	Mild (<3 cm)	Disrupted	Moderate lysis	Mild
III A	Severe (>3 cm)	Intact	Moderate lysis	Moderate
III B	Severe (>3 cm)	Disrupted	Severe lysis	Severe

nance of component alignment, and stability and achievement of fracture union [21]. Simple intraoperative fractures are treated with stable fixation of the implant and the fracture [7]. More complex intraoperative fractures require major reconstruction and stabilization of the columns. Postoperative fractures associated with well-fixed implants are typically treated with open reduction and internal fixation. In a postoperative fracture with unstable component, options ranging from revision of the acetabular component to fracture stabilization and implant fixation may be necessary. The treatment goal is not always anatomical reduction when there is significant bone loss involvement. Preservation of native bone stock to allow stable implantation of acetabulum component takes priority in certain cases. In Peterson and Lewallen [12] study, 11 patients with periprosthetic acetabular fractures were treated based on stability of the component. The two unstable fractures were treated with revision surgeries and one subsequently had to have additional revision with supplemental plate fixation due to nonunion. The six of eight stable fractures had bony union after nonoperative treatment consisting of non-weight-bearing, partial weight-bearing, or other type of modification of activity. However, four of these six patients ultimately had to have revision surgeries because of pain and component loosening. The fracture or remodeling occurred after bony union may have altered stability of acetabulum or component which resulted in high rate of revision. The study of 13 patients with periprosthetic acetabular fractures by Sharkey et al. [4], six patients were treated with additional acetabular screw fixation either via holes within the cup or peripheral to the cup, two patients had stable implants and did not need further fixation or a change in postoperative rehabilitation and one patient did not require additional fixation but was treated with an 8-week postoperative non-weight-bearing period. Fracture union was observed in all nine patients. The four remaining postoperative fractures had evidence of loosening on follow-up radiographs. Two required subsequent component revision. Failure often occurs if an unstable fracture is not stabilized or unrecognized.

Intraoperative acetabular fractures during total hip arthroplasty has been well reported in literature. Although rare, the potential catastrophic complications associated with acetabular fractures have been presented in case reports. It is a daunting task to many surgeons to manage the fractures during total hip arthroplasty surgeries. There is a lacking of established universal guidelines or classification systems that can potentially aid diagnosis and treatment. Definitive management of the fractures has been very controversial and variable outcomes have been reported in previous literatures. Most common cause of intraoperative acetabular fractures is forceful impaction during cup insertion of cementless prosthesis. Study has shown that acetabular fracture could occur with oversizing by 2 mm. Callaghan et al. [13] and Curtis et al. [9] reported acetabular fractures when oversized by 4 mm. It should be noted that the 2 mm rule is appropriate for average size of acetabular implant but when very large cups are used, it may be oversized by more than 2 mm. This should be determined on case-by-case base and clinical circumstances, as well as quality of the bone should be all taken into consideration. Kim et al. [6] found the significant impaction forces needed to insert an acetabular component that was oversized by 2 mm led to fracture of 4 of 15 acetabula. Components oversized by 4 mm led to fracture of 14 of 15 acetabula. Kim and his colleges also found that fractures of the rim of the acetabulum were more commonly seen in the larger specimens, whereas the fractures seen in the smaller acetabula often involved the acetabular columns which lead to more devastating effect. If the fractures were recognized during surgery, the stability of the implant can be assessed right then. Haidukewych et al. [5] reported 21 periprosthetic acetabular fractures. Seventeen of the twenty-one fractures were noted to have stable acetabular components. Stability of component can be judged by surgeons' estimation of the quality of "press-fit" and lack of motion when pressing on the periphery of the implanted cup. Stable fracture with acetabular implant can be left alone without any additional treatment, and it has shown to have excellent outcome. All 17 fractures had bony union at the time of most recent follow-up. However, if the instability of acetabular component was found with the intraoperative fractures, then supplemental fixation has to be considered. Acetabular component can be exchanged to designs with supplemental screw fixations. At least two to three screws, ideally at either end of the fracture line. Callaghan et al. [13] recommended to have bicortical screw fixation within the acetabular component for greater stability. Weight-bearing status can be adjusted to partial initially in order to protect screw fixations and weight-bearing can be advanced until healing occurs (normally 8 to 12 weeks).

Della Valle et al. [14] also made recommendation for treatment of intraoperative acetabular fractures. According to the review, if a nondisplaced fracture with stable component is encountered, the prosthesis can be left in situ and standard total hip arthroplasty rehabilitation protocols may be applied. If the component is unstable, the structural integrity of the anterior and posterior column must be assessed and supplemental screw fixation should be used. Consideration should be given to the use of jumbo revision cup if there is significant instability and bone loss that necessitates the use of a larger acetabular component. Bone grafting should also be used for these fractures and patient should maintain protected weight-bearing postoperatively until the fracture has healed. If there is substantial motion at the fracture site, including the presence of pelvic dissociation, the posterior column should be treated with open reduction and internal fixation (with posterior column plating). After the pelvis has been stabilized, the acetabulum may be reconstructed with standard techniques with caution. For displaced fractures, some suggested that the component should be removed in order to assess the fracture extent and location. Displaced fracture with or without pelvic discontinuity can be treated with supplemental plate fixations, bone grafting and screw-augmented fixation of cementless component. In patient with severe osteoporotic bone stock, antiprotrusio reconstruction cages with or without posterior plate augmentation, bone grafting or cementing of all-polyethylene cup into augmentation cage can be considered. The reconstruction case will bridge from inferiorly to superiorly and allow temporary stabilization of the fracture while the bone grafting incorporates and fracture healing occurs.

Postoperative periprosthetic acetabular fractures present different challenges for surgeons. Fractures can be categorized based on time of onset: early postoperative or acute fractures versus late postoperative fractures. Treatment options are generally based on fracture displacement, component stability, and also columnar stability. For early postoperative periprosthetic acetabular fractures, minimal displaced fractures with stable component can be successfully treated with conservative treatment which includes 10–12 weeks of protected weight-bearing and possible cast immobilization [13]. Radiographs should be used judiciously to determine stability of component. Displaced fractures with component loosening require revision with wall or columnar fixation. Fracture fixation typically involves posterior column plating with bone grafting. Revision of cementless acetabular component with screw options is usually considered. Potty et al. [7] suggested using reconstruction cage and subsequent bone grafting may be appropriate. If severe acetabular bone loss encountered and standard hemispheric cementless cup cannot provide reliable biological fixation and bone ingrowth, large trabecular metal cup can be considered to acquire rigid stability and more predictable bone ingrowth [22]. Late postoperative acetabular fractures are managed in similar fashion. Surgery is almost always required. With clear radiographic evidence of acetabular component loosening, component revision is required. If columns are involved with fractures, revision with combined column fixation is recommended. In patients with severe fracture patterns, large acetabular bone loss or severe osteolysis, the use of antiprotrusio cage, trabecular metal augments, or allograft augments, jumbo cup with plate fixation may be needed. If significant bone loss is not amendable for any reconstruction along with pelvic dissociation/discontinuity, custom triflange implant may be warranted. Cemented acetabular component fractures tend to occur late because of osteolytic lesions over time. Callaghan et al. [13] reported initial nonoperative treatment can be considered in non-displaced fractures to allow fracture healing before revision surgery. Then large cementless acetabular component with screw augmentation or antiprotrusio cage construct can be used without stripping posterior column. Della Valle et al. [14] proposed classification for postoperative acetabular fractures is based on etiology of fractures. Traumatic fractures vary significantly in terms of mechanism of injury, but the treatment principle of periprosthetic acetabular fractures generally remain the same. The goal is to restore the structural integrity of the columns and restore bone stock with bone graft, allowing for stable reimplantation of the acetabular prosthesis. Although very rarely reported in literature, major vascular injuries have been found to be associated with periprosthetic acetabular fractures. Harvie et al. [23] reported in their case report a rare incidence of periprosthetic acetabular fracture with hip dislocation that was associated with major vascular injury. The elderly patient suffered from low energy motor-vehicle accident and patient demonstrated significant hemodynamic instability. After minimal response to fluid/blood resuscitation, subsequent urgent CAT scan demonstrated large hematoma around the pelvic region. Emergent angiography showed bleeding from both anterior and posterior branches of internal iliac artery. Patient was successfully stabilized after embolization. High index of suspicion and early recognition are the key to achieve the best outcome possible.

If the component is stable, initial nonsurgical treatment is recommended with toe-touch weight-bearing for approximately 3 months or until radiographic evidence of fracture union seen but it is associated with high revision rate even with complete bony union [12]. Unstable component requires immediate component revision with supplemental fracture fixation with plate and screws. Exchange of hemispherical acetabular component with screw fixation should be avoided in this scenario because of high rate of failure [12]. Spontaneous fractures or fractures associated with osteolytic lesions are managed depending on the amount of remaining host bone available for reconstruction. Often times the exact bone stock can only be assessed intraoperatively. Radiographic indicators of severe bone loss include superior component migration of more than 2 cm (lack of superior support), ischial lysis (posterior column deficiency), destruction of the radiographic acetabular teardrop (destruction of the inferior portion of the anterior column), and a break in the ilioischial line (anterior column deficiency) [24]. Porous-coated hemispherical acetabular component with screw fixation with bong grafting in conjunction with fixation of the fracture (with plate and screws) or an antiprotrusio cage construct with bone grafting and plate-screw fixation of the factures were described. Paprosky and Magnus [25] reported failure of reconstruction if hemispherical porous-coated acetabular component is used when there is a break in the ilioschial line.

Acetabular bony defect is one of the most challenging problems surgeons face during pelvic reconstruction surgeries, especially in the setting of pelvic discontinuity. Pelvic discontinuity is defined as a complete separation of the superior and inferior hemipelvis. An increasing number of fractures associated with pelvic dissociation are seen during acetabular reconstruction of cemented and cementless that have been in vivo for many years [26]. Posterior column internal fixation alone may not be sufficient for some pelvic dissociation cases. Fixation with reconstruction cage and bone grafting may be appropriate. Hemispherical cementless cup and trabecular metal cup are also being used. Tanzer et al. [27] reported on three pelvic discontinuities that were treated with a hemispherical porous-coated acetabular component fixed with screws. Two of these three reconstructions failed and accounted for the only two failures in their series of 140 cases. Similarly, Moreland and Bernstein [28] described that in the two patients with a pelvic discontinuity in their series of acetabular revision treatment with a hemispherical porous-coated acetabular component was unsuccessful. Springer et al. [22] reported on seven women who had a delayed transverse fracture of the acetabulum after undergoing a revision total hip arthroplasty with a trabecular metal cup. The authors thought these fractures were not caused intraoperatively but were related to the weak remaining bone stock which failed after resumption of activity. The occurrence of these fractures and their displacement suggest that a cup that bridges from superiorly to inferiorly and has a high bone ingrowth potential may not be sufficient in cases of severe bone loss. Thus, pelvic discontinuity should not be treated with hemispherical cup alone. Instead, stability may be achieved by using antiprotrusio cage that fits within the cup which also spans to the ischium and ilium. An all-polyethylene cup can then be cemented into the cage regardless of the position of the cup or cage. Boscainos et al. [29] reported good early results in 14 patients treated with the cup-cage technique although the rate of recurrent dislocation was high, with 2 of 14 patients requiring revision to a constrained acetabular liner. Both Springer et al. [22] and Boscainos et al. [29] described the use of this cup-cage technique in revision THA. The use of this technique for intraoperative acetabular fractures has not been reported. From the Mayo clinic study by Berry et al. [18], all of the eight patients with pelvic discontinuity treated with a reconstruction cage and bone grafting had a stable acetabular component at a mean of 3.1 year postoperative follow-up, early revision due to instability occurred in one patient. Four of eight patients had reconstructions associated with definite healing of the discontinuity and possible healing in the other four. In the same study, the four patients with pelvic discontinuity associated with prior pelvic irradiation who were treated with a reconstruction cage and or a plate on the posterior column had a stable implant whereas one patient treated with a cemented acetabular component and two plates required repeated revision.

Extra-large sockets or jumbo cups have been gaining popularity over the years due to its potential to improve bony contacts and achieve biological fixation. Jumbo cup is defined as having a minimal outside diameter of 66 mm for men and 62 mm for women [30] or 10 mm greater than contralateral normal acetabulum. This definition was based on the fact that there sizes were 10 mm greater than the mean implant diameters (56.9 mm for men and 51.9 mm for women) used for primary total hip arthroplasties. Jumbo cups can be useful in revision acetabular component when large bony defect becomes an issue. They are also be used in fracture scenario. Multiple studies have reported excellent survivorship at 10 to 20 years with success rate well over 90% [30–35]. Certain risk factors must be taken into consideration if hip arthroplasty is being used to treat an acute acetabular fractures: incompetent columns, particularly the posterior column and when pelvic discontinuity presents; loss of medial wall, disruption of the quadrilateral plate; early loosening due to lack to bony structural support. "If a particular acute acetabulum fracture can be identified as having a poor prognosis irrespective of the initial method of treatment, then the role for a therapeutic alternative such as acute THA merits consideration" [36]. In a biomechanical analysis of three different acetabular revision constructs, Gililland et al. [37] compared traditional unicolumnar fixation: a cup-cage construct, a posterior column plate with cup to bicolumnar fixation: a posterior column plate with cup and anterior column screw to determine the most stable construct. The bicolumnar construct provided the most stable construct with least bone-cup interface micromotions.

Nwankwo et al. [38, 39] demonstrated in both computer simulation and radiographic findings that the hip center shifted 0.27 mm superiorly and 0.02 mm anteriorly, and anterior column bone removal increased 0.86 mm for every 1 mm increase in reamer diameter when jumbo cup technique is used for revision THA. The results indicated hip center elevation despite placement of the jumbo cup adjacent to the inferior acetabulum. For a hypothetical increase from a 54 mm socket to a 72 mm socket, an elevation of the hip center of approximately 5 mm and loss of approximately 15 mm of anterior column bone are expected. This suggests an increased in femoral head length or neck size may be necessary to compensate the hip center elevation and potential limb length shortening when jumbo cup is used. Changing of hip center raises many potential problems. Elevated hip center will lead to ipsilateral leg shortening which has shown in the study by Dou et al. [40]. Delp et al. [41] demonstrated that superolateral or superior placement of hip center significantly decreases the moment arms of the hip abductor muscles. For example, a 2 cm superior and 2 cm lateral placement of the hip center will cause an average of 28% of decrease of moment arms. In almost all studies of jumbo acetabular components, the most frequent complication was postoperative dislocation, with reported rates ranging from 2.4% to 21%. Lachiewicz and Soileau [33] reported 10% (12 of 120 patients) rate of dislocation which is similar to Whaley et al. [30], 12% (11 of 89 patients). The reasons for the increased risk of dislocation with jumbo acetabular cup are likely multifactorial: surgical approach used, prior revision surgeries, amount of bone loss, and femoral head size. There was a significant association between a head size of smaller than 32 mm and the risk of dislocation reported by Lachiewicz and Soileau [33]. Iliopsoas tendon impingement was also reported when hip center was changed excessively [42].

Historically, bulk bone grafts (e.g., femoral head) has been used frequently in management of severe acetabular bone loss. However, there has been significant variability in terms of complications and outcome. The most significant complication that is affecting the survival rate is potential of graft subsidence which subsequently leads to component loosening and failure. Short-term graft survival rate is generally described as good [43], but other studies have shown the contrary [44]. Mid-term results are also shown good survival rates [45]. However the long-term results have been showing most of the inconsistency. Lee et al. [46] have shown high percentage of failure of acetabular fixation. Recent paper by Delimar et al. [47] had a total of 72 hips that underwent total hip arthroplasty with bone autograft or allograft. Variable radiographic parameters were assessed after operations, 6 months and 1, 2, 3, and 10 years after operation. All measured parameters in all patients and in patients with autograft and those with allograft separately showed significant changes consistent with graft failure and acetabular cup instability. Authors raised significant concerns of long-term endoprosthesis stability with bulk bone grafts.

The use of cup-cage reconstruction models remains an area of increased research focus. The roof ring and antiprotrusio cage (reconstruction ring) have been used to address acetabular bone loss in revision total hip arthroplasty surgeries over the years. This roof rings have been largely replaced by cementless cups fixed with supplemental screws. The antiprotrusio cages are larger metallic constructs that achieve purchase via multiple screws and flanges in the ilium and ischium. They are used for more extensive bone defects. The concept is to protect the extensively grafted acetabulum by transferring load from acetabular bed to the ilium and ischium. With this technique, the failure rates of up to 50% have been reported and mainly attributed to nonbiological fixation of the cages and relying on the screws and flanges for fixation [48]. W. Paprosky et al. [49] also reported a 50% failure rate in a series of 16 pelvic discontinuities treated by a range of different cages. The use of trabecular metal cup-cage reconstruction is a relatively new technique to address pelvic discontinuity. The trabecular metal shell is inserted with a mixture of bleeding host bone and morselized allograft. An antiprotrusio cage is then placed in conjunction of the shell to provide early load sharing for the acetabular component while bone ingrowth and stabilization occur. The recent biomechanical study by Gililland et al. [37] has shown that the stiffness of fixation of a pelvic discontinuity in a cup-cage construct in similar to a combined cage and posterior column plate. Abolghasemian et al. [50] evaluated the use of the cup-cage construction compared with standard ilioischial cage for those in pelvic discontinuity. The cup-cage constructs had a significant higher 7-year survivorship of 87.2% (95% CI: 71–103%) compared with 49.9% (95% CI: 15–84%) for the cage only group. The rate of radiological healing of the pelvic discontinuity was also better with the cup-cage construct rather than cage alone. The functional outcome, however, was similar for the successful cases in both groups. The long-term follow-up studies remains lacking in current literature.

Sporer et al. [51] described the acetabular distraction with using porous tantalum component an alternative technique for reconstruction in cases of severe bone loss with associated pelvic discontinuity. It involves using porous tantalum components (jumbo cup) with or without augments placed into a distracted pelvic discontinuity. In theory, the construct should provide initial mechanical stability for bone ingrowth to occur into the prosthesis both superiorly and inferiorly to bridge the discontinuity in a biologic fashion. Suboptimal outcomes from existing management approaches were the drive for the development of the new surgical technique. They reviewed 20 patients who underwent acetabular distraction with minimum 24-month follow-up. They reported excellent results on pain and walking with only one revision for aseptic loosening at 9 months following the initial procedure. Four components showed initial radiographic migration but no additional migration seen over a mean of 49 months. Four major complications were encountered including an iatrogenic colonic perforation, femoral artery injury, superficial infection, and a greater trochanteric fracture. This technique was then thoroughly described and advocated by Sheth et al. [52] and Brown et al. [53]. Though the novel method has provided another option to address pelvic discontinuity with severe acetabular bone loss, there is no large series study with long-term follow-up to date. The high rate of early implant migration in the previous study could still be statistically significant in larger series. The potential high complication rate associated with this technique remains controversial and the recommendation remains unclear.

Case Presentations

Nonoperative Cases

Postoperative periprosthetic acetabular fractures. Column stability verified with X-rays and CT. Patient can be managed with progressive weight-bearing starting with non-weight-bearing for 4–6 weeks then partial weight-bearing for 4 weeks. Close follow-up should be maintained with new X-rays to prevent failure of the implant or worsening of fractures. Literature has shown good clinical outcomes for patients who had nondisplaced or minimally displaced peripheral fractures of the acetabulum.

LS: failed fracture fixation
NL: failed HHA with posterior superior incompetence fracture
DY: pelvic discontinuity failed HHA
CM: failed THA with osteolysis

Tips, Tricks, and Avoiding Pitfalls

Thorough preoperative planning is the key to minimize the risk of periprosthetic acetabular fractures. A detailed patient history and physical examinations should be documented. Adequate preoperative radiographs and advanced imaging studies should be obtained to assess risk factors and evaluate any deformity or bony deficiency. All potential reconstruction options should be carefully planned and taken into consideration. Templating of preoperative full length radiographs is also helpful to anticipate component sizes. Infection should always be taken into consideration while evaluating postoperative periprosthetic fractures. Appropriate laboratory and nuclear studies can be useful in this scenario. Prevention of intraoperative acetabular fractures during insertion of implant is the key to avoid component failure [4]. Meticulous reaming should be performed, carefully exposing the acetabular floor without violating/blowing out the anterior/posterior/medial walls of the socket [10]. Care should be taken to assess the anterior and posterior wall intraoperatively to avoid eccentric reaming. During component insertion, failure of the prosthesis to advance with repetitive impaction should alert surgeons for oversized implant or significant underreaming. Additional reaming should be considered and forceful impaction should be absolutely avoided. Although no specific guideline of oversizing the acetabular component exists, one should avoid underreaming more than 2 mm unless an unusually large component is being inserted. Line-to-line reaming should be strongly considered when significant osteoporotic bone or revision surgeries involved. Adequate soft tissue releases are necessary to achieve sufficient surgical exposure. Minimal invasive type of incision should be avoided during revision surgeries. If necessary, variants of trochanteric osteotomy should be considered to gain the best exposure of acetabuli.

Authors' Preferred Method and Take-Home Points

- Preoperative planning and ruling out concomitant infection are of paramount importance; any question of infection, one should be ready to perform and explant and placement of an antibiotic spacer, one that allows for immediate mobilization and at least partial weight-bearing.
- Goals of fixation, even in the acute period, is to allow for immediate weight-bearing, and this can be achieved with utilizing a revision acetabular component, which often requires posterior column plating for increased stabilization/neutralization.
- Avoid medialization whenever possible, and even in the acute setting, an off-the-shelf cage can offer columnar stability to allow for appropriate reconstruction and restoration of anatomic parameters.
- For chronic fractures with complete discontinuity, again after ruling out infection, restoration of the columnar support is the goal; this can be achieved with distraction osteogenesis techniques, cup-cage constructs, off-the-shelf cage constructs, as well as custom cage constructs for larger more complex defects.

References

1. Kurtz S, Ong K, Lau E, Mowat F, Halpern M. Projections of primary and revision hip and knee arthroplasty in the United States from 2005 to 2030. J Bone Joint Surg Am. 2007;89(4):780–5. https://doi.org/10.2106/JBJS.F.00222.
2. Miller AJ. Late fracture of the acetabulum after total hip replacement. J Bone Joint Surg Br. 1972;54(4):600–6.
3. McElfresh EC, Coventry MB. Femoral and pelvic fractures after total hip arthroplasty. J Bone Joint Surg Am. 1974;56(3):483–92.
4. Sharkey PF, Hozack WJ, Callaghan JJ, Kim YS, Berry DJ, Hanssen AD, LeWallen DG. Acetabular fracture associated with cementless acetabular component insertion: a report of 13 cases. J Arthroplasty. 1999;14(4):426–31.
5. Haidukewych GJ, Jacofsky DJ, Hanssen AD, Lewallen DG. Intraoperative fractures of the acetabulum during primary total hip arthroplasty. J Bone Joint Surg Am. 2006;88(9):1952–6. https://doi.org/10.2106/JBJS.E.00890.
6. Kim YS, Callaghan JJ, Ahn PB, Brown TD. Fracture of the acetabulum during insertion of an oversized hemispherical component. J Bone Joint Surg Am. 1995;77(1):111–7.
7. Potty AG, Corona J, Manning BT, Le A, Saleh KJ. Acute periprosthetic fractures of the acetabulum after total hip arthroplasty. Instr Course Lect. 2014;63:199–207.
8. Adler E, Stuchin SA, Kummer FJ. Stability of press-fit acetabular cups. J Arthroplasty. 1992;7(3):295–301.
9. Curtis MJ, Jinnah RH, Wilson VD, Hungerford DS. The initial stability of uncemented acetabular components. J Bone Joint Surg Br. 1992;74(3):372–6.
10. Haddad FS, Masri BA, Garbuz DS, Duncan CP. The prevention of periprosthetic fractures in total hip and knee arthroplasty. Orthop Clin North Am. 1999;30(2):191–207.
11. Chatoo M, Parfitt J, Pearse MF. Periprosthetic acetabular fracture associated with extensive osteolysis. J Arthroplasty. 1998;13(7):843–5.
12. Peterson CA, Lewallen DG. Periprosthetic fracture of the acetabulum after total hip arthroplasty. J Bone Joint Surg Am. 1996;78(8):1206–13.
13. Callaghan JJ, Kim YS, Pederson DR, Brown TD. Periprosthetic fractures of the acetabulum. Orthop Clin North Am. 1999;30(2):221–34.
14. Della Valle CJ, Momberger NG, Paprosky WG. Periprosthetic fractures of the acetabulum associated with a total hip arthroplasty. Instr Course Lect. 2003;52:281–90.
15. Hozack WJ, Mesa JJ, Carey C, Rothman RH. Relationship between polyethylene wear, pelvic osteolysis, and clinical symptomatology in patients with cementless acetabular components. A framework for decision making. J Arthroplasty. 1996;11(7):769–72.
16. Helfet DL, Ali A. Periprosthetic fractures of the acetabulum. Instr Course Lect. 2004;53:93–8.
17. Davidson D, Pike J, Garbuz D, Duncan CP, Masri BA. Intraoperative periprosthetic fractures during total hip arthroplasty. Evaluation and management. J Bone Joint Surg Am. 2008;90(9):2000–12. https://doi.org/10.2106/JBJS.H.00331.
18. Berry DJ, Lewallen DG, Hanssen AD, Cabanela ME. Pelvic discontinuity in revision total hip arthroplasty. J Bone Joint Surg Am. 1999;81(12):1692–702.

19. D'Antonio JA, Capello WN, Borden LS, Bargar WL, Bierbaum BF, Boettcher WG, et al. Classification and management of acetabular abnormalities in total hip arthroplasty. Clin Orthop Relat Res. 1989;243:126–37.
20. Paprosky WG, Perona PG, Lawrence JM. Acetabular defect classification and surgical reconstruction in revision arthroplasty. A 6-year follow-up evaluation. J Arthroplasty. 1994;9(1):33–44.
21. Masri BA, Meek RM, Duncan CP. Periprosthetic fractures evaluation and treatment. Clin Orthop Relat Res. 2004;420:80–95.
22. Springer BD, Berry DJ, Cabanela ME, Hanssen AD, Lewallen DG. Early postoperative transverse pelvic fracture: a new complication related to revision arthroplasty with an uncemented cup. J Bone Joint Surg Am. 2005;87(12):2626–31. https://doi.org/10.2106/JBJS.E.00088.
23. Harvie P, Gundle R, Willett K. Traumatic periprosthetic acetabular fracture: life threatening haemorrhage and a novel method of acetabular reconstruction. Injury. 2004;35(8):819–22. https://doi.org/10.1016/S0020-1383(03)00218-3.
24. Paprosky WG, Sekundiak TD. Total acetabular allografts. Instr Course Lect. 1999;48:67–76.
25. Paprosky WG, Magnus RE. Principles of bone grafting in revision total hip arthroplasty. Acetabular technique. Clin Orthop Relat Res. 1994;298:147–55.
26. Mahoney CR, Garvin KL. Periprosthetic acetabular stress fracture causing pelvic discontinuity. Orthopedics. 2002;25(1):83–5.
27. Tanzer M, Drucker D, Jasty M, McDonald M, Harris WH. Revision of the acetabular component with an uncemented Harris-Galante porous-coated prosthesis. J Bone Joint Surg Am. 1992;74(7):987–94.
28. Moreland JR, Bernstein ML. Femoral revision hip arthroplasty with uncemented, porous-coated stems. Clin Orthop Relat Res. 1995;319:141–50.
29. Boscainos PJ, Kellett CF, Maury AC, Backstein D, Gross AE. Management of periacetabular bone loss in revision hip arthroplasty. Clin Orthop Relat Res. 2007;465:159–65. https://doi.org/10.1097/BLO.0b013e3181560c6c.
30. Whaley AL, Berry DJ, Harmsen WS. Extra-large uncemented hemispherical acetabular components for revision total hip arthroplasty. J Bone Joint Surg Am. 2001;83-A(9):1352–7.
31. Gustke KA, Levering MF, Miranda MA. Use of jumbo cups for revision of acetabulae with large bony defects. J Arthroplasty. 2014;29(1):199–203. https://doi.org/10.1016/j.arth.2012.11.010.
32. Kremers HM, Howard JL, Loechler Y, Schleck CD, Harmsen WS, Berry DJ, et al. Comparative long-term survivorship of uncemented acetabular components in revision total hip arthroplasty. J Bone Joint Surg Am. 2012;94(12):e82. https://doi.org/10.2106/JBJS.K.00549.
33. Lachiewicz PF, Soileau ES. Fixation, survival, and dislocation of jumbo acetabular components in revision hip arthroplasty. J Bone Joint Surg Am. 2013;95(6):543–8. https://doi.org/10.2106/JBJS.L.00758.
34. Park DK, Della Valle CJ, Quigley L, Moric M, Rosenberg AG, Galante JO. Revision of the acetabular component without cement. A concise follow-up, at twenty to twenty-four years, of a previous report. J Bone Joint Surg Am. 2009;91(2):350–5. https://doi.org/10.2106/JBJS.H.00302.
35. Skytta ET, Eskelinen A, Paavolainen PO, Remes VM. Early results of 827 trabecular metal revision shells in acetabular revision. J Arthroplasty. 2011;26(3):342–5. https://doi.org/10.1016/j.arth.2010.01.106.
36. Mears DC, Velyvis JH. Acute total hip arthroplasty for selected displaced acetabular fractures: two to twelve-year results. J Bone Joint Surg Am. 2002;84-A(1):1–9.
37. Gililland JM, Anderson LA, Henninger HB, Kubiak EN, Peters CL. Biomechanical analysis of acetabular revision constructs: is pelvic discontinuity best treated with bicolumnar or traditional unicolumnar fixation? J Arthroplasty. 2013;28(1):178–86. https://doi.org/10.1016/j.arth.2012.04.031.
38. Nwankwo C, Dong NN, Heffernan CD, Ries MD. Do jumbo cups cause hip center elevation in revision THA? A computer simulation. Clin Orthop Relat Res. 2014;472(2):572–6. https://doi.org/10.1007/s11999-013-3169-2.
39. Nwankwo CD, Ries MD. Do jumbo cups cause hip center elevation in revision THA? A radiographic evaluation. Clin Orthop Relat Res. 2014;472(9):2793–8. https://doi.org/10.1007/s11999-014-3632-8.
40. Dou Y, Zhou Y, Tang Q, Yang D, Liu J. Leg-length discrepancy after revision hip arthroplasty: are modular stems superior? J Arthroplasty. 2013;28(4):676–9. https://doi.org/10.1016/j.arth.2012.08.009.
41. Delp SL, Wixson RL, Komattu AV, Kocmond JH. How superior placement of the joint center in hip arthroplasty affects the abductor muscles. Clin Orthop Relat Res. 1996;328:137–46.
42. Dora C, Houweling M, Koch P, Sierra RJ. Iliopsoas impingement after total hip replacement: the results of non-operative management, tenotomy or acetabular revision. J Bone Joint Surg Br. 2007;89(8):1031–5. https://doi.org/10.1302/0301-620X.89B8.19208.
43. Harris WH, Crothers O, Oh I. Total hip replacement and femoral-head bone-grafting for severe acetabular deficiency in adults. J Bone Joint Surg Am. 1977;59(6):752–9.
44. Mulroy RD Jr, Harris WH. The effect of improved cementing techniques on component loosening in total hip replacement. An 11-year radiographic review. J Bone Joint Surg Br. 1990;72(5):757–60.
45. Gerber SD, Harris WH. Femoral head autografting to augment acetabular deficiency in patients requiring total hip replacement. A minimum five-year and an average seven-year follow-up study. J Bone Joint Surg Am. 1986;68(8):1241–8.
46. Lee BP, Cabanela ME, Wallrichs SL, Ilstrup DM. Bone-graft augmentation for acetabular

deficiencies in total hip arthroplasty. Results of long-term follow-up evaluation. J Arthroplasty. 1997;12(5):503–10.
47. Delimar D, Aljinovic A, Bicanic G. Failure of bulk bone grafts after total hip arthroplasty for hip dysplasia. Arch Orthop Trauma Surg. 2014;134(8):1167–73. https://doi.org/10.1007/s00402-014-2006-8.
48. Goodman S, Saastamoinen H, Shasha N, Gross A. Complications of ilioischial reconstruction rings in revision total hip arthroplasty. J Arthroplasty. 2004;19(4):436–46.
49. Paprosky W, Sporer S, O'Rourke MR. The treatment of pelvic discontinuity with acetabular cages. Clin Orthop Relat Res. 2006;453:183–7. https://doi.org/10.1097/01.blo.0000246530.52253.7b.
50. Abolghasemian M, Tangsaraporn S, Drexler M, Barbuto R, Backstein D, Safir O, et al. The challenge of pelvic discontinuity: cup-cage reconstruction does better than conventional cages in mid-term. Bone Joint J. 2014;96-B(2):195–200. https://doi.org/10.1302/0301-620X.96B2.31907.
51. Sporer SM, Bottros JJ, Hulst JB, Kancherla VK, Moric M, Paprosky WG. Acetabular distraction: an alternative for severe defects with chronic pelvic discontinuity? Clin Orthop Relat Res. 2012;470(11):3156–63. https://doi.org/10.1007/s11999-012-2514-1.
52. Sheth NP, Melnic CM, Paprosky WG. Acetabular distraction: an alternative for severe acetabular bone loss and chronic pelvic discontinuity. Bone Joint J. 2014;96-B(11 Supple A):36–42. https://doi.org/10.1302/0301-620X.96B11.34455.
53. Brown NM, Hellman M, Haughom BH, Shah RP, Sporer SM, Paprosky WG. Acetabular distraction: an alternative approach to pelvic discontinuity in failed total hip replacement. Bone Joint J. 2014;96-B(11 Supple A):73–7. https://doi.org/10.1302/0301-620X.96B11.34316.

"Pearls in Revision Total Hip Arthroplasty: Addressing the Periprosthetic Fracture About the Proximal Femur—Loose or Well-Fixed?"

6

Erik N. Kubiak

Introduction and General Remarks

Periprosthetic fractures of the proximal femur occur in multiple settings and, like all trauma, tend to occur either as the result of lower energy trauma in the setting of compromised bone or as a result of high-energy trauma in patients with relatively normal bone. This has important consequences on the choice of retaining or replacing stems and the method of bone fixation. Classically, proximal femoral periprosthetic fractures occurred in low energy settings as the result of bone insufficiency that arises, in part, as a result of particle disease in combination with stress shielding of the proximal femur (Fig. 6.1) [1, 2].

This group of injuries requires that the femoral stem be replaced, often in combination with revision of the severely worn acetabular component. Revision of both components made more difficult by lack of bone and the unreconstructability of the femoral fracture and acetabular bone defects.

More recently, we have observed an increase in the number of proximal femoral periprosthetic fractures that arise either as the result of high-energy mechanisms with contemporary biologically fixed components (non-cemented) [3–6] (Fig. 6.2). These injuries differ from the classic periprosthetic injuries arising as a result of bone deficiency and particle disease in the fact that there is often of good quality. The proximal femur can be anatomically reconstructed using modern fracture fixation methods. Femoral stem revision is reserved in these injuries to only those stems, which are frankly loose (Fig. 6.1). We will spend much of this chapter focusing on the techniques require to achieve good results with this group of injuries. In-depth discussion of how to deal with insufficiency fractures has been exhaustively discussed in other texts and will not be the focus of this discussion.

Wedge style ingrowth stems have become the most popular stems in the United States. They have their own special considerations that must be taken into account when discussing periprosthetic fracture reconstruction. We, and others, have observed a recent increase in the incidence of proximal femur fractures around these "wedge" style femoral stems. These fractures occur throughout the life of implantation but are most common in the acute setting before ingrowth. There is some debate as to whether these are iatrogenic fractures that occur during implantation or are the result of femoral component settling during mobilization. The currently favored wedge style ingrowth femoral stems are particularly prone to settling and femoral fracture when used in patients with osteopenia. Current recommenda-

E. N. Kubiak (✉)
UMC/UNLV Department of Orthopedic Surgery, University Medical Center of Southern Nevada, Las Vegas, NV, USA

University of Nevada Las Vegas, Las Vegas, NV, USA

R. S. Yoon et al. (eds.), *Trauma and Infection Control in Revision Hip and Knee Arthroplasty*, https://doi.org/10.1007/978-3-031-71971-4_6

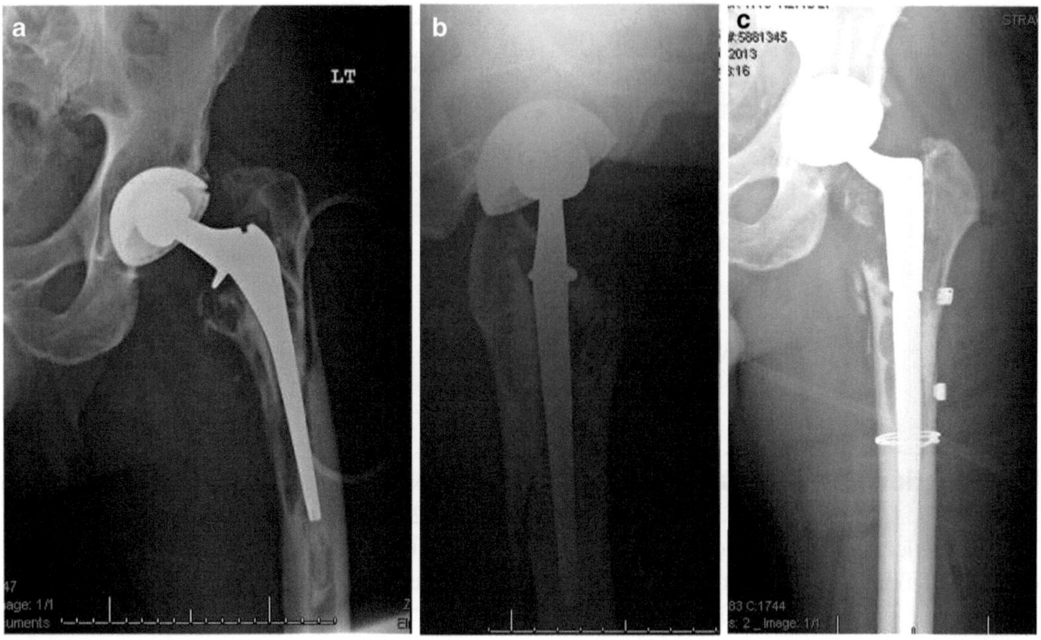

Fig. 6.1 (**a**) 58 year old male 8 years sp primary THA with 3 years of antecedent thigh pain falls trout fishing and must be air lifted out of the wilderness. (**b**) Note the asymmetry of the head in the acetabulum indicative of polyethelene wear. (**c**) Cerclage cables are used to prevent fracture propagation and likely loss of the abductor insertion to the proximal femur. Careful removal of the cement and maintenance of the isthmus while causing minimal iatrogenic damage to the abductor attachments to the proximal femur assures a successful outcome

tions are not to use these stems in patients with osteopenia [7, 8]. These stems create long spiral multifragmentary fractures of the proximal femur that often require reconstruction of the femur provisionally before stem reimplantation.

Regardless of the mechanism of failure, the surgeon must be able to establish the presence of an intact isthmus or the reconstructability of the femoral isthmus before settling on the most appropriate stem design. Modern fixation techniques allow the retention of well-fixed stems in almost all cases. Though it can be hard to determine definitely if the stem is well fixed. Moreover, modern approaches to fixation allow for the reconstruction of a femur wherein the isthmus cannot support a stem without subsidence prior to ORIF of the femur which reconstitutes the isthmus [9–11]. In the setting of a reconstructable femur fracture, we tend to err on the side of stem retention when stem is questionably loose. Stem revision is reserved for situations where the stem is frankly loose or the femur unreconstructable due to poor bone quality.

We will describe in detail the reconstruction constructs that have been most successfully employed for the fixation of common patterns of periprosthetic fracture using the Vancouver classification of periprosthetic fractures as a guiding framework for the discussion.

When Do You Keep the Stem? When Do You Revise the Stem?

We retain well-fixed femoral stems regardless of whether they are biologically fixed stems or cemented stems. If there is some doubt as to the stability of the stem we make sure that revision options are available prior to entering the operating theater. Signs of a loose stem are broken cement mantle, associated greater and lesser trochanter fracture, change on position of the stem relative to the medial and lateral femur compared to preoperative films, and radiolucent line around the stem. All loose stems are routinely revised. It is important to not only have revision stems avail-

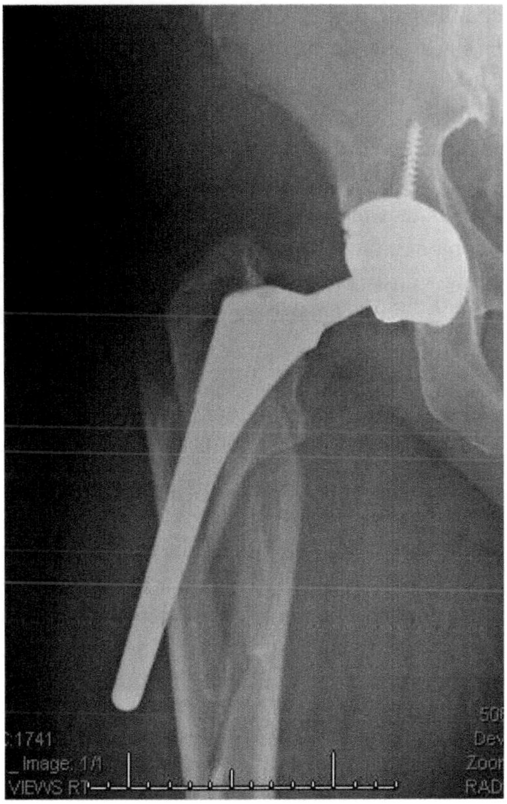

Fig. 6.2 56 year old female sustained a Vancouver B1 fracture of the femur in a road traffic accident. Stem is still well ingrown to the proximal femoral metaphysis

able but also heads and a plan for revision of the acetabular component if the need arises.

What Drives the Stem Design?

Our revision stem design of choice in the setting of a periprosthetic fracture is a "wagner style" modular splined tapered stem. The modularity is employed to adjust limb length. We routinely assemble the stem in the patient. This allows the modular stem component to function as a splint around which to assemble the proximal femur and also allows the stem to protect the femoral construct during any indicated acetabular work. Long cemented revision stems are avoided when possible secondary to the tendency of the cement to escape through the fracture gaps, potential thermal injury to fracture bone, and the high incidence of premature loosening.

How Do You Manage Incompetent Isthmus Due to Fracture?

A reconstructed or intact isthmus is necessary to prevent femoral stem settling regardless of whether or not a cemented or biological ingrowth femoral component is selected. Therefore when the isthmus is disrupted by fracture, it is routinely reconstructed. In those circumstances that the isthmus is not reconstructable, proximal femoral replacing tumor prosthesis is selected.

Do You Plate the Entire Femur?

Plating the entire femur is typical to maximize the chance of a successful fixation construct as real estate for screw fixation will frequently be compromised by the presence of the femoral stem. Conversely, as we see more and more total knee replacements ipsilateral to total hips, we will employee long plate constructs to improve distal fixation and reduce the risk of subsequent intraprosthetic fracture. The general rule of thumb is to fix the femur from the greater trochanter to the lateral femoral condyle [12, 13]. There is nothing worse than scrutinizing your final fluoroscopic images only to discover a previously unrecognized fracture propagation into the distal "stable" fragment. Do not leave the operating room hoping that this will get better with time. The time to increase the length of the femoral plate is before the patient is in post op recovery or on the floor. As general rule, we require three points of fixation in both the proximal and distal fragments.

When and What Is Used to Augment the Fixation of Poor Quality Bone?

Not infrequently when treating periprosthetic fractures, the treating surgeon is faced with the terrible triumvirate of poor host, poor bone quality, and fracture comminution. When presented with this combination. Fixation needs to be able to withstand early patient mobilization; much of this will in the end be dependent on purchase in pour quality bone. At present, the best strategies will employ long fixation constructs and fixed angle screws placed in a bicortical fashion around stems. Biomechanical studies have demonstrated that cortical struts and cerclage cables confer additional fixation strength benefits [14–16]. Unfortunately, the constructs used in biomechanical studies are often impractical or frankly impossible to create clinically due to anatomic constraints. In general, we find that cerclage wires are best deployed to constrain complex spiral fractures and facilitate their compression with clamps, can be excellent provisional fixation under locked plates, can prevent distal fracture propagation during canal preparation for distal fragment reaming, and are useful for the fixation of extended trochanteric osteotomies. Allograft struts are infrequently used our preference to use long plates and long femoral stems en lei of allograft struts which are frequently too short to be of sufficient benefit.

Fracture Classification

The most frequently employed classification system for periprosthetic fractures of the proximal femur is the Vancouver classification. This divides fracture types by location and stem stability [17] (Table 6.1).

Vancouver type A fractures are generally treated in a closed fashion and are most commonly the result of eccentric loading of compromised bone or direct impact. Iatrogenic fractures of the greater trochanter are fixed acutely when they compromise stem stability or represent greater than 50% of the insertion of the gluteus medius. Beware of Vancouver A3 fractures where the lesser and the greater trochanters are both fractured. When both trochanters are broken, the stem most of the time has settled (Fig. 6.3). This is particularly true with wedge-type stems.

Vancouver type B fractures are the most commonly surgically treated fractures of the proximal femur. Current fixation techniques employing a combination of locked plates and cerclage wires allow most of these fractures to be fixed (Fig. 6.4a–c) and the anatomy of the proximal femur to be preserved.

The most difficult thing to determine when treating these fractures is stem stability. The excellent stability of current fixation techniques has led us to err to fixing these fractures even when the stem stability is questionable. Obviously loose stems are revised to splined tapered Wagner style stems (Fig. 6.5a, b). When these fractures occur in the perioperative period as the result of wedge type femoral stem settling, we often have to provisionally reconstruct the femur to reestablish a femoral isthmus prior to stem reimplantation.

Vancouver type C fractures are in most circumstances supracondylar femur fractures or at least distal third femur fractures and are treated like supracondylar femur fractures. These injuries are going be plated. The surgeon needs to decide whether or not a plate designed for fixation of the distal femur is necessary to provide sufficient fixation of the most distal femoral fracture fragment (Fig. 6.6a, b). In general, three cortical screws spread over a minimum of five holes are the minimal and if this is not possible in the intact distal femur before the metaphysis is encountered, a distal femoral supracondylar plate should be selected.

Table 6.1 Vancouver fracture periprosthetic fracture classification

Fracture type	Incidence, %	Location	Subtype
A	44	Trochanteric	A(G): Greater trochanter
			A(L): Lesser trochanter
B	87	Around the stem tip	B(1): Prosthesis stable (18%)
			B(2): Prosthesis loose (45%)
			B(3): Bone stock inadequate (37%)
C	9	Well below the stem tip	

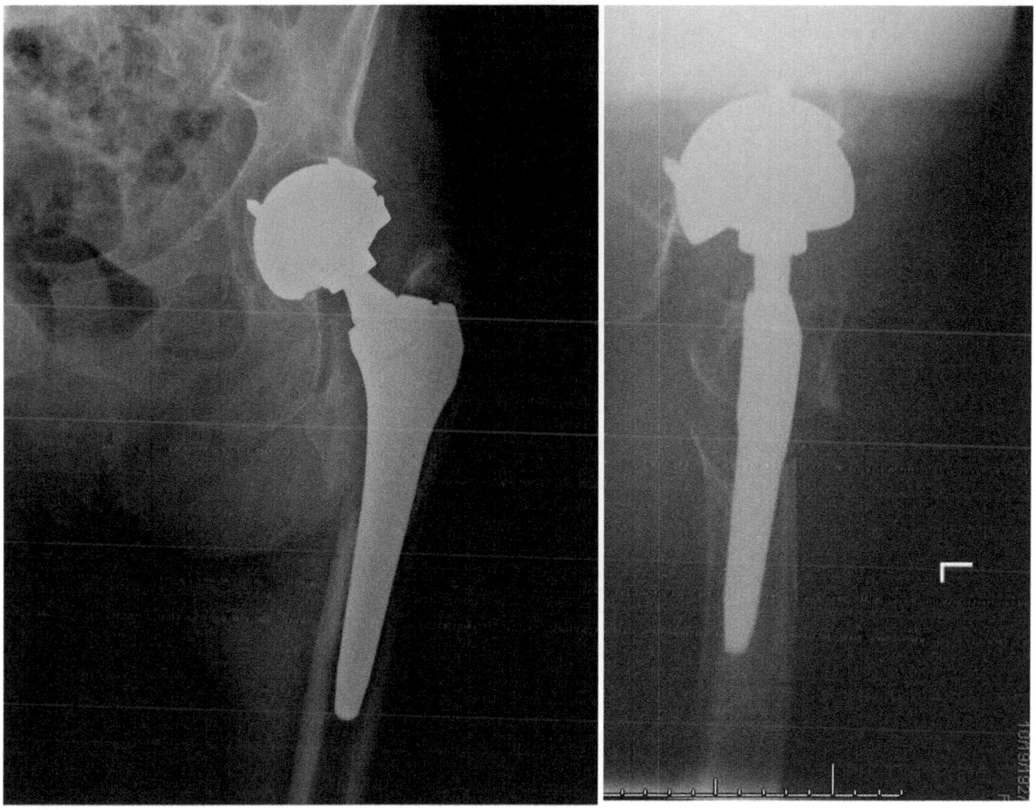

Fig. 6.3 84 year old female pain in left leg after fall, exhibiting fractures of both greater and lesser trochanter indicative of a loose stem

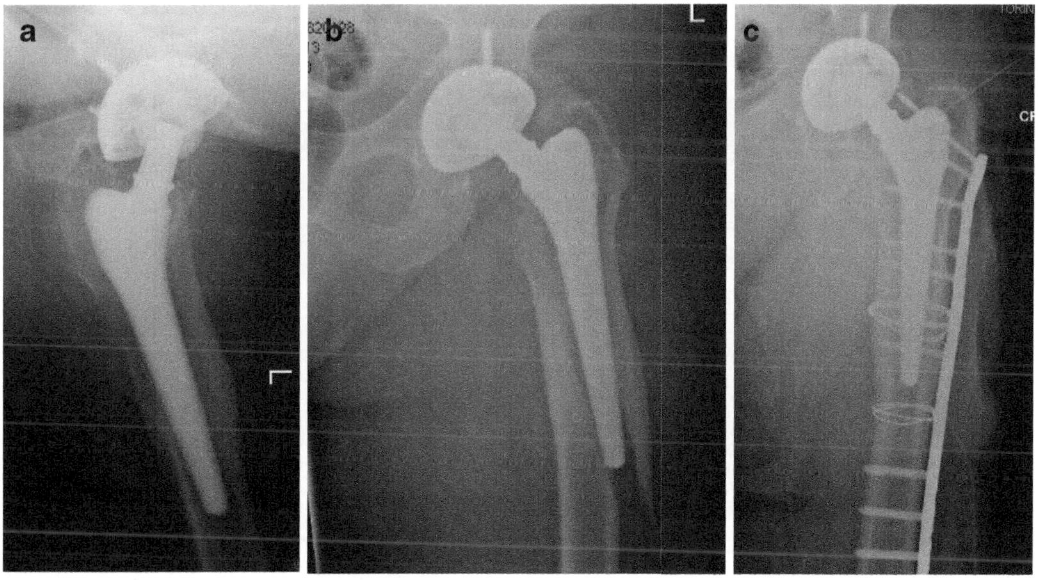

Fig. 6.4 (**a, b**) 52 year old male with Vancouver B1 fracture: excellent bone and a well-fixed stem. (**c**) Modern ORIF with screws placed anterior and posterior to stem provides excellent fixation and allows for abductor muscle insertion sparing fixation

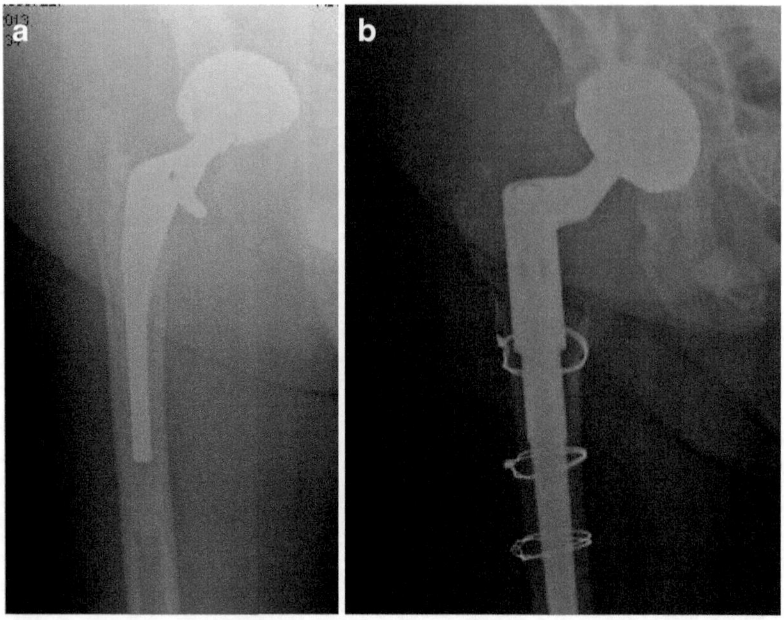

Fig. 6.5 (**a**) 54 year old male with 2 years of thigh pain presents with fracture that occurs while walking down the street. Key is to remove the cement and maintain the isthmus while causing minimal iatrogenic damage to the abductor attachments to the proximal femur. (**b**) Revision to a diaphyseal fitting stem offers the most stable construct and immediate mobilization

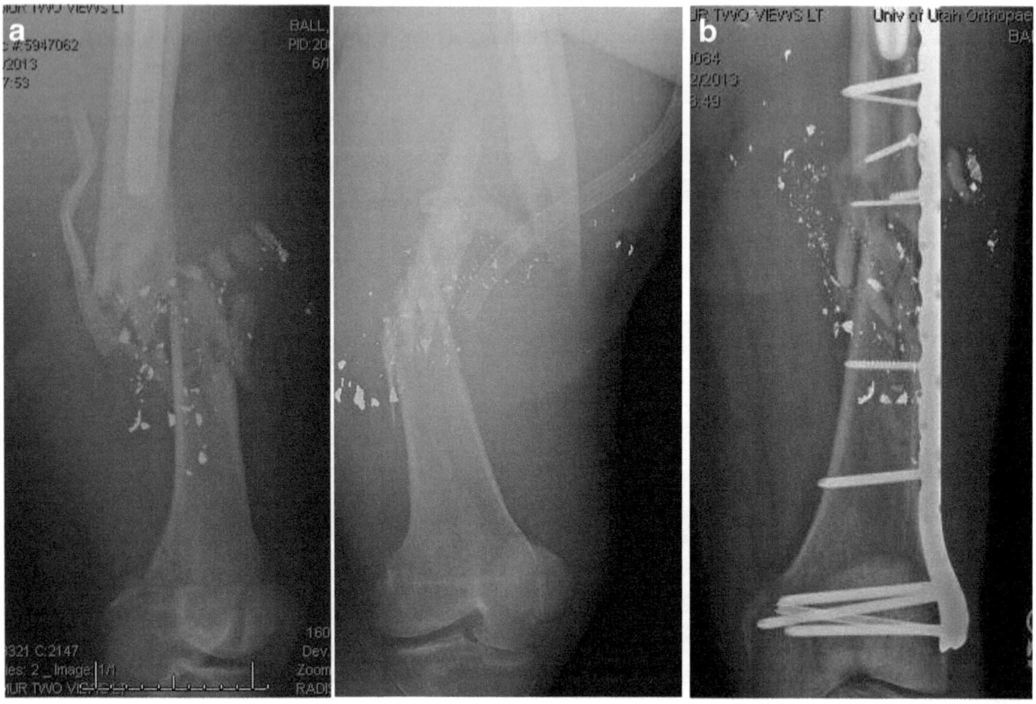

Fig. 6.6 (**a**) 67 year old male accidental gunshot to the thigh and a resultant Vanc C1 fracture. (**b**) ORIF with a supracondylar plate to maximize metaphyseal fixation in the distal femoral segment. No bone graft was necessary; note, the attachment plates provide for bicortical fixation around the well fixed femoral hip stem

Fracture Specific Treatment Plans

Vancouver A Type Fractures General Remarks

Closed management is reserved for isolated greater or lesser trochanter fractures and patients who are too sick to undergo surgery. Beware of combined fractures of the lesser and the greater trochanter as they almost always arise as the result of a subsided loose femoral stem (Fig. 6.7). These patients moreover will almost all be unable to bear weight on the injured side.

Non-operative Treatment

Vancouver A1 fractures have a checkered history when it comes to fixation most fractures are given a trial of closed management [18]. Closed management consists of protected weight bearing and reassurance that short-term discomfort is normal but that long disability is not normal. Isolated Vancouver A2 fractures—isolated fractures of the lesser trochanter—are rare and treated almost universally in a closed fashion.

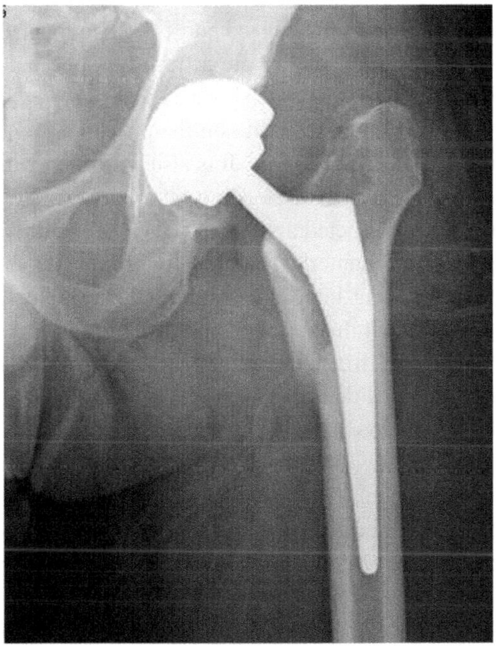

Fig. 6.7 Subsided stem following concurrent greater and lesser trochanter fracture

Operative Treatment

We reserve operative intervention for Vancouver A1 fractures in patients who have a new onset of hip instability after the fracture and/or unresolving pain and a pronounced adductor lurch. Inability to mobilize after sustaining an A1 fracture is not in and of itself a reason to attempt ORIF of the greater trochanter acutely. If the patient continues to have difficulty ambulating after 2 to 4 weeks of closed management, one must consider the possibility that the stem is loose in addition to the fractured greater trochanter. A thorough scrutinization of the films must be undertaken to rule out distal stem migration. If this is present, then revision of the stem is indicated +/− ORIF of the greater trochanter.

Cerclage wires, cerclage suture, and hook plates have been used to treat Vancouver A1 fractures with mixed results [19–21]. Some authors have advocated for the excision of the painful fractured greater trochanter. We reserve excision for painful fractures of the greater trochanter in two circumstances: (1) those greater trochanters which are small and fragmented and (2) when it is not possible to fix the biological viable greater trochanter fragment to viable bleeding distal bone—this often occurs when distal bone has been losing during revision surgery. Figure 6.8a, b demonstrates a typical situation of modern fixation techniques that are able to achieve a united fracture.

The workhorse for greater trochanter fixation in our hands has been locked (fixed angle) trochanteric fixation plate [21]. This plate enables us to fix the proximal trochanter fragment with multiple fixed angle screws much like the proximal humerus. With this plate, we are then able to secure the greater trochanter to the distal femoral fragment securely with compression in a tension band position. In order for this to be successful, living bleeding trochanter must be compressed directly to living bleeding distal femur.

To achieve this end, we first approach the proximal femur through a direct lateral approach with the patient in a lateral decubitus position. When the prior surgery was performed via a modified Kocher-Langenbeck approach, we will routinely extend the vertical limb of the incision

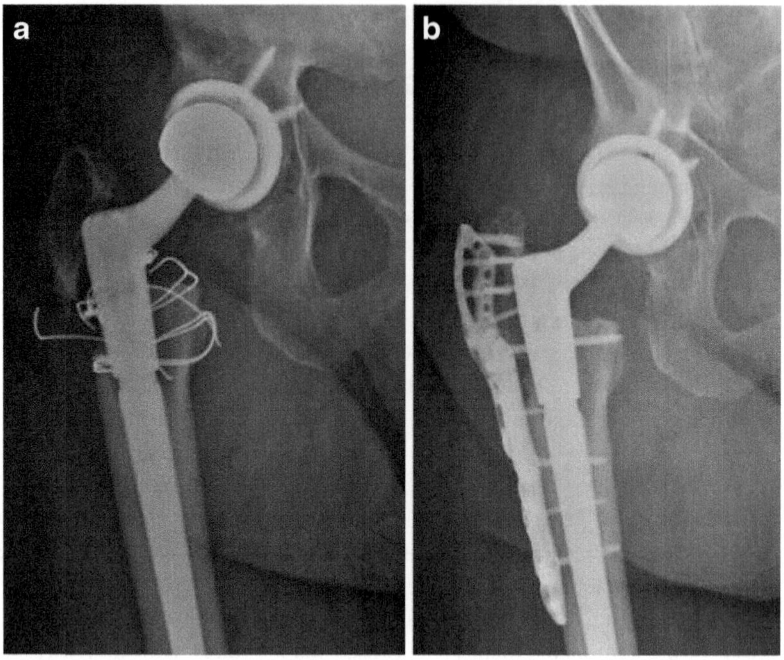

Fig. 6.8 (**a**) Greater trochanteric periprosthetic fracture fixed with (**b**) modern fixation techniques that offer the ideal situation for united fracture

centered over the iliotibial band as proximal as necessary. If alternative approaches were employed like a Hueter approach, we will make a new midline incision centered over the greater trochanter and complete the approach through a split of the iliotibial band as below.

Soft tissues are divided into the IT band. The IT band is split in line with the fibers; the split is centered over the middle aspect of the greater trochanter. Once the greater trochanter fragment is identified, it is freed of interposed fibrous tissue. Mobility of the greater fragment is assessed; in most circumstances of long standing non-united trochanteric fracture, the fragment will have migrated proximally and posteriorly. The fragment is carefully freed of fibrous tissue. The gluteus medius is mobilized off the ilium gently with respect to its blood supply. This blood supply arises from the superior gluteal artery as it passes posterior to anterior through the greater sciatic notch. Attention must be paid to not disrupt the superior gluteal neurovascular bundle during the mobilization of the gluteus medius.

The superficial myofascia of the gluteus medius is lengthened by pie-crusting. Make sure that the cuts are perpendicular to the muscle fiber orientation taking care not to cut the underlying muscle. Next we fix the greater trochanteric fragment to the trochanteric plate. Using the plate to evaluate the mobility of the greater trochanter fragment avoids the problem of iatrogenic fracture of the fragment that is all too common when clamps are used to hold the fragment. The greater trochanter fragment is everted and a high-speed burr is used to roughen its undersurface and create a fresh bleeding bone bed. Try to keep as much bone as possible.

Next the recipient site on the proximal femur is freed of fibrous tissue. It is also freshened with the burr to create a bleeding bone surface. Now the leg is abducted and flexed. The plate with the greater trochanteric fragment is brought to the femur. Living bone must contact living bone at this point. (If this is not possible, then excision of the greater trochanter and constraining of the total hip if it demonstrated preoperative instability should be strongly considered.) The plate is provisionally held to the femur with pointed reduction clamps +/− cerclage. Additional clamps or the AO tensioning device are used to distalize the greater trochanter. Once positioning of the plate, greater trochanter and the docking of living bone to living bone are confirmed final fixation of the plate to the femur with bicortical screws (at least three) on both sides of the femoral stem completes the fixation construct. It is best to employ multiple clamps that are sequentially tightened to preform the reduction. Use of a single clamp increases the risk of fracturing the greater trochanter into multiple fragments and ruins any chance of a successful repair.

Normal postoperative protocols for revision total joints are followed. If the patient required abduction and flexion to achieve reduction, they are placed in a brace and gradually allowed to extend and adduct their leg over the ensuing 3–5 days post op under the supervision of a licensed therapist. Postoperative weight bearing protocol is weight of leg with a walker.

Vancouver A3 fractures are almost universally indicative of a loose femoral stem especially in the presence of a wedge style stem. These injuries will often fail non-operative management with protective weight bearing and require revision. When proceeding with these revisions, strong consideration for constraining the acetabular component must be entertained when secure fixation and eventual union of the greater trochanteric fragment are not expected.

Vancouver B Type Fractures: General Remarks

Vancouver B periprosthetic femur fractures represent a heterogenous group of injuries. In all but the most medically unstable patients, surgical intervention will be required. Preoperative planning is dependent on a thorough understanding of stem stability and bone quality. We will discuss strategies for all circumstances.

We will discuss the operative treatment Vancouver B type fractures according to the subclassifications. In general, two factors come into play with B type fractures and this directs the treatment. Most important and hardest thing to determine is the stability if the femoral stem; thankfully contemporary fixation techniques have been successful in treating marginal stems.

Non-operative Treatment

The closed management of Vancouver B fractures is reserved for patients who are not medically unable to undergo surgery.

Operative Treatment

Preservation of the adductor mechanism is paramount to the long-term success of operative fixation of Vancouver B periprosthetic femur fractures. We therefore tend to err on the side of ORIF unless the stem is obviously loose. Keys evidence of loosening is the change of position of the stem relative to the greater and lesser trochanters on post injury films as compared to preinjury films. The second factor guiding treatment is the condition of the femoral isthmus. An intact or reconstructable femoral isthmus allows for stem revision and ORIF, whereas the lack of an isthmus or an unreconstructable isthmus will necessitate proximal femoral replacement. I will now discuss treatment strategies for the subtypes of B fractures individually through cases.

Vancouver B1

Vancouver B1 by definition is a well-fixed stem with +/– good bone stock. ORIF will be the mainstay of treatment for these injuries. The type of ORIF will be dictated by the quality of bone and the degree of fracture comminution. The mainstays for ORIF are respect for the soft tissue envelope, maintenance of bone fragment blood supply, and restoration of preinjury femoral anatomy. Figures 6.9 and 6.10 are illustrative of these principles.

At present, there are two ways to place screws on both sides of a femoral stem. Firstly, there are plates designed with multiple rows of screw holes that will facilitate screws anterior and posterior to a femoral stem (Fig. 6.9a, b). Secondly, there are plates designed to attach to an existing plate that will facilitate screw placement anterior and posterior to the femoral stem. The benefit of this design is that they can be used with different large fragment locking plates, where the large

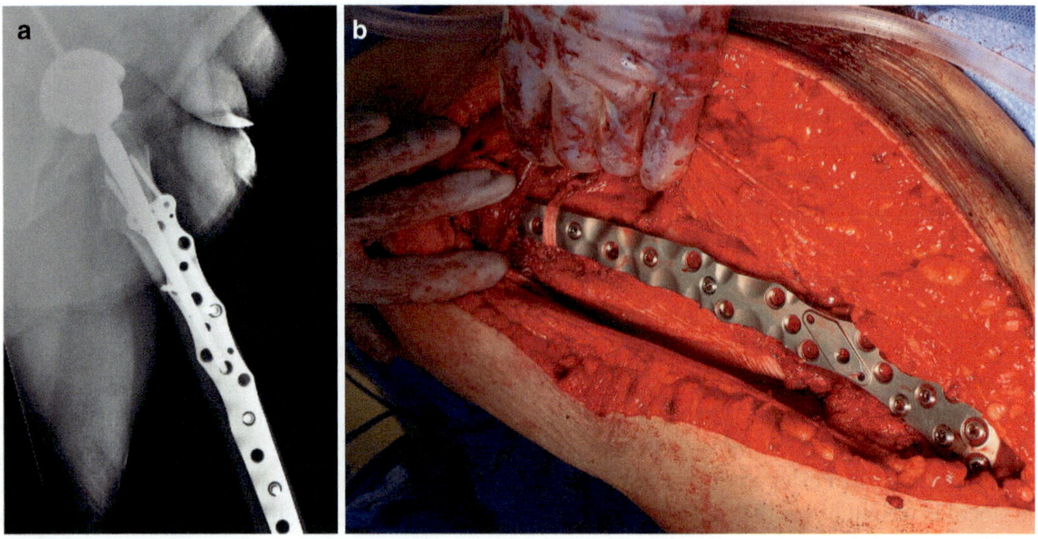

Fig. 6.9 (**a**, **b**) One type of plate design has different rows of screw holes that allow for anterior or posterior placement of screws

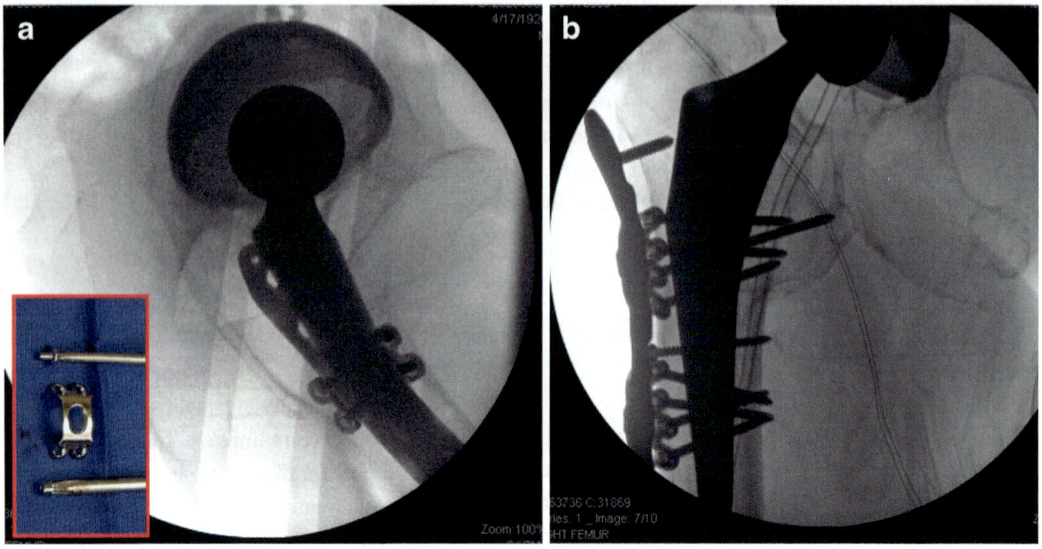

Fig. 6.10 (**a**, **b**) Locking attachment plates can be utilized in conjunction with any large fragment plate and allow for anterior or posterior placement of screws around any femoral stem

fragment locking plates designed for the proximal and distal femur as well as other large fragment plates designed for other anatomic locations (Fig. 6.11a, b).

General guidelines for placement of screws around a stem are based on my clinical experience and biomechanical investigations. General rules for the use around stems are as follows: Smaller 2.7–4.0 mm screws should be used (take care to not over torque by taping if resistance is too high and risk stripping the head or worse shearing off the screw head), screws should be equally distributed anterior and posterior to the stem, three well-placed 4.0 mm screws will fail after the plate has undergone plastic deformation; therefore, three well-placed 4.0 mm screws are

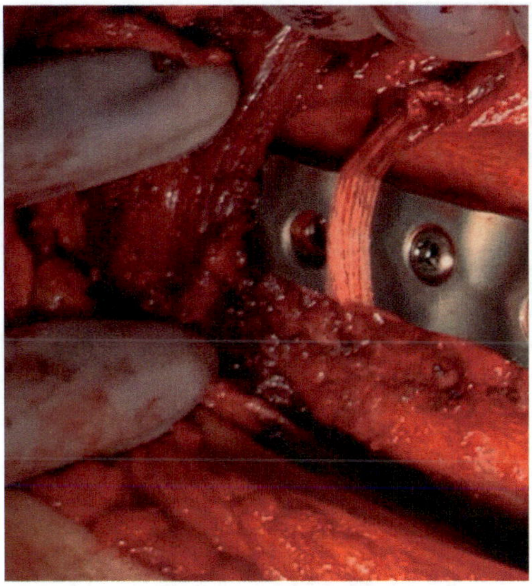

Fig. 6.11 Radio-opaque UHMWPE sutures are an evolution if fixation. They provide excellent security, fatigue resistance, ability to retighten, and no risk of third body wear

the minimal screw number, use plates designed to place screws anterior and posterior to the stem, use long plate constructs when possible (six available screw holes should overlap both the distal and proximal fracture fragment). When there is a distal stem as with a distal revision total knee over lap the distal stem with the plate when possible—this is an excellent time to use a construct with modular supplementary fixation plates. I seldom see a reason to use cortical strut allografts in this circumstance (Side note: I only use allograft struts as pads to prevent cerclage wires from cutting through severely osteopenic bone).

Vancouver B2

Vancouver B2 fractures are a heterogenous group of injuries that on the one hand can be treated much like B1 injuries with the addition of revising the femoral stem and the other hand are in fact essentially B3 three injuries that will require proximal femoral replacement. To understand how to best treat the B2 fracture, it is crucial to know why the stem is loose—is it due to osteolysis (Fig. 6.5a) or fracture (Fig. 6.12)—and what is the condition of the femoral isthmus. When the isthmus is intact, proceed with stem revision and ORIF of the proximal femur (Fig. 6.5b). When this isthmus is not intact, the surgeon must be able to ascertain can it be reconstructed—if the isthmus is not reconstructable, then proceed as for a B3 injury.

Approach will generally be posterior lateral extended Kocker-Langenbeck. Patient should be placed in the lateral decubitus position. Often we will employ the positioning tunnel that we use for calcaneus fractures to support the fractured femur and provide a flat stable surface to work on. Having the leg supported facilitates work on the femur and makes re-establishing the femoral anatomy much easier. Most of the time iliotibial band will need to be divided distally and the vastus lateralis elevated off the femur. Care should be taken to maintain the blood supply to the fracture fragments.

The femoral stem and any residual cement must be removed from the femur. If possible I will remove the stem without taking down the capsule. I remove the stem by using the fracture to gain access to the acetabulum and the loose stem. To do this, I rotate the proximal femur superiorly as one does in a direct lateral approach or when using an extended trochanteric osteotomy leaving the abductors and the capsule attached to the proximal fragment as much as possible.

Often the greater trochanter needs to be split to remove the stem despite the presence of the periprosthetic fracture. This has been called a "clamshell osteotomy."

The "clamshell osteotomy" is performed as follows: Elevate vastus lateralis from posterior intermuscular septum by carefully lifting the muscle with a Cobb elevator. Ligate with suture or clips all septum perforators from the profound femoris. Take care to not divide the perforators too close to the linea aspera. They can retract medial to the linea aspera becoming very difficult to ligate. Flex the knee to remove tension from profunda femoris and the sciatic nerve.

Gently distract fracture. If proximal femur can be mobilized anteriorly off the stem, great! If not perform vertical split mid greater trochanter in

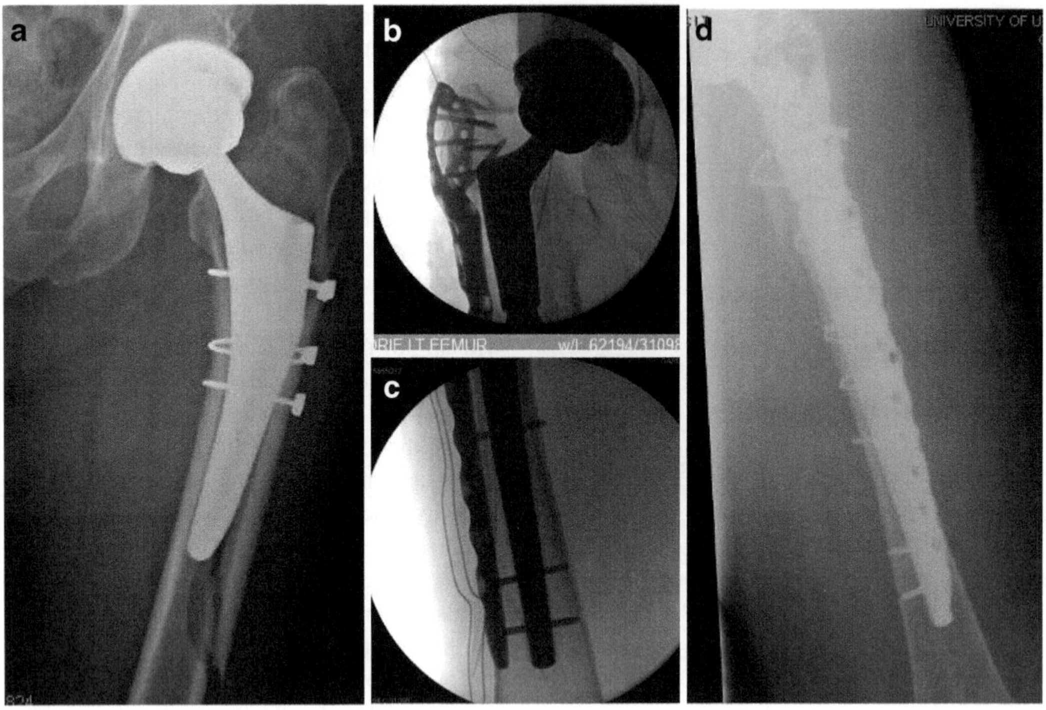

Fig. 6.12 (**a**) 63 year old female with severe osteoporosis and a Van C1 periprosthetic fracture. She developed an infected nonunion after an attempted ORIF of her Van C femur fracture. (**b**) The femoral isthmus was polished and insufficient after the successful treatment of the infection the femoral isthmus was insufficient. (**c**) At one year post revision she complained of knee pain and crepitus the result of the femoral stem settling into knee. (**d**) 5 years s/p revision to proximal femoral replacing prosthesis she had returned to her previous functional level. (**e**) Later view of healed fracture fixation which demonstrates the principles of: Balance of fixation around the hip stem, maximized proximal fixation, minimum of three screws and over a minimum of fives holes in the distal femoral segment

the coronal plane. This is done with microsagittal saw. Preserve muscle attachments and use a laminar spreader to distract fracture in a controlled fashion.

Knock the head off the femoral stem with a bone tamp while elevating stem to disengage head from stem. Remove stem from femur and patient. Perform an inferior capsule and release only as much as needed to remove the head from the cup when preserving the cup and polyethylene.

Cerclage cable around proximal end distal fragment. Minimum one cable if not two.

Cable ends are left in place for elevation of the femur during reaming and so that cables can be retensioned prior to potting of the final femoral stem.

Conically ream distal femur. Be very conservative with reaming especially in Dorr C bone. Retain what femoral isthmus is left. This is what will prevent stem subsidence. Need at least one cortical diameter above isthmus to support wedge tapered stem.

Once at desired reamer size. Reamer should be centered over acetabulum so that the +20–30 cm body mark is in the center of the hip socket. Select stem one size greater than reamer and impact into position. Select the stem length based stem in the distal fragment and should be roughly equivalent to the exposed stem and body proximally.

Prior to impaction of the final stem, re-tension the distal fragment cerclage wires. Stem should be impacted to one body less than was measured at the time of final reaming. The trial body and neutral head are attached to the impacted body and reduced to the acetabulum. This will place tension on the quadriceps and hamstrings. If the hip capsule is redundant and not retensioned, then trialling with the high offset femoral body is performed to retension the capsule appropriately.

Trial the leg through ROM. Hip should be stable when flexed 90 degrees and internally rotated 20 degrees.

If this is so, remove the trial proximal body and prepare to place the final body. If the hip is not stable confirm length and rotation are correct. Trial with a longer body if necessary. Impact the final proximal body into position—with 20 degrees of anteversion. Place and tension the locking bolt. Trial with the neutral head. Small adjustments can be made with head size. Avoid skirted heads if possible. Impact the final femoral head into position and reduce the hip.

Reduce the proximal anterior and posterior trochanteric fragments around the proximal body of the stem. It is often useful to remove cortical medial calcar femorale fragment and lateral superior neck cortices with the high-speed acorn burr to facilitate boney contact of the anterior and posterior fragments once they are clamped around the proximal femoral stem body. This process is repeated until the reduction is satisfactory. Elevate vastus lateralis from posterior intermuscular septum. Careful lifting with Cobb elevator. Ligate with suture or clips all septum perforators from the profound femoris. Take care to not divide to close to the septum. Flex the knee to remove tension from profunda femoris and the sciatic nerve.

Gently distract fracture. If proximal femur can be mobilized anteriorly off the stem, great! If not perform vertical split mid greater trochanter in the coronal plane. This is done with microsagittal saw. Preserve muscle attachments. Laminar spreader to distract fracture.

Bone tamp against head at head neck junction while elevating stem to disengage head from stem. Remove stem from femur and patient. Capsule releases inferiorly only as much as needed to remove the head from the cup when preserving the cup and polyethylene. Most of the time the stem comes out with little trouble. Any residual bone attachments are removed from the stem with osteotomes and or a pencil tipped burr on the midas rex. Again, care should be taken to preserve bone stock as much as possible and to protect the abductor muscle mass. Next the residual cement must be removed—this is done through the fracture with osteotomes and an acorn burr on the midas. Make sure that the distal plug is removed—it is also important to remove the distal pedestal that arises with some ingrowth stems.

Cerclage cable around proximal end distal fragment. Minimum one cable if not two.

Cable ends are left in place for elevation of the femur during reaming and so that cables can be retensioned prior to potting of the final femoral stem. The placement of this cerclage is critical and must be performed before proceeding with reaming, trialing, and stem reimplantation we always place a cerclage wire around the most proximal end of the distal stable fragment regardless of whether or not the isthmus is intact.

Conically ream distal femur. Be very conservative with reaming especially in Dorr C bone. Retain what femoral isthmus is left. This is what will prevent stem subsidence. Need at least one cortical diameter above isthmus to support wedge tapered stem.

Once at desired reamer size. Reamer should be centered over acetabulum. +20–30 cm body mark. Select stem one size greater than reamer and impact into position. Select the stem length based stem in the distal fragment and should be roughly equivalent to the exposed stem and body proximally.

Trial the leg through ROM. Hip should be stable when flexed 90 degrees and internally rotated 20 degrees. If the hip is stable with the trial, remove the trial proximal body. Impact the final proximal body into position—with 20 degrees of anteversion. Place and tension the locking bolt. Trial with the neutral head. Small adjustments can be made with head size. Avoid skirted heads if possible. Impact the final femoral head into position and reduce the hip.

Reduce the proximal anterior and posterior trochanteric fragments around the proximal body of the stem. It is often useful to remove cortical medial calcar femorale fragment and lateral superior neck cortices with the high-speed acorn burr to facilitate boney contact of the anterior and posterior fragments once they are clamped around the proximal femoral stem body. This process is repeated until the reduction is satisfactory.

The reduction is completed, and the fracture and osteotomy are clamped around the stem. Cerclage cables are passed around the proximal fracture fragments, osteotomy pieces, and femoral stem. These are sequentially tightened and retightened. The hip is put through several arches of motion, and the cerclage cables retightened.

Our preference is to use UWMPE sutures or other similar non-metallic cerclage cables when reducing and stabilizing the proximal femur to minimize metallic third body particle generation contamination of the femoral acetabular articulation when/if cerclage cables fail (Fig. 6.11).

The IT band is closed with interrupted nonabsorbable suture. The skin re-approximated with interrupted sub-suture.

Patients are made weight bearing as tolerated during the 6 to 12 week convalescent period during which time fracture healing and stem integration are occurring.

Isthmus Intact

When the isthmus is intact and the cerclage placed, the distal femur is conically reamed. Care is taken not to overream and destroy the isthmus. The conical distal spined distal component is impacted into the femur [22–24]. Trial proximal bodies are trialed to establish the correct femoral length. In general, I select the smallest diameter proximal body. This will ease reconstruction of the femur. The appropriate proximal body is attached to the distal splined component according to manufacturer instructions. The head is impacted into place, and the hip reduced. The proximal femoral fragments are reconstructed around the stem provisionally with Luque wires. Often the insides of the fragments will need to be sculpted to fit the new stem—this is done carefully with the burr. Finally the fracture is neutralized with a long lateral plate with screws placed around the stem into the proximal fragments. A minimum of three screws distributed over six holes should be used in the distal fragment. A minimum of four bicortical screws should be placed proximally. Cerclage cables are placed as deemed necessary. Ultimate success of the construct is dependent on the viability of the bone and the lack of fracture gaps. Small malreductions are tolerated to prevent fracture gaps.

Isthmus Disrupted: Reconstructable

When the isthmus can be reconstructed than we provisionally ORIF the femur first then place the femoral stem and complete the ORIF with the femoral stem in place. The provisional fixation and reconstruction of the proximal femur restore femoral anatomy. The restoration of femoral anatomy restores the abductor mechanism and allows easier understanding of rotation and limb length.

Using the plate to splint the reconstructed fractured femur is the key to making this work. A combination of unicortical, bicortical screws, cerclage wires are used to securely hold the reduced fractured femur. Reconstruct the proximal femur to the plate; make sure use screws that will not impede the passage of the reamers, broaches, and the eventual stem. Our preferred screw is a 3.5 or 4.0 mm screw placed anterior and posterior to future stem trajectory—these screws can be placed in an intracortical fashion. Then proceed with preparing the femoral canal for the future stem by reaming and broaching.

The revision stem choice is determined by the condition of the femoral isthmus. This is important for the simple reason that without a competent isthmus, the risk for stem subsidence is high. When the isthmus is incompetent, the surgeon must decide is this is due to osteopenia or bone loss (A Door C femur) or if this is secondary to distal fracture propagation. When the isthmus is compromised as a result bone loss we prefer to treat with proximal femoral replacement. If the isthmus is incompetent as a result of fracture comminution, the surgeon must determine if after the femur is reconstructed will there be an isthmus—when the isthmus is reconstructable, we proceed with reconstruct as we would for a B2 fracture with a competent isthmus.

The hallmark of the Vancouver B3 injury is the lack of proximal bone and the incompetence of the femoral isthmus. This can arise either as a result of fracture comminution, iatrogenic bone after multiple revisions, osteolysis, and/or osteopenia. Most of the time a combination of these factors are at work.

Vancouver C Type Fractures: General Remarks

Vancouver C periprosthetic femur fractures in many ways resemble supracondylar femur fractures. They are treated in much the same way as discussed in the chapter on supracondylar femur fractures with the added complexity of working around the stem in the proximal femur. There is essentially no circumstance where a Vancouver C fracture can be treated without overlapping the femoral stem proximally with the plate. Fixing the plate to the proximal femur with the stem in place has been made much simpler now that we have plates designed to place screws around the femoral stem. In most circumstances, I will choose to use a supracondylar femoral plate for these fractures to maximize fixation options in the distal femoral segment.

Non-operative Treatment

The closed management of Vancouver C fractures is reserved for patients who are not medically able to undergo surgery.

Operative Treatment

Vancouver C type fractures are generally open reduced and internally fixated with the patient in a supine position on a radiolucent table. A bump is placed under the ipsilateral posterior superior iliac spine to compensate for normal femoral external rotation. The ipsilateral arm is brought across the chest. The injured leg is placed on stacked blankets or sheets so that a lateral image can be obtained without the other leg confusing the image.

Generally a direct lateral approach to the femur is desirable. We will often open distally as for a supracondylar femur fracture and slide the plate proximally under the vastus lateralis. The proximal fixation can be accomplished through small incisions (Fig. 6.13). The easiest way to do this has been to place a Holman retractor anterior and posterior to the femur using them like goal posts and sliding the plate between the retractors. This facilitates centering the plate over the femur and makes placing screws anterior and posterior to the femoral stem easier.

Supracondylar plates that can be used with supplementary fixation plates allow for management of complex fractures (Fig. 6.7). The supracondylar plates design will accommodate distal fragment comminution, total knee implants, and the presence of a distal stemmed revision knee component.

Atypical Periprosthetic Fractures

There are recent reports of bisphosphonate-related stress fractures occurring below well-fixed well-functioning femoral prosthesis [25–27]. These patients often present with thigh pain or hip pain after a period of normal hip function. Careful evaluation of the entire femur radiographically is indicated. We have not found the routine use of computed tomography necessary. Both femurs should be evaluated. The fixation proceeds as for the treatment of Vancouver B1 fractures. The treating physician needs to understand that bone remodeling in these patients is arrested so classical compression techniques are not indicated. We use dynamic fixation constructs to treat these fractures: near cortex overdrill and far cortical locking [28–30].

The Dreaded Broken Stem

As patients get younger and more active after arthroplasty of the hip, we see the occasional broken femoral stem. These fractures occur with monobloc and modular stems. They have many challenges, but we fail back to the same principles that we use in the management of Van B3 fractures: (1) removal of stem with as much bone preservation as possible, (2) conical reaming of the isthmus after placement of prophylactic cerclage cables, (3) revision of the acetabular component as necessary with preservation of the hip capsule (clamshell technique), and (4) secure fixation of the proximal femoral osteotomy with cerclage and plates as indicated. Figure 6.14 illustrates that despite these principles being followed the proximal femoral replacement needs to be in the surgeons' armamentarium when tackling these difficult cases.

Postoperative Management

Postoperative management consists of drain placement with removal when outputs are below 30CC in 8 h. DVT prophylaxis with the institutions preferred drug is performed for six weeks post operatively. Most importantly all of our patients are out of bed as soon as possible and weight bearing as

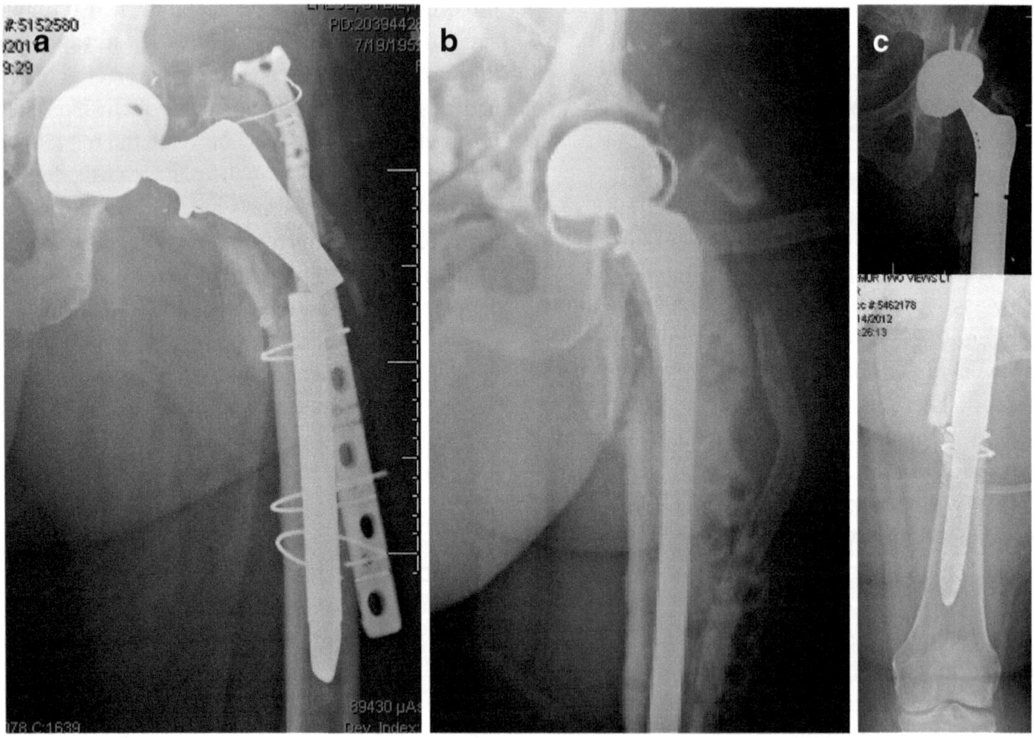

Fig. 6.13 (**a**) 38 year old morbidly obese female with a broken femoral stem, revised to modular stem which was then complicated by infection necessitating an antibiotic eluding spacer. (**b**) Later, after a proper course of treatment with IV antibiotics, she to a proximal femoral replacement (**c**)

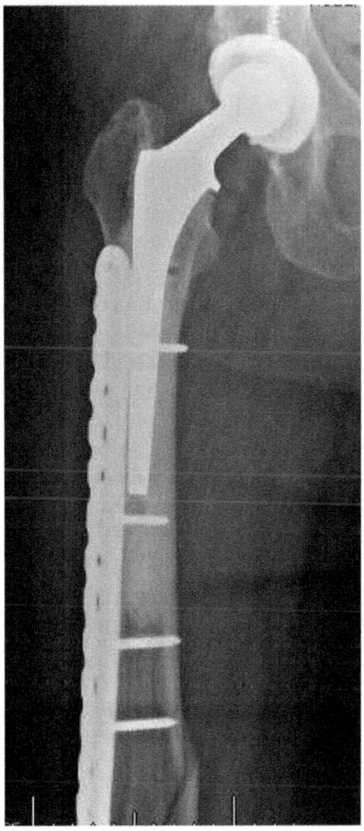

Fig. 6.14 Proximal fixation of a Vancouver C fracture, fixation around the well fixed stem via a limited proximal incision

tolerated. I firmly believe that in all but the most desperate of circumstances the patients operation should afford weight bearing as tolerated or a different operation should be selected.

Conclusion

The treatment of periprosthetic fracture is both challenging and rewarding. We continue to evolve our techniques in the pursuit of safe operations, more predictable results, and better functional outcomes for our patients. It is important to (1) establish the mode of failure, (2) preserve bone stock, (3) reduce the risk postoperative complications, and (4) restore the biomechanics of the hip to reduce the risk of dislocation and preserve patient function.

Authors Preferred Method/Take Home Points

Take Home

- Be prepared for big surgery. Blood loss. Fluid shifts. Hemodynamic instability.
- Revise stems before catastrophic failure occurs.
- Never trust the diaphysis.
- Preserve the hip capsule when you can revising the acetabulum.
- Use of the extended trochanteric osteotomy or clamshell osteotomy are critical for removal of femoral stems with minimal damage to the native femur.
- Be ready to replace the proximal femur in severe Vancouver B2 and B3 fractures.

Technique

- Lateral position on a radiolucent flattop table is preferred so that imaging is easy.
- Imagining should be in the room and on.
- General anesthesia with the patient relaxed.
- Mid coronal incision if virgin field of incorporating the previous posterior approach if not completely useless.
- Trochanteric osteotomy with B1 burr on a high-speed drill for making bone cuts.
- Understand clamshell osteotomy and use it when possible.
- Extract all foreign material, stems, old suture, cables, plates, screws, and cement if removing stem.
- If keeping the stem do as little as possible to achieve an anatomical reduction of the fracture.
- Use provisional and prophylactic cerclage cables.
- Protect the isthmus.
- Use a modular spine tapered stem.
- Use plates that allow for fixation around the well-fixed stem.
- Weight bear as tolerated revision stems with great isthmus.
- Wight of leg weight bearing ORIF.
- Posterior hip precautions.

References

1. Trousdale WH, et al. Seasonality of periprosthetic femur fractures in 12,700 primary and revision total hip arthroplasties. J Arthroplast. 2017;32(6):2000–4.
2. Abdel MP, et al. Epidemiology of periprosthetic fracture of the femur in 32 644 primary total hip arthroplasties: a 40-year experience. Bone Joint J. 2016;98-B(4):461–7.
3. Gromov K, et al. Risk factors for post-operative periprosthetic fractures following primary total hip arthroplasty with a proximally coated double-tapered cementless femoral component. Bone Joint J. 2017;99-B(4):451–7.
4. Carli AV, Negus JJ, Haddad FS. Periprosthetic femoral fractures and trying to avoid them: what is the contribution of femoral component design to the increased risk of periprosthetic femoral fracture? Bone Joint J. 2017;99-B(1 Supple A):50–9.
5. Berend KR, et al. Risk of periprosthetic fractures with direct anterior primary total hip arthroplasty. J Arthroplast. 2016;31(10):2295–8.
6. Lim SJ, et al. High incidence of stem loosening in association with periprosthetic femur fractures in previously well-fixed cementless grit-blasted tapered-wedge stems. Int Orthop. 2015;39(9):1689–93.
7. Kolisek FR, et al. Outcomes of second-generation tapered wedge femoral stem. Surg Technol Int. 2016;28:275–9.
8. Cho SH, Cho HL, Cho H. Primary cementless hip arthroplasty in unstable intertrochanteric femur fracture in elderlys: short-term results. Hip Pelvis. 2014;26(3):157–65.
9. Shin YS, Han SB. Periprosthetic fracture around a stable femoral stem treated with locking plate osteosynthesis: distal femoral locking plate alone versus with cerclage cable. Eur J Orthop Surg Traumatol. 2017;27(5):623–30.
10. Lewis GS, et al. Tangential bicortical locked fixation improves stability in Vancouver B1 periprosthetic femur fractures: a biomechanical study. J Orthop Trauma. 2015;29(10):e364–70.
11. Graham SM, et al. Periprosthetic femoral fracture fixation: a biomechanical comparison between proximal locking screws and cables. J Orthop Sci. 2015;20(5):875–80.
12. Stoffel K, et al. The influence of the operation technique and implant used in the treatment of periprosthetic hip and interprosthetic femur fractures: a systematic literature review of 1571 cases. Arch Orthop Trauma Surg. 2016;136(4):553–61.
13. Kubiak EN, et al. Does the lateral plate need to overlap the stem to mitigate stress concentration when treating Vancouver C periprosthetic supracondylar femur fracture? J Arthroplast. 2015;30(1):104–8.
14. Thes A, et al. Cortical onlay strut allograft with cerclage wiring of periprosthetic fractures of the humerus without stem loosening: technique and preliminary results. Eur J Orthop Surg Traumatol. 2017;27(4):553–7.
15. Kim YH, et al. Use of locking plate and strut onlay allografts for periprosthetic fracture around well-fixed femoral components. J Arthroplast. 2017;32(1):166–70.
16. Yeo I, et al. High union rates of locking compression plating with cortical strut allograft for type B1 periprosthetic femoral fractures. Int Orthop. 2016;40(11):2365–71.
17. Brady OH, et al. Classification of the hip. Orthop Clin North Am. 1999;30(2):215–20.
18. Brun OC, Maansson L. Fractures of the greater trochanter following total hip replacement. Hip Int. 2013;23(2):143–6.
19. Sariyilmaz K, et al. Comparison of fixation techniques in Vancouver type AG periprosthetic femoral fracture: a biomechanical study. Acta Orthop Traumatol Turc. 2016;50(3):373–8.
20. Lenz M, et al. Plate fixation in periprosthetic femur fractures Vancouver type B1-trochanteric hook plate or subtrochanterical bicortical locking? Injury. 2016;47(12):2800–4.
21. McGrory BJ, Lucas R. The use of locking plates for greater trochanteric fixation. Orthopedics. 2009;32(12):917.
22. Bohm P, Bischel O. The use of tapered stems for femoral revision surgery. Clin Orthop Relat Res. 2004;420:148–59.
23. Ko PS, et al. Distal fixation with Wagner revision stem in treating Vancouver type B2 periprosthetic femur fractures in geriatric patients. J Arthroplast. 2003;18(4):446–52.
24. Bohm P, Bischel O. Femoral revision with the Wagner SL revision stem: evaluation of one hundred and twenty-nine revisions followed for a mean of 4.8 years. J Bone Joint Surg Am. 2001;83-A(7):1023–31.
25. Woo SB, Choi ST, Chan WL. Atypical periprosthetic femoral fracture: a case report. J Orthop Surg (Hong Kong). 2016;24(2):269–72.
26. Robinson Jde D, et al. Periprosthetic atypical femoral fractures in patients on long-term bisphosphonates: a multicenter retrospective review. J Orthop Trauma. 2016;30(4):170–6.
27. Curtin BM, Fehring TK. Bisphosphonate fractures as a cause of painful total hip arthroplasty. Orthopedics. 2011;34(12):e939–44.
28. Moazen M, et al. Application of Far Cortical Locking technology in periprosthetic femoral fracture fixation: a biomechanical study. J Arthroplast. 2016;31(8):1849–56.
29. Ries ZG, Marsh JL. Far cortical locking technology for fixation of periprosthetic distal femur fractures: a surgical technique. J Knee Surg. 2013;26(1):15–8.
30. Ries Z, et al. Healing results of periprosthetic distal femur fractures treated with far cortical locking technology: a preliminary retrospective study. Iowa Orthop J. 2013;33:7–11.

7 Addressing the Periprosthetic Fracture About the Distal Femur: Loose or Well-Fixed?

Kendall M. Masada, Marcelo Batista Bonadio, Neil P. Sheth, and Derek J. Donegan

Introduction

Total knee arthroplasty (TKA) is highly effective as a treatment for disabling degenerative knee arthritis with high success rates and low complication rates. The demand for primary TKA is projected to grow to 3.5 million procedures in 2030, as the population ages and younger patients are considered candidates for the procedure [1]. It is estimated that 0.3% to 5.5% of patients will sustain a periprosthetic fracture as a complication of primary TKA and up to 30% following revision TKA [2–6]. This incidence is expected to increase as patients are living longer, implant survivorship is improving, and more TKA procedures are performed annually.

Supracondylar femur fractures are the most common fracture around TKA with a reported incidence of 0.3–2.5% with a majority of these fractures occurring in patients over age 60 [3–7]. Most fractures result from low velocity/energy falls on a flexed knee, especially in older osteoporotic patients, but occasionally result from high-energy trauma in young patients. Several risk factors have been identified, such as osteoporosis, rheumatoid arthritis, osteolysis, chronic use of steroids, female gender, and frequent falls [7–9]. Violation or notching of the anterior cortex of the femur intraoperatively has also classically been associated with supracondylar fractures. Culp et al. [10]. performed a biomechanical study demonstrating that a 3 mm anterior cortical notch decreased the torsional strength by 29.2%; however, another large clinical series of 660 patients undergoing TKA revealed that only 2 (1.1%) patients out of 180 who had anterior femoral notching sustained a fracture [4].

Various methods of internal fixation have been described for the treatment of these injuries. The use of locked plates, inserted percutaneously, intramedullary nails designed to be used with TKAs, and dual implant fixation strategies have revolutionized the fixation of these fractures and currently fractures with well-fixed implants are considered for reduction and internal fixation, whereas fractures around a loose prosthesis are candidates for revision total knee arthroplasty.

The economic impact and disability associated with these fractures are substantial [11]. Therefore, an effective treatment strategy to manage these challenging injuries is crucial. This chapter provides a treatment approach to periprosthetic fractures of the distal femur above a TKA, with a focus on decision-making and contemporary techniques, using illustrative cases.

K. M. Masada · N. P. Sheth · D. J. Donegan (✉)
University of Pennsylvania, Philadelphia, PA, USA
e-mail: Kendall.Masada@Pennmedicine.upenn.edu

M. B. Bonadio
University of São Paulo, São Paulo, Brazil

R. S. Yoon et al. (eds.), *Trauma and Infection Control in Revision Hip and Knee Arthroplasty*,
https://doi.org/10.1007/978-3-031-71971-4_7

Classification

Periprosthetic fractures above a TKA are classified based on anatomic location and component involvement. There has been multiple classification schemes proposed for supracondylar femur fractures after TKA (Table 7.1). The most widely used classification system in the literature for supracondylar periprosthetic fractures is that of Lewis and Rorabeck [15], in which type I is a non-displaced fracture with an intact prosthesis; type II is a displaced fracture with an intact prosthesis; and type III is a displaced fracture associated with a loose prosthesis.

Table 7.1 Classifications for periprosthetic femur fractures around TKA

Study	Type/group	Description
Neer et al. [12]	Type I	Undisplaced (<5 mm displacement and/or <5° angulation)
	Type II	Displaced >1 cm
	Type IIa	With lateral femoral shaft displacement
	Type IIb	With medial femoral shaft displacement
	Type III	Displaced and comminuted
DiGiola and Rubash [13]	Group I	Extra-articular, undisplaced (<5 mm displacement and <5° angulation)
	Group II	Extra-articular, displaced (>5 mm displacement and >5° angulation)
	Group III	Severely displaced (loss of cortical contact) or angulated (>10°); may have intercondylar or t-shaped component
Chen et al. [14]	Type I	Non-displaced (Neer type I)
	Type II	Displaced and/or comminuted (Neer type II and III)
Lewis and Rorabeck [15]	Type I	Undisplaced fracture; prosthesis intact
	Type II	Displaced fracture; prosthesis intact
	Type III	Displaced or undisplaced fracture; prosthesis loose or falling

Treatment Options

Treatment of supracondylar femoral periprosthetic fractures can be divided into three major categories: non-surgical, open reduction and internal fixation (ORIF), and arthroplasty solutions.

Non-surgical

Usually, patients that are candidates for non-surgical treatments have some contraindication for surgical intervention due to significant co-morbidities, putting them at high risk for intra and postoperative complications. Another scenario amenable to non-operative treatment is a patient with very low level of activity (e.g., non-ambulatory for extended time), where the benefit of surgery doesn't outweigh the risk.

Although non-operative treatment does avoid surgical- and anesthesia-related complications, there is a high risk for venous thromboembolic disease, decubitus ulcer formation, pneumonia, urinary tract infection, and muscle atrophy associated with prolonged recumbence [16].

Open Reduction and Internal Fixation

The option of ORIF is appropriate for the situation of a supracondylar femoral fracture above a well-fixed, well-functioning TKA, with adequate distal bone stock for fixation. These fractures are typically treated with retrograde intramedullary (IM) nailing, locking plates, or dual implant constructs.

Retrograde Intramedullary Nail

Retrograde IM nailing represents a good option when there is adequate distal bone stock. The advantage is that it limits soft-tissue disruption and allows utilization of the previously placed incision for the TKA. The disadvantage includes that retrograde nailing can only be performed in TKA with preservation of the posterior cruciate ligament or an open box. In addition, the location of the box may alter the starting point of the retrograde nail leading to sagittal plane deformity. Compatibility relies on discerning the femoral component design and intercondylar distance of specific TKAs [17]. Challenges to successful union with IM techniques include marginal distal fixation provided by locking screws for the typically comminuted, osteopenic distal bony fragments. Multi-planar distal interlocking screws in retrograde nails can then be used to enhance stability of the construct. In situations where the distal segment is long enough, anterograde femoral nailing can be used for the treatment of periprosthetic fractures. However, in our experience, these fractures are rarely encountered.

Maneghini et al. in a retrospective study with 22 supracondylar femoral periprosthetic fractures, treated with retrograde IM nails, had 2 (9%) nonunion, with a mean of 3.8 distal locking screws [18].

Distal Femoral Locking Plate

Locking plates have revolutionized our ability to treat periprosthetic fractures in severely osteoporotic bone. They permit multiple fixed-angle points of fixation, increasing the biomechanical strength, and can be inserted with minimally invasive techniques [19]. This type of access minimizes the need for additional large incisions around the knee and potentially minimizes soft-tissue complications and stiffness associated with traditional exposures used for ORIF [20]. A minimally invasive osteosynthesis also preserve the local bone biology, what is even more important in elderly patients, who are already compromised hosts [21]. When minimally invasive techniques are used, vigilance is required to avoid malalignment, typically valgus and hyperextension, of the distal fragment.

The use of locking plates for the management of complex periarticular injuries has demonstrated excellent clinical results with reliable distal fixation. Multiple studies have reported a high union rate with the use of locked plating for periprosthetic fractures with low complications rates [22–24]. When compared with retrograde IM nailing, the standard of care remains controversial as there is a lack of strong prospective evidence.

Ristevskc et al. in a systematic review of the literature with 44 studies of level IV of evidence, providing a total of 719 fractures, didn't find differences between the two methods with regard to nonunion rates or rate of secondary surgical procedures; however, retrograde nailing demonstrated significant higher malunion rate when compared with locked plating [25]. In another systematic review of 1188 patients, Shah et al. re-demonstrated no difference in union rate but found ORIF demonstrated a statistically significant decrease in the overall complication rate and reoperation rate when compared with IMN [26]. When examining patient-reported outcome assessments, such as the Knee Society Score, ORIF and IMN are equivalent [27]. Bong et al. demonstrated IM nailing to be superior to locked plating biomechanically in a cadaver model of periprosthetic fractures of the distal femur [28]. Theoretically, the IM nailing has a mechanical advantage, as bearing a load-sharing device, permitting an earlier weight bearing [18]. However, it does appear that locked plating has its advantages particularly when the fracture is distal to the anterior flange and there is a concern about distal fixation [19, 24].

Dual Implant Constructs

Recent additions to the ORIF toolbox are dual implant constructs with medial and lateral locking plates (dual plating), and nail plate combinations (NPC), with a locking plate augmented by an IMN. The benefit of dual constructs is more even distribution of the stress between the bone and the implants allowing for immediate weight bearing [29]. Andring et al. found the patients who underwent dual plating compared to those who received single plating but were more likely to be weight bearing immediately after surgery and had improved return to baseline ambulatory status [30]. Biomechanical studies have shown both dual constructs are more resistant to failure in axial and torsional load tests, and load-to-failure tests compared with both locking plate and IMN alone [31, 32]. In a study comparing dual plating and NPC, dual plating provided stiffer fixation to axial and torsional loading. The study hypothesized the difference was due to an inability to use all distal interlocking bolt positions within the nail or all distal screw positions within the plate in the NPC construct [33].

The advantages of dual plating are the ability to address medial side comminution and deformity and the compatibility with any TKA prosthesis. This allows for greater reduction control and avoids the extension deformity sometimes created by an IMN posterior start site due to the prosthesis. However, this comes at additional soft-tissue cost with a second surgical incision and potential effect on fracture healing.

Arthroplasty Solutions

When supracondylar periprosthetic fractures are associated with a loose femoral component or with minimal residual bone for stable fixation of the distal fragment, revision arthroplasty is the treatment of choice. For most clinical scenarios, either standard revision components with a stem bypassing the fracture or a distal femoral replacement are used.

It is unusual, however, to have distal femoral bone stock that is inadequate for internal fixation yet adequate for formal revision. In general, the decision to perform a revision TKA is based on a loose femoral component with adequate remaining bone stock and the ability to bypass the fracture by at least two cortical diameters, with a long femoral stem [34]. Quality of the proximal segment cortices should also be factored into the decision process, assuming that a thick enough cortex can accept cementless stem fixation. Cemented stems may be used, but care must be taken to prevent extrusion of cement into the fracture site, preventing fracture healing.

Knowing the type of implant plays an important role in performing the revision TKA for a periprosthetic distal femur fracture. If the type of prosthesis is known, the tibial component may be maintained, assuming it is well-fixed and appropriately positioned. Also, the tibial tray must be able to accept the planned femoral component size and the planed degree of constraint, in the event that a more constrained polyethylene may be required. A scenario that may necessitate the removal of the tibial component is a very large extension and flexion gap. In situations where a very large polyethylene is necessary for adequate balance, removal of the tibial component allows placement of tibial block augment, which decreases the flexion and extension space, and permits for greater versatility for the reconstruction using a smaller polyethylene and fine tuning of both gaps.

Few studies in the literature have focused on clinical outcomes following revision of components for periprosthetic distal femoral fractures. Cordeiro et al. reported that in a series of ten periprosthetic supracondylar femur fractures, above a TKA, they had five (50%) of the patients treated with revision to a curved, long stem intramedullary cemented component [35]. All patients were allowed to weight bear and start range of motion 10 days postoperatively. Four of the patients (80%) obtained 90° of knee flexion, and only one (20%) required a second surgical procedure for development of a secondary varus deformity. However, all patients were considered to have a good clinical outcome following revision of components.

Distal femoral replacement (DFR) has been used as a salvage option for complex arthroplasty and failed internal fixation of periprosthetic distal femur fractures, but can also be used acutely for periprosthetic fractures. The decision to perform a DFR is based on a loose femoral component and/or poor distal fragment bone quality. Other considerations are a lack of dependence on fracture healing and immediate unrestricted weight bearing in lower-demand and/or more medically complex patients [36].

DFR is considered a salvage option due to poor long-term survivorship with high rates of revision. Wyles et al., with a retrospective cohort of 144 patients, showed 10-year cumulative incidences of revision for aseptic loosening, all-cause revision, and any reoperation were 17.0%, 27.5%, and 46.3%, respectively [37]. Among patients who had DFR performed for fracture, the most common failure mechanism was aseptic loosening, with a 5-year risk of 10.2%. The use of DFRs for periprosthetic distal femur fractures shows good short-term outcomes, but longer term outcomes are not yet well-defined, partially due to the high mortality of the patient population. Jassim et al., retrospectively studied 11 patients who underwent DFR for periprosthetic femur fracture and found 90% survival of the implants at a mean of 33 months follow-up [38]. In contrast, Rahman et al. found a 25% complication rate and 12.5% rate of revision at a mean of 33.9 months [39].

When compared to ORIF, DFR is considered an acceptable alternative based on similar complication rates and functional outcomes. While single-center retrospective study shows mixed results, such as higher revision rates with ORIF in Darrith et al., larger studies show no significant differences [40]. In a multi-center retrospective cohort of 370 patients, Joseph et al. demonstrated that the propensity-matched ORIF and DFR groups had no difference in reoperation rate, 1-year mortality, and functional status [41]. A meta-analysis found that ORIF was comparable to DFR with respect to overall morbidity and functional outcomes [42]. These results are limited by the heterogeneous groups being studied, and further prospective studies are needed.

Algorithmic Approach to Choosing a Treatment Option

Pre-operative Patient Evaluation

Patients sustaining periprosthetic fractures are typically older, fragile and have considerable co-morbidities. Pre-operative planning requires proper evaluation of the clinical condition and the associated surgical risks of the patient through a multidisciplinary team approach. A fast evaluation of the patient's clinical status, associated with a well-planned surgery strategy, allows a rapid surgical intervention. This is essential to decrease the risk of complications, similar to the management of hip fractures in elderly.

Determining If the Prosthesis Is Loose or Well-Fixed

The first step to determine if the implants are well-fixed is adequate radiographs. Pre-operative radiographic assessment includes an antero-posterior knee, cross table lateral of the involved knee, as well as full-length femur and tibia. Full-length X-rays assist in identifying other implants that may be in place. For example, a long stem total hip arthroplasty above the involved TKA needs to be taken into account in the pre-operative planning phase. A series of previous radiographs, if available, can be used for comparison to determine if the implant is currently loose and show any implant loosening prior to the trauma.

Additional information for determining if the implants are loose includes pre-fracture history and symptoms. A poorly functioning TKA or symptoms such as pain, instability, and stiffness may indicate loose components, chronic periprosthetic infection, or other conditions requiring components revision. If there is any suspicion of chronic infection, laboratory analysis should be conducted with a sedimentation rate and C-reactive protein.

Additional imaging modalities such as computed tomography and magnetic resonance imaging are not often required. While, CT scans can be used to better evaluate bone stock, but metal artifacts can jeopardize the evaluation.

Bone Stock and Prosthesis Type

Radiographic assessment is essential for understanding the fracture pattern and evaluating the residual bone stock of the distal segment. Plain radiographs reveal the personality of the fracture and identify the location of the fracture, the degree of displacement, the proximity of the femoral component to the location of the fracture, and the stability of the components. Bone quality can be estimated by the thickness of the cortices and the amount of distal femoral stress shielding.

As stated above, understanding the type of prosthesis is important. The radiographs can help to identify the type of implant but the access to

Table 7.2 Treatment algorithm based on implant fixation and available bone stock

	Well-fixed implant	Loose implant
Adequate distal bone stock	Reduction and internal fixation (locked plate/retrograde nailing/nail plate combo)[a]	Revision TKA
Inadequate distal bone stock	Distal femoral replacement	Distal femoral replacement

[a]Deciding between locked plate and retrograde nailing depends on the type of femoral component for the passage of the nail and the capacity of the used plate or nail for distal fixation

the previous surgical reports is a more reliable method, providing more information as the size of the implants, surgical exposure, and intraoperative complications. Implant types are important especially when considering the use of retrograde intramedullary nailing, since an understanding if the femoral component can accept a nail is needed for this procedure.

Once that all that information is placed together, the adequate option of treatment can be determined as presented in Table 7.2.

Illustrative Cases

Case 1: ORIF with Lateral Plate

An 87-year-old female with history of hypertension sustained a low-energy fall on her flexed knee 10 years following TKA. Prior to her fall, the patient was a community ambulatory and ambulates with the assistance of a cane. She sustained her fall at home and was brought to the ED via ambulance. She presented to the ED with edema and gross deformity of the distal femur. There was no evidence of an open injury, and this was identified as an isolated injury. The initial radiographs demonstrate a distal femoral fracture proximal to a TKA, with enough bone to accommodate a plate fixation. The TKA does not present any sign of loosening (Fig. 7.1). Prior operative reports identify the implant of TKA as a posterior-stabilized implant with close box in the femoral component.

Particular attention needs to be paid to the assessment of bone stock in the distal part of the fracture to judge whether it is sufficient bone to allow screw fixation. Appropriate radiographs are usually sufficient to determine whether the distal portion of the fracture is of sufficient bone stock for attachment to locked plates.

Based on the previous function of the patient, the amount of distal bone stock, and a stable femoral component of a closed box TKA, the decision was made preoperatively to perform and open reduction and internal fixation using a laterally based locked plate through a minimally invasive technique.

Surgical Technique

The patient is positioned supine on a radiolucent flat top Jackson table, with a bump under the ipsilateral hip. The C-arm will enter from the contralateral side, perpendicular to the OR table. For better positioning of the extremity, a black ramp can be placed under the ipsilateral leg. For difficult fractures to reduce sterile skeletal traction can be placed and weight hung off the end of the bed over a pipe bender.

A standard lateral approach to the distal femur can be used, and if necessary can be extended proximally. Mark out the landmarks of joint line and femoral shaft/condyle. Mark the incision in line with the femoral shaft, starting at the Gerdy's tubercle and extending proximally as necessary for the reduction and insertion of the plate. Incise the skin down to the level of the iliotibial band fascia, and then incise the fascia in line with the skin incision, exposing the lateral of the femoral condyle.

The exposure of the fracture site is not recommended if you plan to bridge the fracture, but otherwise is mandatory if an anatomical reduction is being performed.

With the use of fluoroscopy, the length, alignment, and rotation are assessed to achieve the reduction with a different set of maneuvers. There is a strong tendency for the distal fragment to tip into hyperextension because of pull of the

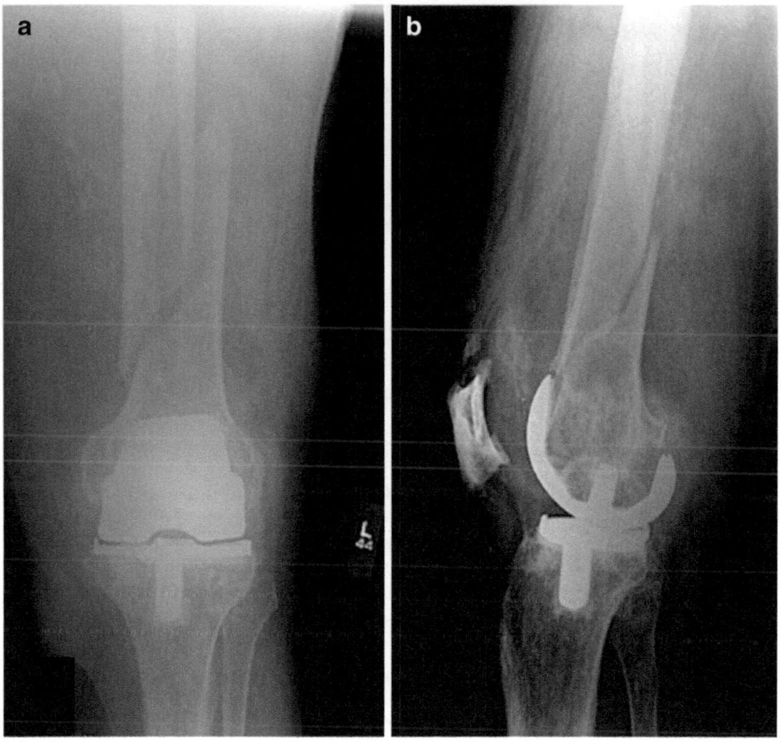

Fig. 7.1 Displaced fracture with enough distal bone stock for plate fixation

gastrocnemius muscles. For counteract the forces of the gastrocnemius, a bump can be placed strategically under the distal portion of the femur. Traction either manually or with the use of a skeletal traction guarantees the maintenance of the correct length. Alternative adjuncts include the large femoral distractor and pointed reduction clamps (Fig. 7.2).

Once adequate reduction is achieved, the appropriate length plate is determined. The goal is to have a plate length that is at least 2–3 times the length of the comminuted area and allow for a proximal screw to whole ratio of 1:2 achieving at least 3 points of bicortical fixation proximally. The plate is then slid submusculary, feeling the contact with the femur throughout the entire course. The plate is positioned as distally as possible on the distal fragment and provisionally held with a guide pin. It is critical to place this guide pin parallel to the knee joint to ensure excellent alignment in the coronal plane. A lateral fluoroscopic view is then used to adjust the sagittal positioning of the plate, and a second pin is used to fix the plate in the proximal segment of the femur through a stab incision. Fluoroscopy is then used to confirm the plate height and balance, through AP and lateral views (Fig. 7.3).

A non-locked screw is then placed immediately proximal to the fracture site as well as distal to the fracture, through the plate, to bring the plate to bone and make fine adjustments to the coronal balance. The plate can then be further secured distally, with the placement of locking screws, taking care not to use screws that are too long, understanding that the trapezoidal shape of the distal femur makes it difficult to evaluate it in the AP view. Typically, screws can pass just posterior to the anterior flange of the femoral component or just above the box of a posterior-stabilized housing. Fixation of the proximal segment is performed with placement of four non-locking screws spread out over the proximal holes of the plate. Once the construct is complete, the non-locking screw that was originally placed just proximal to the fracture should be removed to assure adequate working length of the construct (Fig. 7.4). The wound is closed in a routine layered fashion over a suction drain.

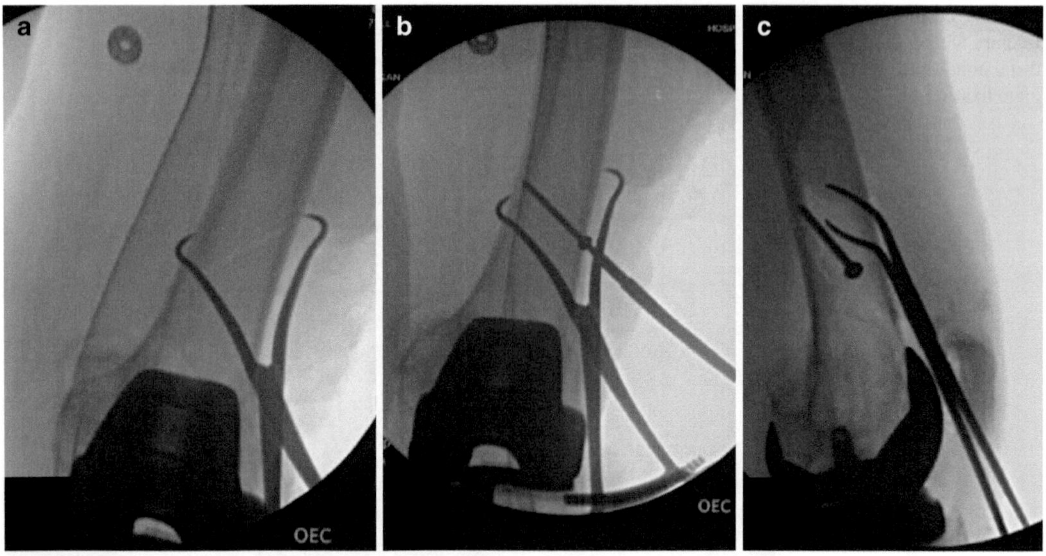

Fig. 7.2 Fracture reduction: (**a**) use of a clamp for fracture reduction, (**b**) use of a lag screw for fragments compression and hold reduction, (**c**) sagittal plane reduction

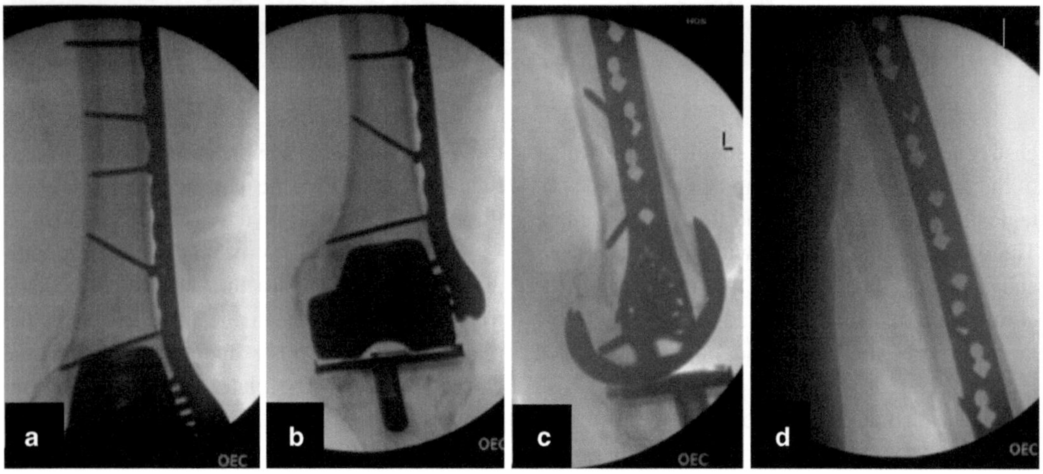

Fig. 7.3 Plate fixation: (**a, b**) AP view, (**c, d**) lateral view

Case 2: Dual Plate

An 81-year-old patient with history of rheumatic arthritis, insulin-dependent diabetes complicated by peripheral neuropathy sustained a low-energy fall 11 years after right TKA. Prior to her fall, the patient was a community ambulator without assistive device. She presented to the ED with pain and swelling to the distal femur with notable shortening of the extremity. There was no evidence of open injury. She also sustained an ipsilateral closed trimalleolar ankle fracture. The initial radiographs demonstrate a distal femoral fracture proximal to a TKA, with stable prior implant, and adequate distal femur for fixation (Fig. 7.5).

Based on the previous function of the patient, the amount of distal bone stock, and a stable posteriorly stabilized femoral component, the decision was made preoperatively to perform open reduction internal fixation with dual medial and lateral plates.

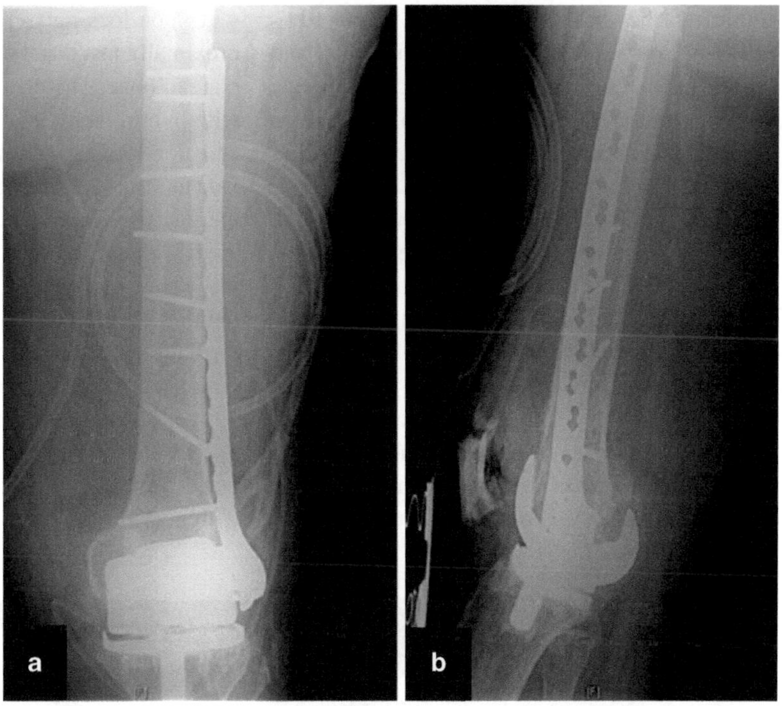

Fig. 7.4 Locking plate final radiographs

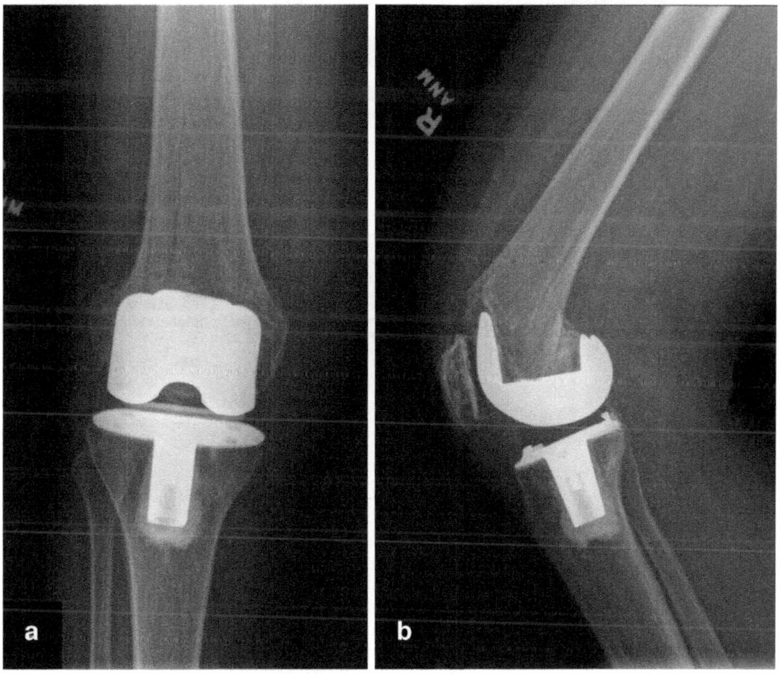

Fig. 7.5 Displaced fracture with enough distal bone stock and a well-fixed implant with a closed box

Surgical Technique

The patient was then positioned supine on the radiolucent table with all bony prominence padded. The affected extremity was prepped and draped in usual sterile fashion over a foam ramp. The C-arm entered from the contralateral side, perpendicular to the OR table. The femur was then approached via the previous midlateral incision over the distal femur based off Gerdy's tubercle. Sharp dissection was taken down, and the IT band was identified and incised in line with the incision. The vastus lateralis was then lifted off the intermuscular septum exposing lateral aspect of the femur. Care was taken to cauterize the perforators that were encountered. The fracture site was identified, and a reduction was performed using a manual manipulation restoring length, alignment, and rotation. The reduction was held with multiple k-wires (Fig. 7.6a). A distal femur lateral locking plate was then placed submuscular of the lateral aspect of the femur showing appropriate overlap with the knee prosthesis. The plate was balanced with K-wired in place (Fig. 7.6b, c). The plate was then secured with non-locking screw distally, non-locking proximally just distal to the stem to compress the plate to bone. The plate was then further secured with hybrid fixation with locking screws distally and non-locking screw proximally (Fig. 7.6d). Due to the poor bone quality and fracture pattern, the decision was made to place a supplemental medial plate. The right knee was then addressed via a separate medial incision over the distal femur. Sharp dissection taken down. The vastus medialis was lifted off distally, exposing the femur. A proximal humerus plate was place upside down on the medial side through the medial incision and balanced with K-wired in place (Fig. 7.6e, f). The plate was then secured with non-locking screw distally and non-locking

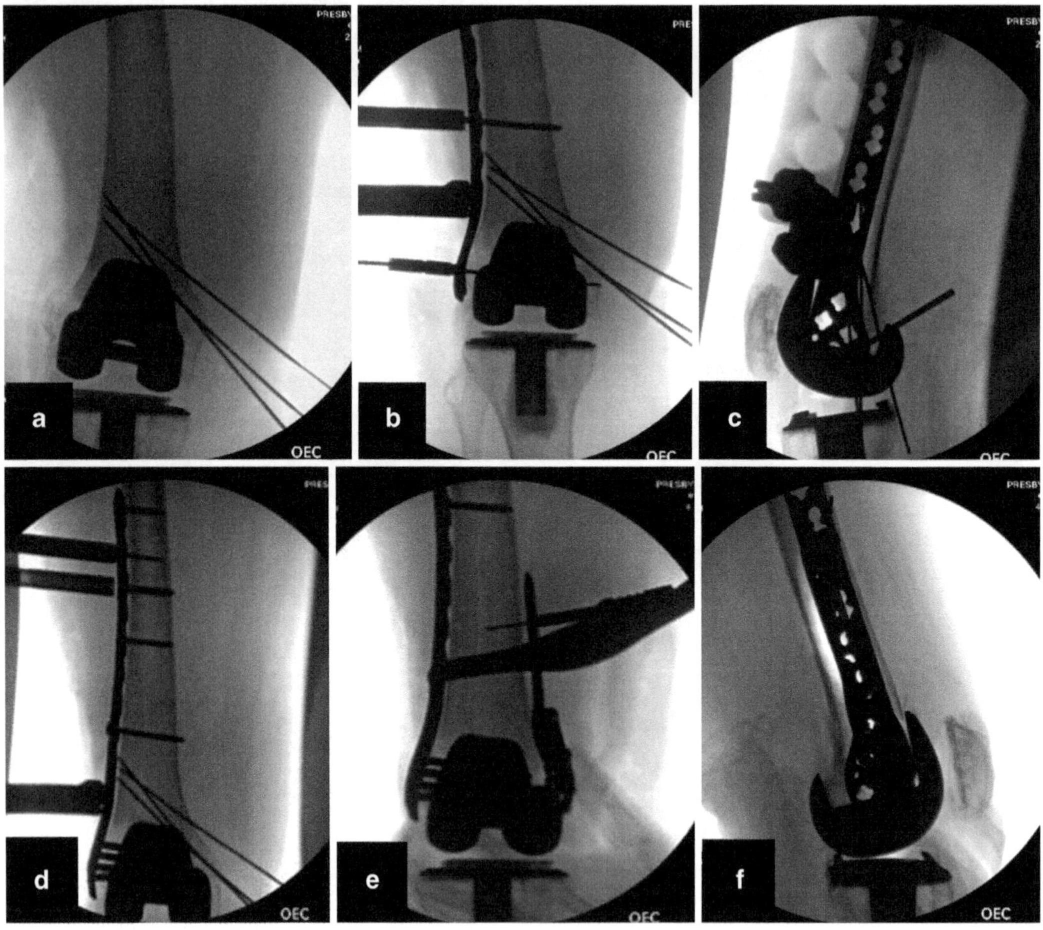

Fig. 7.6 Fracture reduction: (**a**) use of K-wires for fracture reduction, (**b, c**) lateral plate balancing, (**d**) hybrid fixation of the lateral plate, (**e, f**) medial plate balancing

proximally to the fracture to compress the plate to bone. The plate was then further secured with hybrid fixation with locking screws distally and non-locking screw proximally. Final fluoroscopic evaluation revealed good length, alignment, and rotation of the femur with appropriate placed hardware (Fig. 7.7). The wound was then irrigated thoroughly and closed in a standard layered fashion.

Case 3: NPC

A 74-year-old patient with multiple medial comorbidities including insulin-dependent diabetes, congestive heart failure, coronary artery disease, and morbid obesity (BMI 49) sustained a low-energy fall 12 years following bilateral TKAs. Prior to his fall, the patient was a housebound ambulator with a walker. He sustained his fall in his apartment and was brought to an outside ED via ambulance and subsequently transferred. He presented with pain and swelling to the distal femur with notable shortening of the extremity. There was no evidence of open injury, and this was identified as an isolated injury. The initial radiographs demonstrate a distal femoral fracture proximal to a TKA, with stable prior implant, and adequate distal femur for fixation (Fig. 7.8).

Based on the previous function of the patient, the amount of distal bone stock, and a stable cruciate-retaining femoral component, the decision was made preoperatively to perform a nail plate combination with a retrograde femur IMN augmented with open reduction and internal fixation using a laterally based locked plate.

Surgical Technique

The patient was then positioned supine on the radiolucent table with all bony prominence padded. The affected extremity was prepped and draped in usual sterile fashion over a radiolucent triangle. The C-arm entered from the contralateral side, perpendicular to the OR table. The femur was first approached by performing closed reduction. Length, alignment, and rotation were restored. At this point, attention was turned to getting a start point using a medial parapatellar approach. Sharp dissection was taken down. Patella tendon was identified and incised medial to the tendon. Starting point was achieved and

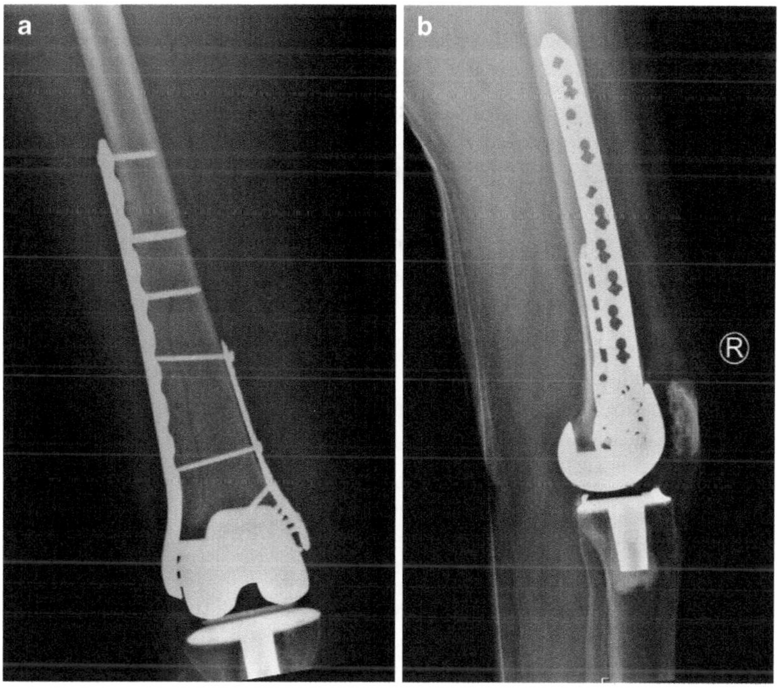

Fig. 7.7 Dual plating final radiographs

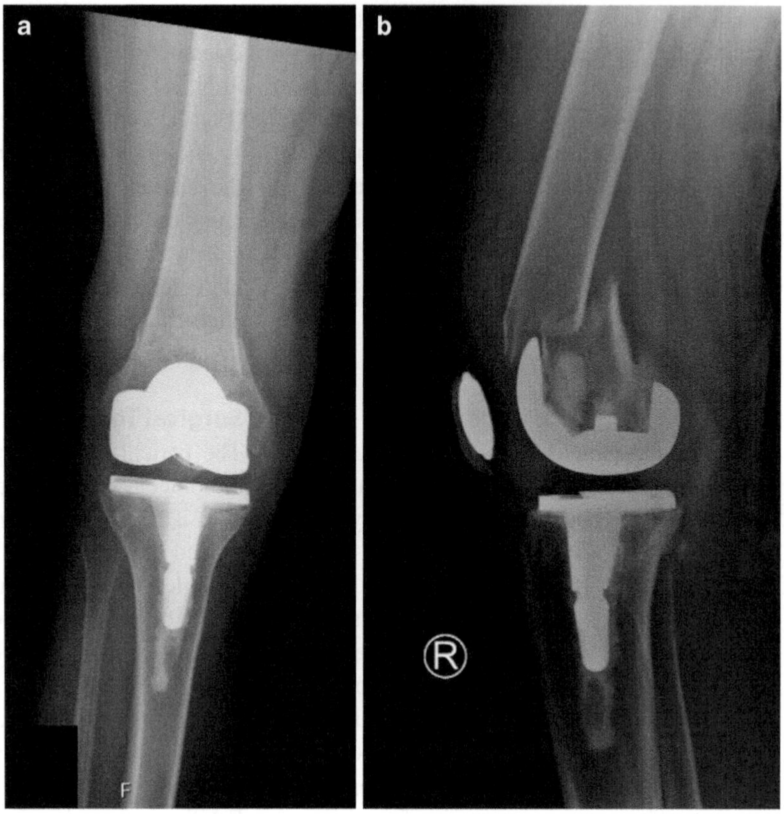

Fig. 7.8 Displaced fracture with enough distal bone stock and a well-fixed implant with an open box

confirmed fluoroscopically (Fig. 7.9a, b). The guidewire was then taken into distal femur in the appropriate trajectory. The distal femur was opened with reamer, and the ball-tip guidewire was then taken into the distal femur across the fracture into the proximal femur. Sequential reaming then began, and the length was measured. The nail was then introduced over the ball-tip guidewire into the distal femur across the fracture and into the proximal femur and seated to appropriate depth and confirmed fluoroscopically (Fig. 7.9c). It was then fixed with one oblique interlocking screw distally through the jig. The most distal interlocking screw was left unfilled in order to link the plate to the nail. Fluoroscopic evaluation revealed good length and rotation of the femur with appropriately placed hardware.

The nail was then supplemented with a laterally based plate via midline incision over the distal femur based off of Gerdy's tubercle. Sharp dissection was taken down to the IT band, which was incised in line with the incision. The femur was identified, and vastus lateralis was lifted off the intermuscular septum exposing lateral aspect of the femur. Care was taken to get hemostasis of the perforators that we countered. A lateral distal femur locking plate was then placed submuscular on the lateral aspect of the femur. The plate was balanced with K-wired in place, ensuring the screws going through the plate could aim around the nail (Figs. 7.9d–f). The plate was then secured with non-locking screws distally through the plate and the nail to link the constructs and a non-locking screw proximally around the nail to compress the plate to bone. The plate was then further secured with hybrid fixation with locking screws distally and non-locking screws proximally. Attention was then turned distally, and one additional oblique interlocking screw was placed through the distal aspect of the nail. Final fluoroscopic evaluation revealed good length, alignment, and rotation of the femur with appropriate placed hardware (Fig. 7.10). The wound was then

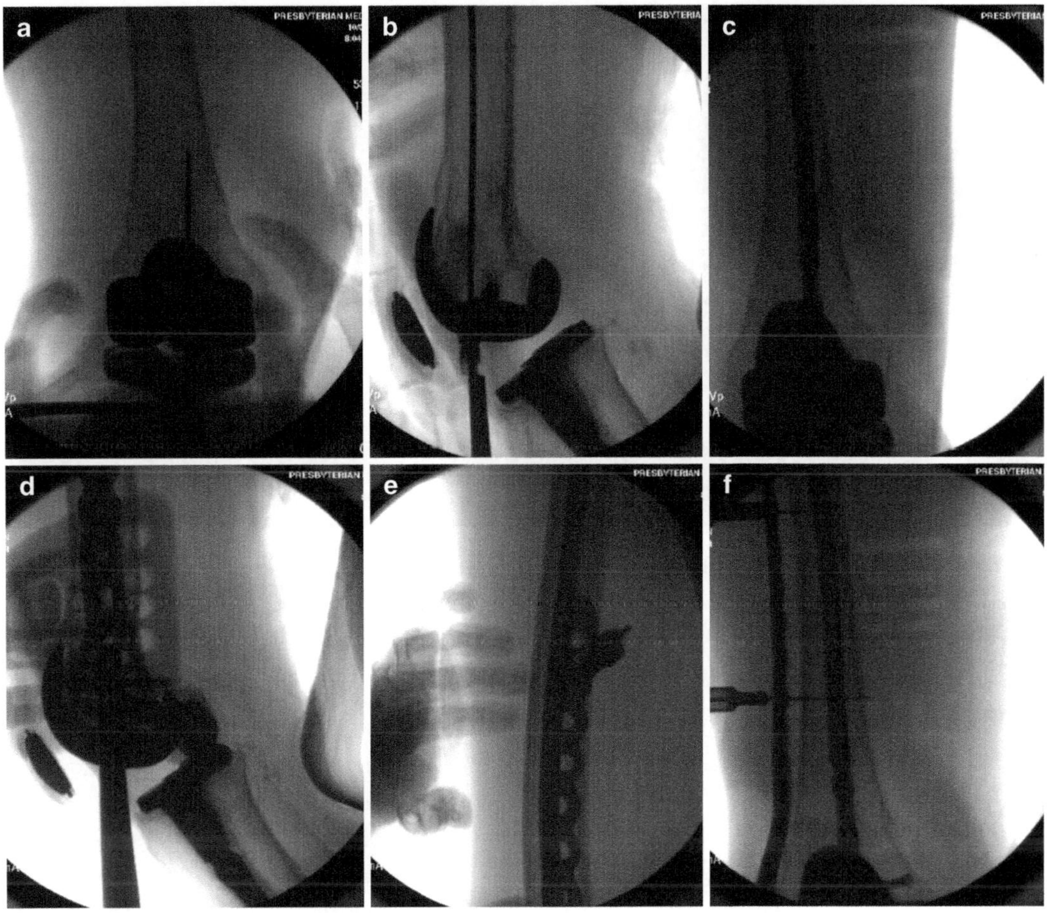

Fig. 7.9 Fracture reduction: (**a, b**) nail starting points, (**c**) nail insertion, (**d–f**) lateral plate balancing around the nail

irrigated thoroughly and closed in a standard layered fashion.

Case 4: DFR

An 80-year-old male with history of insulin-dependent diabetes sustained a low-energy fall on her flexed knee 7 years following TKA. Prior to her fall, the patient was a community ambulator and ambulates with the assistance of a walker. She sustained her fall at an assisted living facility and was brought to the ED via ambulance. She presented to the ED with edema and gross deformity of the distal femur. There was no evidence of an open injury, and this was identified as an isolated injury. The initial radiographs demonstrate a distal femoral fracture proximal to a TKA, with poor bone attached to the implant and signs of loosening of the implant (Fig. 7.11).

Based on the quality of the remaining distal femoral bone and a loose femoral component, the decision was made preoperatively to remove both the femoral and the tibial components along with the distal bone segment and use a distal femoral replacement for the reconstruction. For this patient, the option of reconstruction with the use of a megaprosthesis permits a faster recovery, being able to bear weight sooner and avoid the risk of failure reconstruction due to a poor bone stock.

Surgical Technique

The patient is positioned supine, with a bump under the ipsilateral hip to control the external rotation of the extremity. The surgical approach

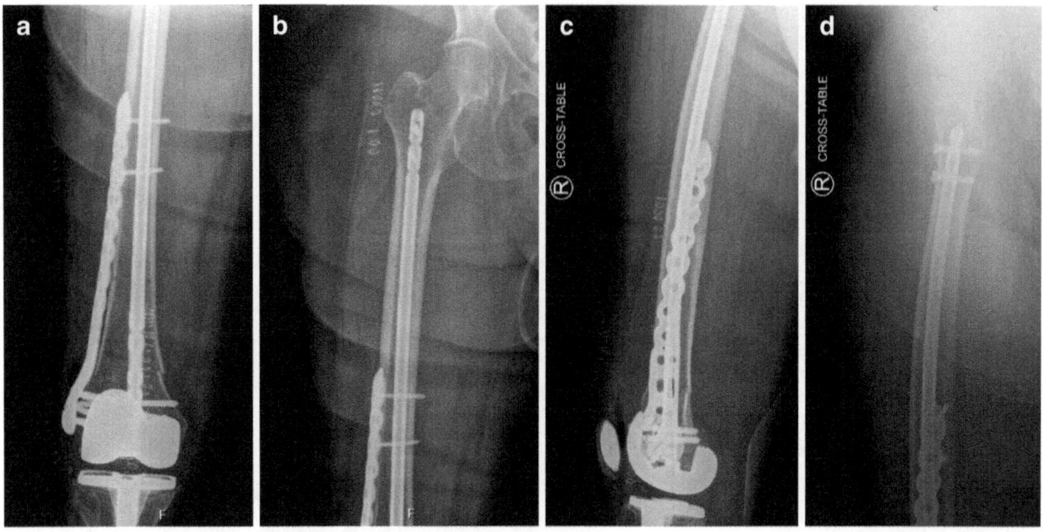

Fig. 7.10 Nail plate combination final radiographs

Fig. 7.11 Displaced fracture with poor bone stock and loose implant

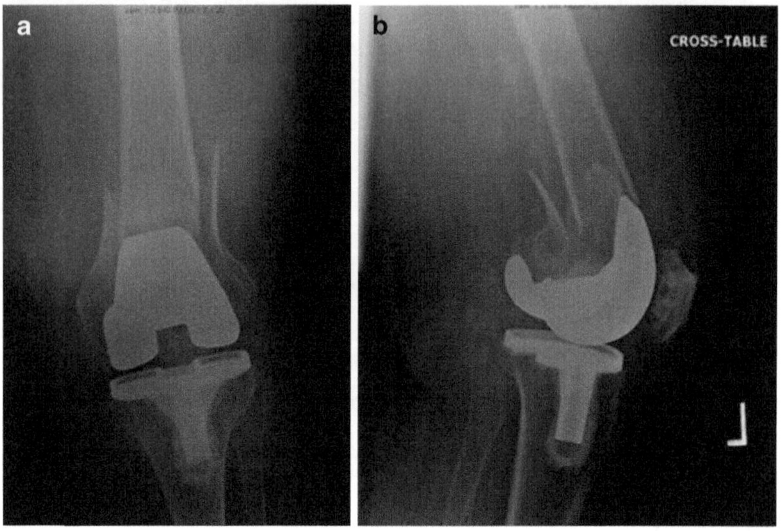

is determined by the presence of a previous incision and surgeon preference or comfort. If the patient has more than one incision in the knee, it is recommended to use the most lateral incision, understanding that the blood supply to the anterior skin of the knee comes from the medial side. If a laterally based incision is used, a full thickness flap deep to the Scarpa's fascia must be made in order to preserve the blood supply to the overlying soft-tissue flap.

An anterior midline incision followed by a medial parapatellar arthrotomy is the most common and utilitarian approach to access the knee for a revision total knee arthroplasty. This access permits a proximal or distal extension to allow adequate exposure of the distal femur or proximal tibia. Following the arthrotomy, a formal synovectomy is performed to reconstitute the medial and lateral gutters, and at this point if there is any suspicion for underlying periprosthetic joint infection, a section of the resected synovia should be sent to frozen section and anaerobic and aerobic cultures should be obtain. A frozen section of less than five neutrophils per high power histologic field is less concerning for deep infection [43]. Eventually, the obtained cultures may return with positive results and should be treated with 6 weeks of microorganism-specific intravenous antibiotics followed by possible oral antibiotic suppression. The accompaniment by an infection disease specialist is critical in this patient scenario.

General orthopedic principle attempts to maintain as much of the host bone as possible. With severely comminuted distal femoral fractures, the femoral resection is performed at level just proximal to comminution such that a stable base remains for fixation of the femoral prosthesis. Before performing the femoral resection, it is important to measure the distance between the planned femoral cut and the tibial tubercle, to avoid elongation of the extremity, once that the collateral ligaments are not present.

The most common technical challenge associated with performing a distal femoral replacement is patella-femoral tracking. Most distal femoral prostheses on the market have a shallow trochlea grove, resulting in an altered patello-femoral biomechanics and thus more emphasis on femoral component rotation. When trial components are appropriately sized and placed in the correct position, rotation of the femoral component can be set by taking the knee trough a range of motion, and the appropriate rotation should be marked on the anterior cortex of the femoral shaft with the electrocautery. As discussed earlier, a lateral release may assist with exposure but also will play an important role in the patellar tracking.

Other bony landmarks that can be used as guide for the femoral component rotation is the linea aspera, that is directly located on the posterior cortex of the femoral shaft. Depending on how much of the distal femur was resected, this landmark may or may not be clearly seen. The amount of external rotation required of the femoral component is usually more than one initially thinks.

The stems of the prosthesis are typically cemented into the femoral and tibial canal, with placement of cement restrictors proximally on the femur and distally on the tibia, to allow for adequate cement pressurization and at least a 2 mm thick cement mantle surrounding the whole stems. After cementing of the components, the distance between the planned femoral cut and the tibial tubercle, measured before, is used as a parameter to decide the thickness of the polyethylene (Fig. 7.12).

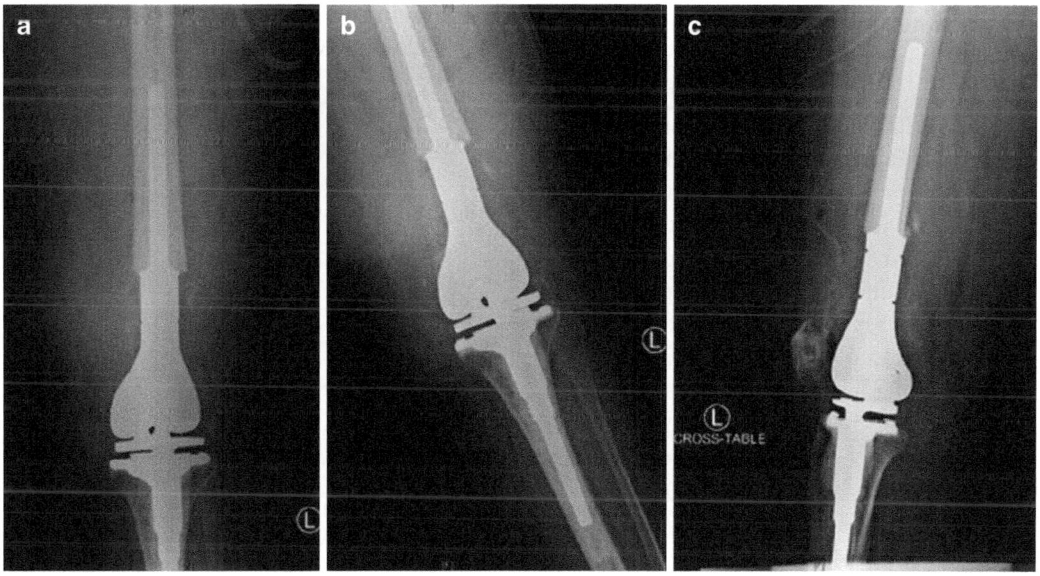

Fig. 7.12 Distal femoral replacement final radiographs

Postoperative Care

The postoperative care varies depending on the option of treatment that was chosen for each patient. Typically patients submitted to ORIF with a locked plate or retrograde intramedullary nail only are not allowed to weight bear immediately, waiting for some degree of fracture union for at a minimum of 6–8 weeks. Those treated with dual implant constructs are often allowed to weight bear immediately. With distal femoral replacement, full weight bearing is generally allowed in the first postoperative day, once that the components are cemented and stable. The ability to weight bear immediately significantly reduces patient immobility and circumvents the inability, related to the dementia, to follow therapy orders, which is paramount in elderly population.

A hinged knee brace can be used postoperatively to protect the reconstruction or to prevent wound complications restricting of the range of motion.

Complications

Many complications following the treatment of a distal femoral periprosthetic fracture above a TKA are similar to those associated with the primary TKA, such as venous thromboembolic disease, cardio respiratory complications, stroke, neuro-vascular injury, loosening, and infection. Other possible complications are more specific to fixation procedures, such as malunion, nonunion, and failure of the fracture fixation.

One of the most devastating complications is a periprosthetic infection. The risk of postoperative infection is higher in patients with co-morbidities such as diabetes, morbid obesity, and any underlying reason for immunocompromise (i.e., prednisone use, previous organ transplant, human immunodeficiency virus, hepatitis C, etc.). The use of intravenous antibiotics 30–60 min prior to the incision as well as intravenous antibiotics administrated for 24 h postoperatively minimizes the risk of infection.

Authors' Preferred Method

- We recommend treatment of all displaced periprosthetic fractures unless the patient is non-ambulatory, without the need for transfers, or is not medically able to tolerate anesthesia.
- Well-fixed implant with adequate distal bone stock: ORIF with plate(s) versus retrograde IMN versus NPC based on fracture pattern.
- Well-fixed implant without adequate distal bone stock: DFR.
- Loose implant: DFR.

Take-Home Points

- Treatment of periprosthetic distal femur fractures around T.KAs remains challenging due to patients' advanced age, osteopenia, and associated medical conditions necessitating early mobilization.
- Treatment requires knowledge of fracture fixation techniques and arthroplasty.
- Key decision points are whether the implant is well-fixed or loose and how much distal bone stock is available.
- If the implant is well-fixed with adequate distal bone stock, consider fracture fixation techniques (IMN, locking plates, or dual implant constructs) based on the fracture pattern.
- If the implant is well-fixed with inadequate distal bone stock, consider DFR.
- If the implant is loose with adequate or poor distal bone stock, consider revision arthroplasty or DFR.
- Ultimate goal of treatment is to restore length, alignment, rotation, and allow for early mobilization.

References

1. Kurtz S, Ong K, Lau E, Mowat F, Halpern M. Projections of primary and revision hip and knee arthroplasty in the United States from 2005 to 2030. J Bone Joint Surg Am. 2007;89(4):780–5.
2. Figgie MP, Goldberg VM, Figgie HE 3rd, Sobel M. The results of treatment of supracondylar fracture above total knee arthroplasty. J Arthroplast. 1990;5(3):267–76.

3. Merkel KD, Johnson EW Jr. Supracondylar fracture of the femur after total knee arthroplasty. J Bone Joint Surg Am. 1986;68(1):29–43.
4. Ritter MA, Faris PM, Keating EM. Anterior femoral notching and ipsilateral supracondylar femur fracture in total knee arthroplasty. J Arthroplast. 1988;3(2):185–7.
5. Healy WL, Siliski JM, Incavo SJ. Operative treatment of distal femoral fractures proximal to total knee replacements. J Bone Joint Surg Am. 1993;75(1):27–34.
6. Inglis AE, Walker PS. Revision of failed knee replacements using fixed-axis hinges. J Bone Joint Surg. 1991;73(5):757–61.
7. COMPOSE Study Team. Epidemiology and characteristics of femoral periprosthetic fractures: data from the characteristics, outcomes and management of periprosthetic fracture service evaluation (COMPOSE) cohort study. Bone Joint J. 2022;104-B(8):987–96.
8. Platzer P, Schuster R, Aldrian S, Prosquill S, Krumboeck A, Zehetgruber I, et al. Management and outcome of periprosthetic fractures after total knee arthroplasty. J Trauma. 2010;68(6):1464–70.
9. Wang CJ, Wang JW, Weng LH, Hsu CC, Huang CC, Chen HS. The effect of alendronate on bone mineral density in the distal part of the femur and proximal part of the tibia after total knee arthroplasty. J Bone Joint Surg Am. 2003;85-A(11):2121–6.
10. Culp RW, Schmidt RG, Hanks G, Mak A, Esterhai JL Jr, Heppenstall RB. Supracondylar fracture of the femur following prosthetic knee arthroplasty. Clin Orthop Relat Res. 1987;222:212–22.
11. Crutcher JP Jr, Tompkins G, Rollier G, Sypher K, Valderrama R, Duwelius PJ. The economic impact of lower extremity periprosthetic fractures in a large hospital system. J Arthroplasty. 2022;37(7S):S439–43.
12. Neer CS 2nd, Grantham SA, Shelton ML. Supracondylar fracture of the adult femur. A study of one hundred and ten cases. J Bone Joint Surg Am. 1967;49(4):591–613.
13. DiGioia AM 3rd, Rubash HE. Periprosthetic fractures of the femur after total knee arthroplasty. A literature review and treatment algorithm. Clin Orthop Relat Res. 1991;271:135–42.
14. Chen F, Mont MA, Bachner RS. Management of ipsilateral supracondylar femur fractures following total knee arthroplasty. J Arthroplasty. 1994;9(5):521–6.
15. Rorabeck CH, Taylor JW. Classification of periprosthetic fractures complicating total knee arthroplasty. Orthop Clin North Am. 1999;30(2):209–14.
16. Yoon BH, Baek JH, Kim MK, Lee YK, Ha YC, Koo KH. Poor prognosis in elderly patients who refused surgery because of economic burden and medical problem after hip fracture. J Korean Med Sci. 2013;28(9):1378–81.
17. Gerow DE, Ross HL, Bodrogi A, Johnson KJ, Endres TJ. Periprosthetic supracondylar femoral fractures above a total knee replacement: an updated compatibility and technique guide for fixation with a retrograde intramedullary nail. J Orthop Trauma. 2022;36(3):e92–7.
18. Meneghini RM, Keyes BJ, Reddy KK, Maar DC. Modern retrograde intramedullary nails versus periarticular locked plates for supracondylar femur fractures after total knee arthroplasty. J Arthroplast. 2014;29(7):1478–81.
19. Nauth A, Ristevski B, Begue T, Schemitsch EH. Periprosthetic distal femur fractures: current concepts. J Orthop Trauma. 2011;25(Suppl 2):S82–5.
20. Haidukewych GJ. Innovations in locking plate technology. J Am Acad Orthop Surg. 2004;12(4):205–12.
21. Krettek C, Muller M, Miclau T. Evolution of minimally invasive plate osteosynthesis (MIPO) in the femur. Injury. 2001;32(Suppl 3):SC14–23.
22. Kolb W, Guhlmann H, Windisch C, Marx F, Koller H, Kolb K. Fixation of periprosthetic femur fractures above total knee arthroplasty with the less invasive stabilization system: a midterm follow-up study. J Trauma. 2010;69(3):670–6.
23. Kregor PJ, Hughes JL, Cole PA. Fixation of distal femoral fractures above total knee arthroplasty utilizing the Less Invasive Stabilization System (L.I.S.S.). Injury. 2001;32(Suppl 3):SC64–75.
24. Streubel PN, Gardner MJ, Morshed S, Collinge CA, Gallagher B, Ricci WM. Are extreme distal periprosthetic supracondylar fractures of the femur too distal to fix using a lateral locked plate? J Bone Joint Surg. 2010;92(4):527–34.
25. Ristevski B, Nauth A, Williams DS, Hall JA, Whelan DB, Bhandari M, et al. Systematic review of the treatment of periprosthetic distal femur fractures. J Orthop Trauma. 2014;28(5):307–12.
26. Shah JK, Szukics P, Gianakos AL, Liporace FA, Yoon RS. Equivalent union rates between intramedullary nail and locked plate fixation for distal femur periprosthetic fractures—a systematic review. Injury. 2020;51(4):1062–8.
27. Rinehart D, Youngman T, Ahn J, Huo M. Review of patient-reported outcomes in periprosthetic distal femur fractures after total knee arthroplasty: a plate or intramedullary nail? Arthroplasty. 2021;3(1):24.
28. Bong MR, Egol KA, Koval KJ, Kummer FJ, Su ET, Iesaka K, et al. Comparison of the LISS and a retrograde-inserted supracondylar intramedullary nail for fixation of a periprosthetic distal femur fracture proximal to a total knee arthroplasty. J Arthroplast. 2002;17(7):876–81.
29. Liporace FA, Yoon RS. Nail plate combination technique for native and periprosthetic distal femur fractures. J Orthop Trauma. 2019;33(2):e64–8.
30. Andring NA, Kaupp SM, Henry KA, Helmig KC, Babcock S, Halvorson JJ, Pilson HT, Carroll EA. Dual plate fixation of periprosthetic distal femur fractures. J Orthop Trauma. 2024;38(1):36–41.
31. Başcı O, Karakaşlı A, Kumtepe E, Güran O, Havıtçıoğlu H. Combination of anatomical locking plate and retrograde intramedullary nail in distal femoral fractures: comparison of mechanical stability. Eklem Hastalik Cerrahisi. 2015;26(1):21–6.

32. Fontenot PB, Diaz M, Stoops K, Barrick B, Santoni B, Mir H. Supplementation of lateral locked plating for distal femur fractures: a biomechanical study. J Orthop Trauma. 2019;33(12):642–8.
33. Wright DJ, DeSanto DJ, McGarry MH, Lee TQ, Scolaro JA. Supplemental fixation of supracondylar distal femur fractures: a biomechanical comparison of dual-plate and plate-nail constructs. J Orthop Trauma. 2020;34(8):434–40.
34. Rorabeck CH, Taylor JW. Periprosthetic fractures of the femur complicating total knee arthroplasty. Orthop Clin North Am. 1999;30(2):265–77.
35. Cordeiro EN, Costa RC, Carazzato JG, Silva JS. Periprosthetic fractures in patients with total knee arthroplasties. Clin Orthop Relat Res. 1990;252:182–9.
36. Haidukewych GJ. Role of distal femoral replacement for periprosthetic fractures above a total knee arthroplasty: when and how? J Orthop Trauma. 2019;33(Suppl 6):S33–5.
37. Wyles CC, Tibbo ME, Yuan BJ, Trousdale RT, Berry DJ, Abdel MP. Long-term results of total knee arthroplasty with contemporary distal femoral replacement. J Bone Joint Surg Am. 2020;102(1):45–51.
38. Jassim SS, McNamara I, Hopgood P. Distal femoral replacement in periprosthetic fracture around total knee arthroplasty. Injury. 2014;45(3):550–3.
39. Rahman WA, Vial TA, Backstein DJ. Distal femoral arthroplasty for management of periprosthetic supracondylar fractures of the femur. J Arthroplasty. 2016;31(3):676–9.
40. Joseph NM, Zuke W, Sharpe M, Bacharach A, Punjabi N, Zhao C, Sattar A, Emara AK, Piuzzi NS, Ochenjele G, Patterson BM, Vallier HA. Outcomes of geriatric periprosthetic distal femur fractures: comparison of fixation versus reconstruction. J Orthop Trauma. 2023;37(10):480–4.
41. Darrith B, Bohl DD, Karadsheh MS, Sporer SM, Berger RA, Levine BR. Periprosthetic fractures of the distal femur: is open reduction and internal fixation or distal femoral replacement superior? J Arthroplast. 2020;35(5):1402–6.
42. Salazar BP, Babian AR, DeBaun MR, Githens MF, Chavez GA, Goodnough LH, Gardner MJ, Bishop JA. Distal femur replacement versus surgical fixation for the treatment of geriatric distal femur fractures: a systematic review. J Orthop Trauma. 2021;35(1):2–9.
43. Lonner JH, Desai P, Dicesare PE, Steiner G, Zuckerman JD. The reliability of analysis of intraoperative frozen sections for identifying active infection during revision hip or knee arthroplasty. J Bone Joint Surg Am. 1996;78(10):1553–8.

8 Revision Hip Arthroplasty in the Infectious Setting

Richard Kyle and John Kampa

Introduction

Total hip arthroplasty (THA) is an enormously successful operation and has become the mainstay of treatment for end-stage arthritis of the hip. Although relatively rare, deep wound infection remains the most devastating complication with significant socioeconomic burden. In order to achieve an aseptic environment after infection, the local soft tissue and anatomy are often sacrificed making revision surgery difficult. Successful eradication of infection is facilitated with the use of antibiotic cement spacers and prolonged systemic antibiotics. Bone stock at re-implantation is often insufficient and occasionally one must work around prior trochanteric osteotomies, further complicating re-implantation. Successful treatment therefore requires a competent surgeon who is experienced with different reconstructive techniques. This chapter highlights the issues and problems that arise and offer tips and tricks when performing revision hip arthroplasty in the infectious setting. The objectives of this chapter are to review the strategies for infection eradication, highlight the difficulties encountered in revision THA for infection, present pertinent case examples, and share the author's preferred method.

R. Kyle (✉) · J. Kampa
Department of Orthopaedic Surgery, Hennepin Healthcare, Minneapolis, MN, USA

Background

In its infancy in the early 1960s, Sir John Charnley had a 9% infection rate following THA. By the end of the decade, in his next cohort, the infection rate was decreased to 1.3% owing to air cleanliness and body exhaust attire [1, 2]. The incidence of prosthetic joint infection (PJI) following THA in the modern era is approximately 2.18% [3]. In 2003 alone, over 202,000 primary total hip arthroplasties were performed and this number is estimated to grow by 174% by 2030 [4]. Therefore, PJI will continue to place significant burden on the healthcare system.

Prosthetic joint infection often necessitates multiple surgical procedures, prolonged antibiotic use, extended inpatient and outpatient rehabilitation, and frequent clinical follow-up. The total direct medical costs associated with revision THA for infection are 2.8 times higher than the costs associated with revision THA for aseptic loosening and 4.8 times higher than the direct medical costs associated w/primary THA [5]. The average total charge for an infected hip revision was $93,600 in 2009 [3]. Aside from the financial burden, the emotional stress placed upon patients and their families can be significant. Some patients may never return to their pre-infection activity level or recover their independence.

Prevention of infection is paramount and should be the focus when considering this prob-

R. S. Yoon et al. (eds.), *Trauma and Infection Control in Revision Hip and Knee Arthroplasty*,
https://doi.org/10.1007/978-3-031-71971-4_8

lem. Numerous strategies have been devised over the years; however, the benefits have been variable. Probably, the most important is perioperative prophylactic antibiotic use. Cefazolin before and after surgery reduced the risk of infection after THA reduced from 3.3% to 0.9% compared to placebo in a double-blind controlled study [6]. First-generation cephalosporins are often the antibiotic of choice based on the fact that they are bactericidal, effective against commonly infecting pathogens, and relatively inexpensive. Advancement of detecting those who are colonized with Staph aureus has led to preoperative treatment using intranasal antibiotic ointment and chlorhexidine body wash to be used in the days prior to surgery. Furthermore, these patients are usually treated with perioperative vancomycin instead of a cephalosporin. Although this strategy shows only short-term decolonization, the results show a decrease in surgical site infection [7].

Dilute betadine lavage prior to wound closure reduced the infection rate from 0.97% to 0.15% in a consecutive series of primary total hip and knee arthroplasties [8]. In an effort to seal the wound and reduce surgical site infection, commercial dressings have been developed to optimize wound healing. Most of these products contain a layer over the wound that contains antimicrobial properties, a fiber which absorbs moisture, and an outer adherent component which seals to the skin. Cai et al. performed a retrospective case-control study comparing Aquacel Ag dressing to standard gauze dressing. They found a sixfold reduction in PJI; however, during the Aquacel study period, they also implemented the routine use of dilute betadine lavage and dual antibiotic prophylaxis with vancomycin and cefazolin (compared to cefazolin alone for the gauze dressing group) [9]. More obvious prevention strategies include medical optimization prior to surgery, attention to nutrition status, smoking cessation, weight loss in overweight patients, glycemic control in diabetics, cessation of immunosuppressive medications, abstinence from excessive alcohol consumption, and treatment of any active cutaneous lesions or skin infections. Intraoperative considerations include maintenance of normal body temperature and reduced OR traffic, operative time, and blood conservation with attention to avoid unnecessary transfusions. Several risk factors have been identified for PJI, and these are outlined in Fig. 8.1.

Risk factors for PJI
Male
Elevated BMI
Higher ASA score
Rheumatoid arthritis
Uncontrolled diabetes
Malnutrition
Smoking
Nasal carriage of S aureus
Alcohol consumption
Immunocompromised
ASA=American Society of Anesthesiologists

Fig. 8.1 Patient risk factors for prosthetic joint infection

Case Presentations

Case 1

A 55-year-old male with HIV initially underwent primary THA for avascular necrosis in Uganda 4 years prior to presentation. He had continued pain and evidence of component loosening as well as protrusio. Unfortunately, his initial films were no longer available. Infectious workup failed to show active infection, and he underwent revision THA. The prior approach was posterior and we elected to make a separate incision for the anterolateral approach to better expose the acetabulum given his protrusio. No gross purulence was encountered and multiple tissue samples were sent. There were no neutrophils per high power field, and all gram stains were negative for organisms. The femur was grossly loose and easily removed, and the remaining cement was removed as well. Once the cup and cement were removed, there was a defect in the medial wall. After thorough debridement of fibrous tissue, the acetabulum was then reamed up to size 60. A frozen femoral head was cut into a wafer and placed into the medial wall defect. Cancellous croutons were also placed in the medial wall defect with the femoral head allograft and then reverse reamed with the 60 mm reamer. After trialing, the 60 shell was placed and further stabilized with two screws. A size 15 curved, fully coated stem was placed. Postoperative films are shown in Figs. 8.2–8.3.

Unfortunately, two cultures grew out Pseudomonas and he had persistent wound drainage. Eleven days later, he returned to the OR for explant and antibiotic spacer placement. With this exposure, serosanguinous fluid was encountered both superficial to the iliotibial band and deep in the hip joint. Again, tissue as well as fluid cultures was sent and then antibiotics were given. All components were removed and sharp debridement ensued. An Austin Moore prosthesis was coated with antibiotic cement and used for the spacer as seen in Fig. 8.4.

Interestingly, no organisms were isolated from the numerous cultures taken at the time of explant. He was treated with a 6-week course of levofloxacin and re-implanted after an antibiotic holiday with inflammatory lab values within the normal range. Again, the anterolateral approach was utilized. New heterotopic bone was excised along with all fibrous tissue. While extracting the stem, an iatrogenic fracture was found at the calcar for which a wire was passed around the proximal femur. After reaming the acetabulum, a size 62 shell had good fit and this was placed after more cancellous allograft was placed in the medial wall defect. For the femur, a size 16.5 × 240 mm length fully coated curved stem was used. Final images are shown in Fig. 8.5. He was kept on ceftazidime postoperatively, no organisms were isolated from cultures and he was discharged on oral levofloxacin for which he completed a 6-week course. Radiographs taken 4 years postoperatively are seen in Figs. 8.6–8.7. Heterotopic bone is readily visible; however, the patient was doing well.

This case sheds light on numerous learning points. First, repeated hip aspirations should be performed when infection is suspected until the hip is proven aseptic. This is especially true in the immune suppressed patient such as this patient with HIV. Isolation of Pseudomonas may have prevented implantation with the first revision. Secondly, medial wall defects can be managed with large size cups and allograft femoral head and cancellous bone graft if a stable cup can be achieved. Lastly, stabilize all fractures through the calcar region with wires and achieve good cortical fixation with a long stem. In this case, antibiotics were used for 6 weeks after the final revision given the patient's immune susceptibility with HIV. This was based on the recommendations from the infectious disease service and should be determined on a case-by-case basis.

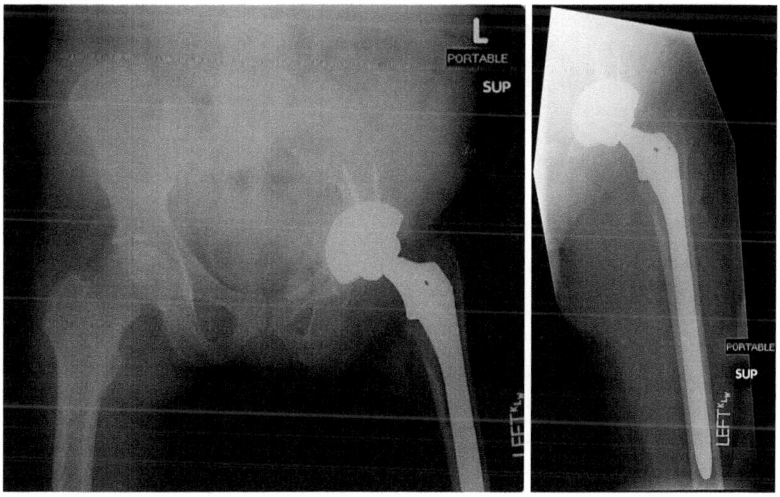

Figs. 8.2–8.3 Postoperative films after revision left THA for loose components. Notice the acetabular protrusion which was present prior to revision. Cancellous allograft croutons were placed in the medial wall defect and are seen on the imaging

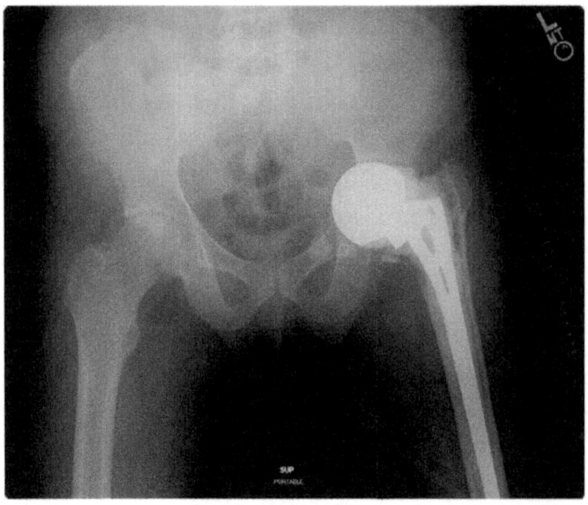

Fig. 8.4 An Austin Moore prosthesis was used to create an antibiotic cement spacer after explant and thorough debridement

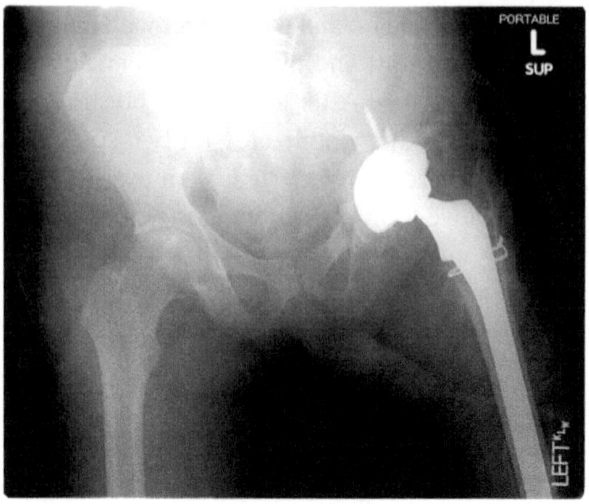

Fig. 8.5 Immediate postoperative AP radiograph after re-implantation

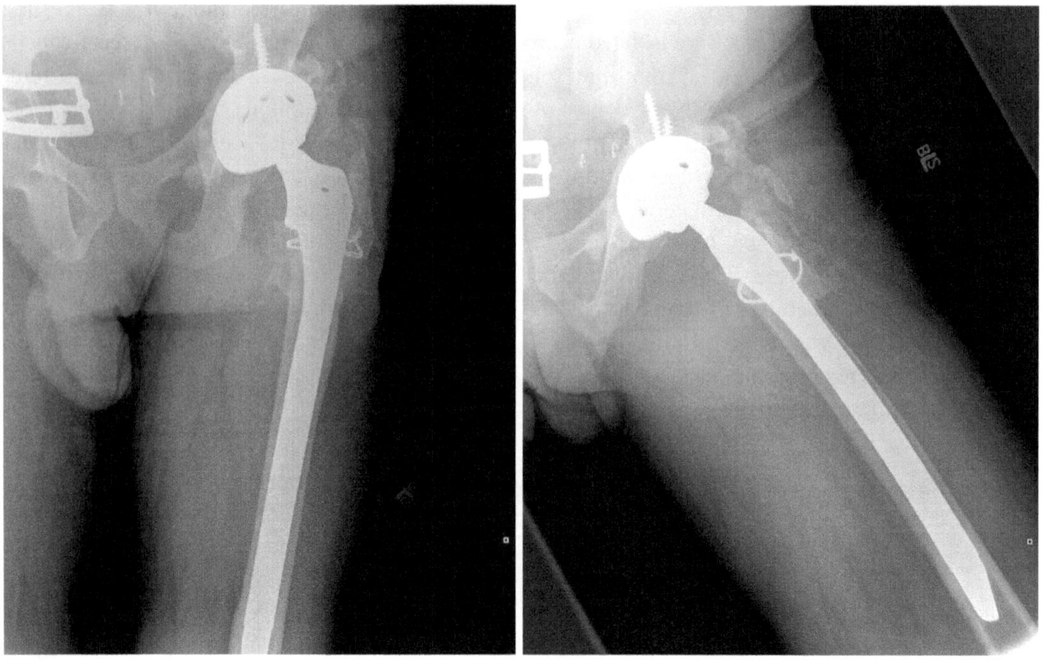

Figs. 8.6–8.7 AP and lateral radiograph taken 4 years after re-implantation

Case 2

A 90-year-old female had previously undergone revision left THA for aseptic loosening in 1997. The stem had been cemented in place. Radiographs taken 3 years later are shown in Figs. 8.8–8.11. This shows varus collapse with subsidence from prior radiographs. She developed bony ectasia on the lateral side of the femur at the tip of the stem. This was revised to an ingrowth stem with cortical allograft struts. Immediate postoperative and 5-year postoperative radiographs are shown in Figs. 8.12–8.13 and 8.14–8.15. This shows excellent incorporation of the struts.

Unfortunately, she later presented with acute onset pain in the left hip and inability to bear weight.

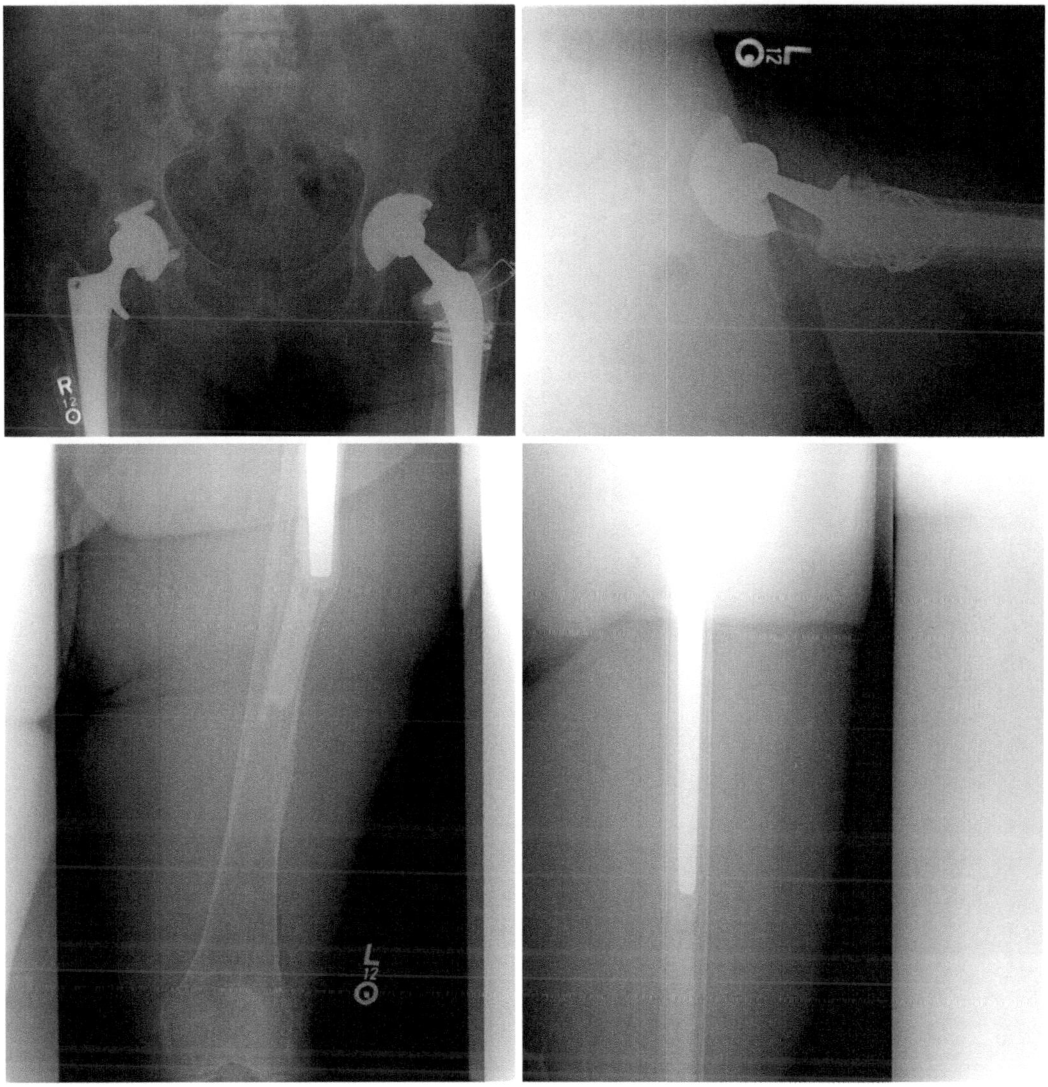

Figs. 8.8–8.11 Radiographs taken 3 years after cemented revision of the left hip for aseptic loosening. Notice the reactive bone formation at the tip of the stem

Laboratory workup showed high normal values but an aspirate of the hip showed gross purulence. She was thus explanted and was found to have purulence deep to the iliotibial band and a loose femoral stem with purulence at the bone stem interface. Tobramycin impregnated antibiotic cement was placed in the acetabulum as seen in Fig. 8.16.

Cultures grew methicillin sensitive Staph aureus (MSSA), and she was treated with ceftriaxone. She did require a repeat I&D for continued erythema and pain, and further purulence was found. Eight weeks after explant she was ready for re-implantation. Mobilizing the femur and attaining appropriate length took extra time in this case since a non-articulating spacer was used. A guide wire was placed under C-arm imaging to confirm intramedullary placement, and reaming was then done over the guide wire. Ultimately, a 60 mm cup and a fully coated 260 mm length bowed stem with a 15 mm calcar segment were placed. Radiographs are seen in Figs. 8.17–8.18. She is doing well at this point, and a radiograph taken 7 years postoperatively is seen in Fig. 8.19.

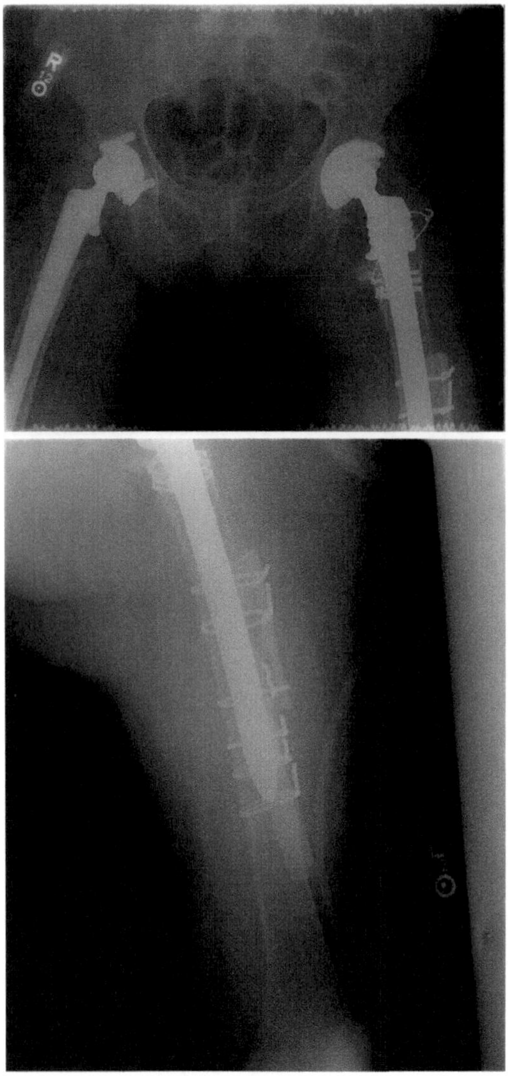

Figs. 8.12–8.13 Immediate postoperative radiographs after revision of the left hip with an ingrowth stem and placement of cortical allograft struts

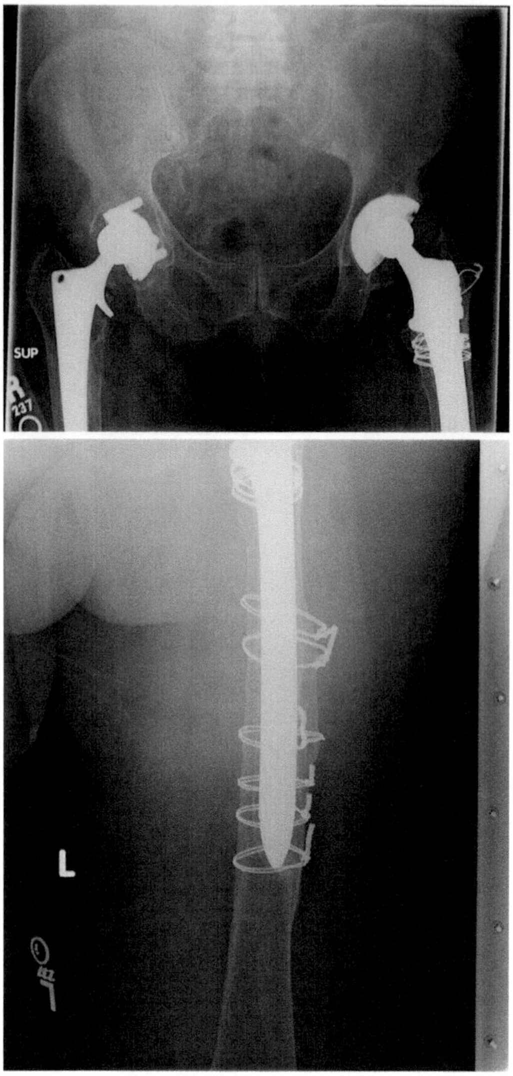

Figs. 8.14–8.15 A 5-year postoperative radiographs showing incorporation of the allograft struts

This case highlights the benefit of an articulating antibiotic spacer to maintain femoral length and allow ease of re-implantation. This was not used in this case, and extra time was spent during the re-implantation to get length back. Debridement and lavage to excise compromised tissue and lessen the bacterial burden must not be overlooked. Despite explant and antibiotics, this patient required a subsequent repeat debridement. Limiting the number of operations is important; however, achieving an aseptic environment is paramount. Lastly, when placing long stems, consider using intraoperative imaging to confirm intramedullary placement of reamers.

Case 3

A 56-year-old female underwent right metal on metal total hip in 2007 at a nearby hospital. She reported serous drainage postoperatively and was treated with a 10-day course of levofloxacin. She had no further follow-up with her surgeon and

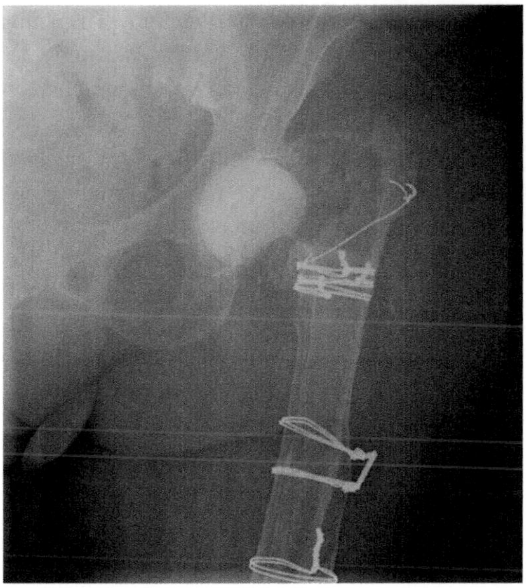

Fig. 8.16 Radiograph taken after explant and placement of an antibiotic cement spacer in the acetabulum

did fine until 3 months prior to presentation. At that time she noticed increasing pain and swelling over the hip and could feel a fluid collection. She presented to our facility when she spontaneously developed a draining sinus tract. She had a nickel-sized area at the distal portion of the incision which had copious purulent and necrotic tissue draining from it. Radiographs are shown in Figs. 8.20–8.22. Notice the endosteal scalloping. Figure 8.23 shows the fluid collection seen on MRI. Abundant necrotic infected tissue was seen along with metallosis at the time of explant.

Despite radiographs demonstrating lucency around the stem and pedestal formation at the tip, the stem was well fixed and unable to be removed with the stem extractor after using flexible osteotomes. An extended trochanteric osteotomy was therefore performed. The acetabular component had little osseous integration and was easily

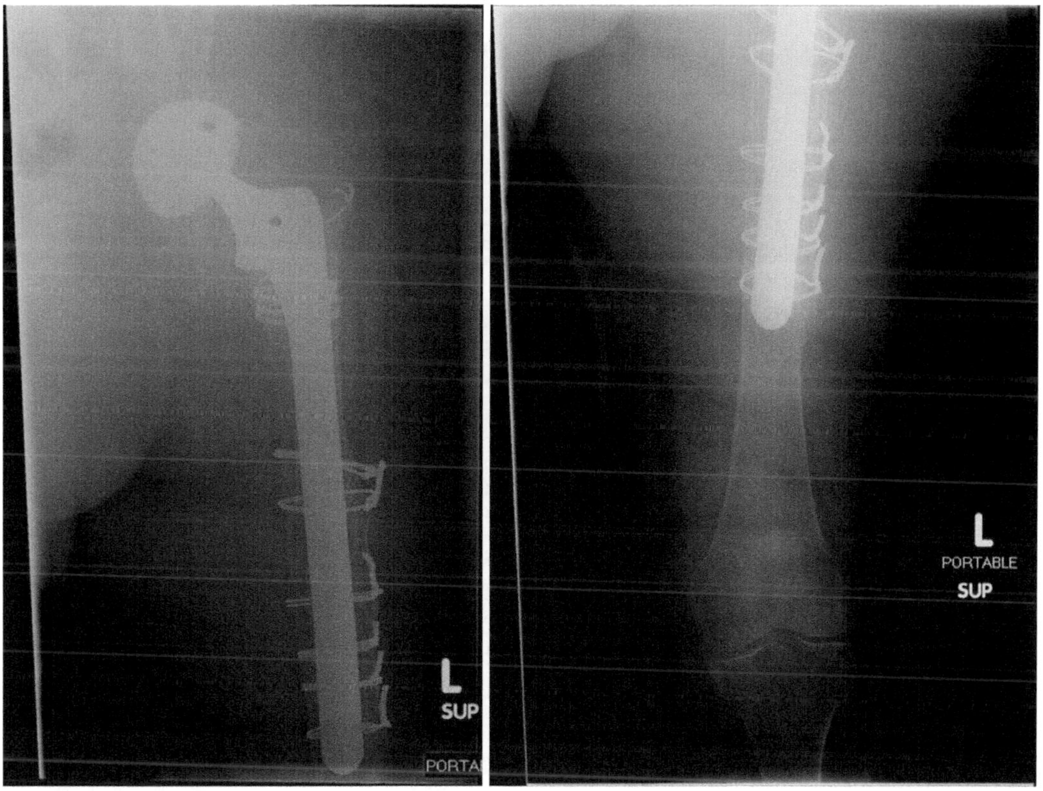

Figs. 8.17–8.18 Postoperative radiographs taken after re-implantation of the left hip

removed. After thorough debridement of all necrotic tissue, the greater trochanter was repaired with cerclage wires. An antibiotic cement nail was placed in the femur, and a ball of cement was left in the acetabulum. The sinus tract was excised, and an incisional wound vacuum was placed. Postoperative radiographs can be seen in Figs. 8.24–8.25.

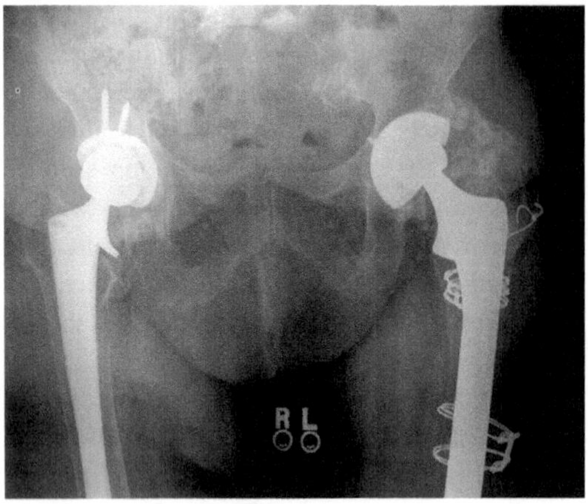

Fig. 8.19 AP radiograph taken 7 years after reimplantation of the left hip

Cultures grew MSSA and coagulase negative Staph. She was treated with ceftriaxone for 6 weeks. She remained on an extended 2 month antibiotic holiday to ensure resolution of her infection. Inflammatory markers remained within normal range. During revision, the antibiotic nail in the femur was unable to be extracted even after extensive debridement of the proximal femur. The trochanteric osteotomy was then re-performed after removing the cerclage cables. A calcar replacing long stem was placed along with a size 52 cup. Preoperative planning and postoperative X-rays are seen in Figs. 8.26–8.29. Postoperatively, she did well but had evidence of subsidence 18 months after surgery (Fig. 8.30) and mild pain consistent with a loose stem.

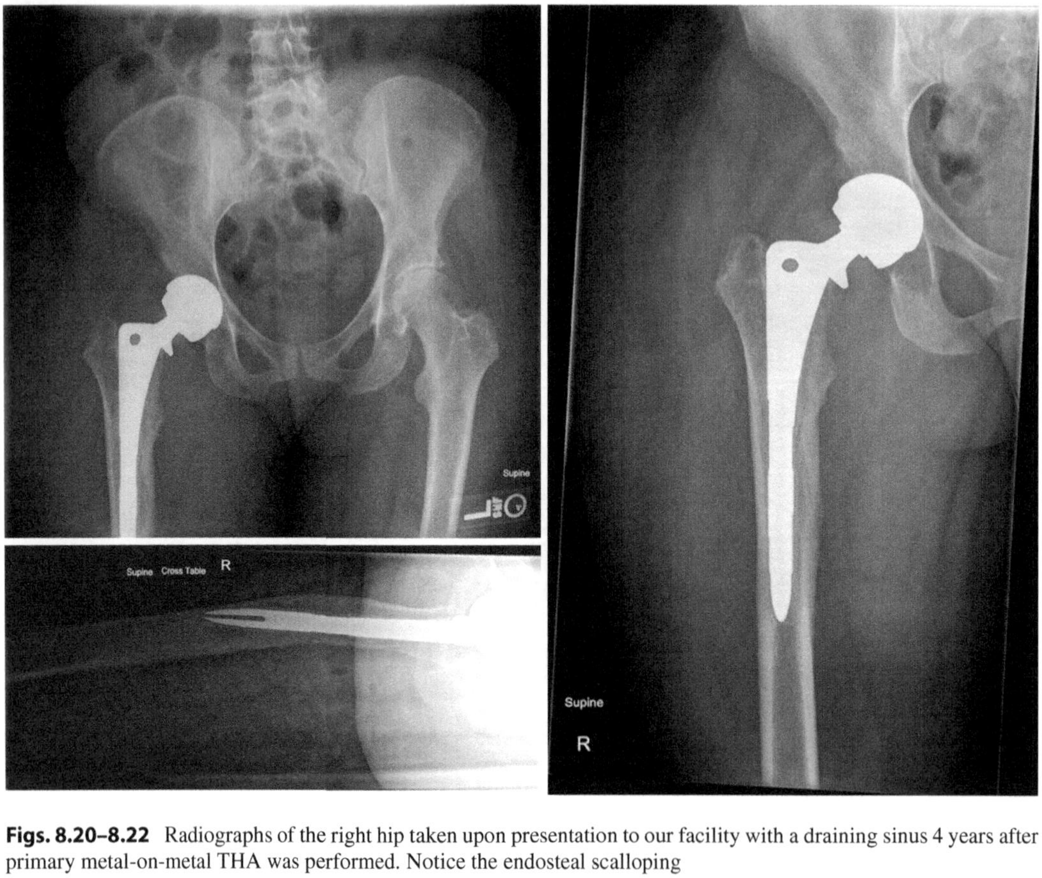

Figs. 8.20–8.22 Radiographs of the right hip taken upon presentation to our facility with a draining sinus 4 years after primary metal-on-metal THA was performed. Notice the endosteal scalloping

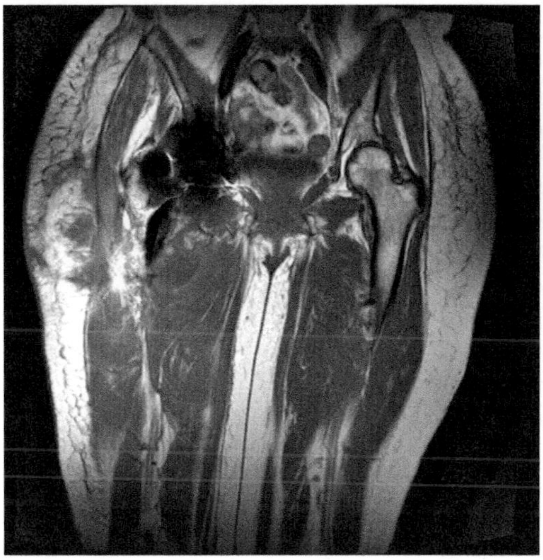

Fig. 8.23 Coronal MRI demonstrating necrotic tissue and debris in the superficial layer of the right hip

Inflammatory markers and a hip aspirate showed no recurrence of infection. She underwent revision of the femur to a fully porous coated stem without complication and had no signs of infection intraoperatively. The femur was loose and was able to be extracted quite easily. Final images are seen in Figs. 8.31–8.32. At this point, she is 1 year out and doing well with minimal pain.

In this case, the use of a partially coated stem leads to subsidence and required revision of the femur. This was salvaged by a tapered, fully porous coated stem which is the author's preferred stem for revisions because of its ease of use and potential for bone ingrowth along the entire length of the prosthesis.

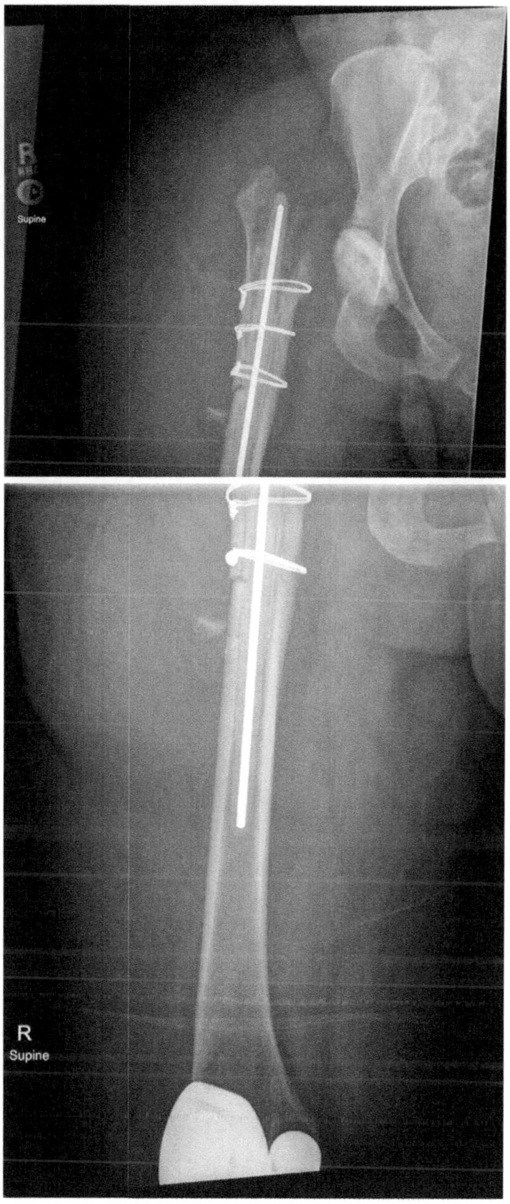

Figs. 8.24–8.25 Radiographs taken after explant of the infected metal on metal prosthesis and placement of a non-articulating antibiotic spacer consisting of an antibiotic cement rod in the femur and an antibiotic cement sphere in the acetabulum. An extended trochanteric osteotomy was required to remove the femoral stem

Case 4

Courtesy of Terry Gioe, MD. Department of Veterans Affairs, VA Medical Center Minneapolis, MN.

A 65-year-old male initially underwent primary THA about 2 years prior. He required irrigation and debridement with head and liner exchange a few weeks after for continued wound drainage. Months later, he underwent explant and antibiotic spacer placement for ongoing infection. It was at this point he transferred his care to our facility. Radiographs are shown in Figs. 8.33–8.35.

Exam of the right hip showed a draining sinus tract in the center portion of the prior incision.

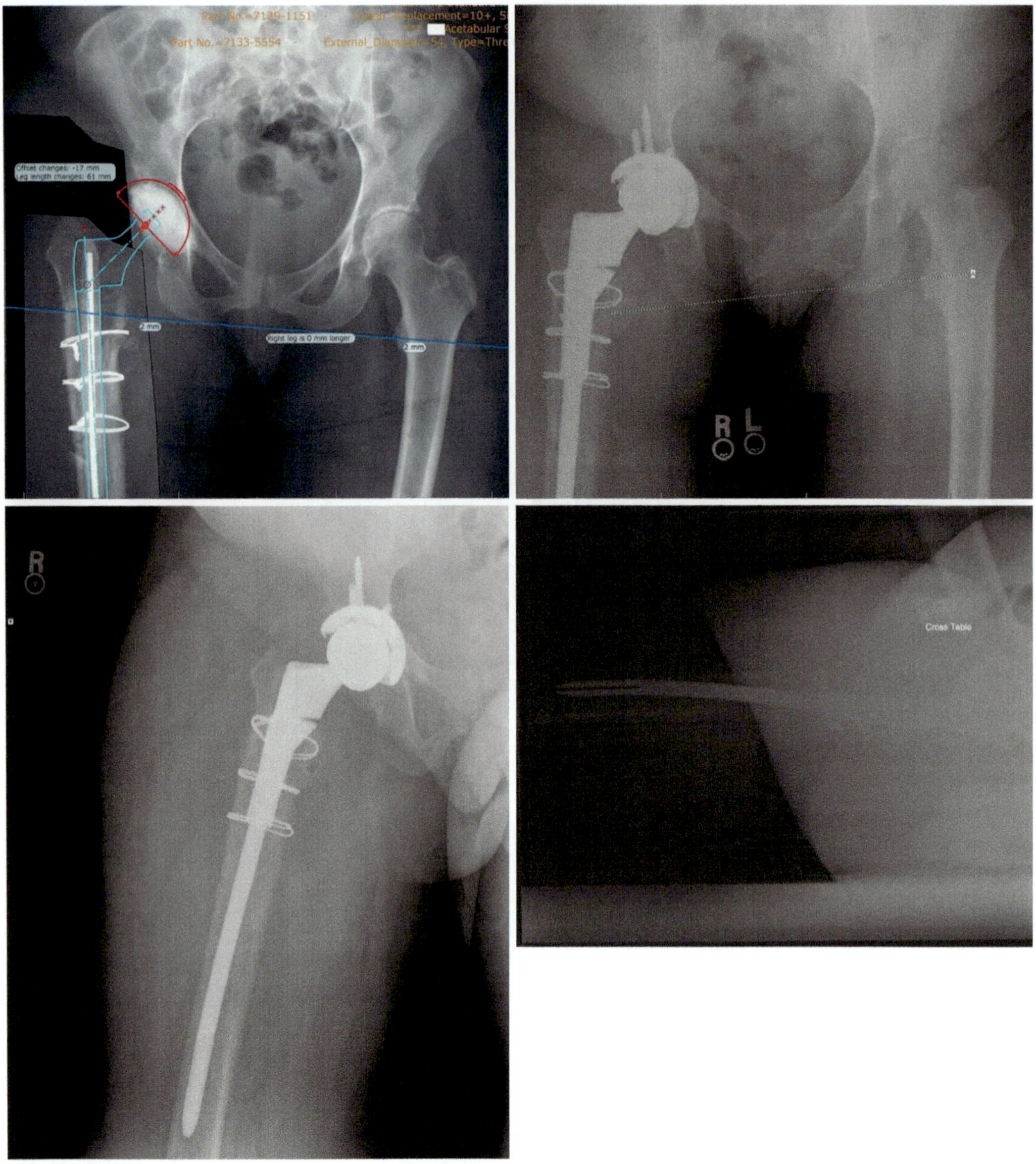

Figs. 8.26–8.29 Preoperative template and immediate postoperative radiographs taken after re-implantation. Restoration of length was achieved despite use of a non-articulating spacer

Aspiration of the hip grew out methicillin resistant Staph aureus (MRSA), so he was treated with vancomycin. He underwent irrigation and debridement and exchange of the antibiotic spacer. The draining sinus tract along with his prior scar was excised. The same posterior approach was used. The femoral stem was extracted but the cement mantle around the stem did not come out with the prosthesis. Using osteotomes and reverse curettes, the proximal cement was removed. The distal cement plug was drilled and reamed over a guidewire (Fig. 8.36). A long pituitary assisted in removing all the distal cement. The cup came out easily. Thorough debridement and lavage ensued. A new prostalac spacer was placed and is seen in Fig. 8.37.

Cultures again grew MRSA, and he was treated with 8 weeks of daptomycin and rifampin.

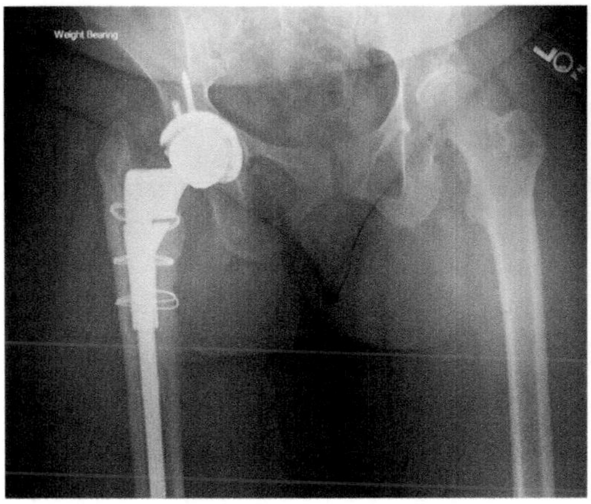

Fig. 8.30 Radiograph taken 18 months after surgery demonstrating subsidence of the stem

After an antibiotic holiday, he was deemed ready for re-implantation. Preoperative planning showed a 3.6 cm limb length discrepancy despite the use of an articulating spacer. Also noteworthy is the disuse osteopenia of the femur which is typical after restricted weight bearing in these patients (Figs. 8.38–8.39).

During re-implantation, a 62 mm cup was placed. A modular tapered revision stem system was used and a +0 neck length was trialed. This had good stability but the leg was still short. A +6 head was placed and reduced with some difficulty. With this, the leg lengths were very close, being only a few millimeters short upon inspection. There was difficulty dislocating the hip despite very careful and cautious attempts. Ultimately with the dislocation, there was gross instability of the distal thigh relative to the proximal thigh. There was clearly an intraoperative fracture of the femur. The incision was extended and the lateral femur was exposed where a spiral fracture was found at the stem tip. An intraoperative radiograph after the fracture was reduced and clamped is seen in Fig. 8.40. A lucent line is still visible in between the clamps. A lateral locking plate with cables and screws was used to stabilize the femur. Immediate postoperative and 4 month postoperative images are seen in Figs. 8.41–8.46.

The two screws distal to the stem were interfragmentary lag screws placed under direct visu-

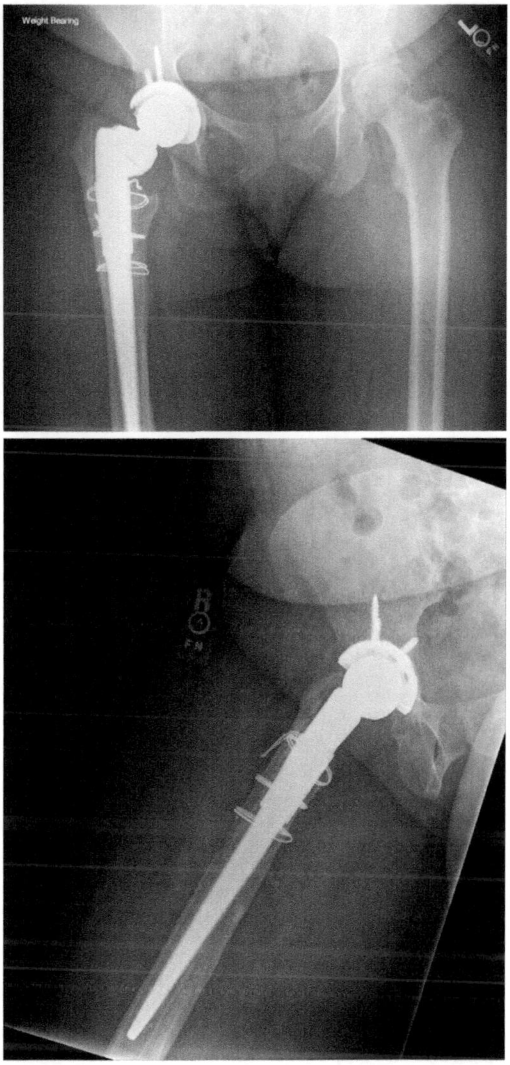

Figs. 8.31–8.32 Radiographs taken 1 year after revision of the femur using a fully porous coated stem

alization of the fracture and placed through the plate. A +3 neck length was ultimately used in this case. Intraoperative cultures showed no growth but he was treated with 3 months of oral moxifloxacin and rifampin. Inflammatory markers at the 3 month postop visit were normal. He is now 4 months out from surgery and doing quite well. He's able to bear full weight and walks with a cane. Current images are seen in Figs. 8.47–8.50.

Notable points in this case include limiting the number of reductions and dislocations during tri-

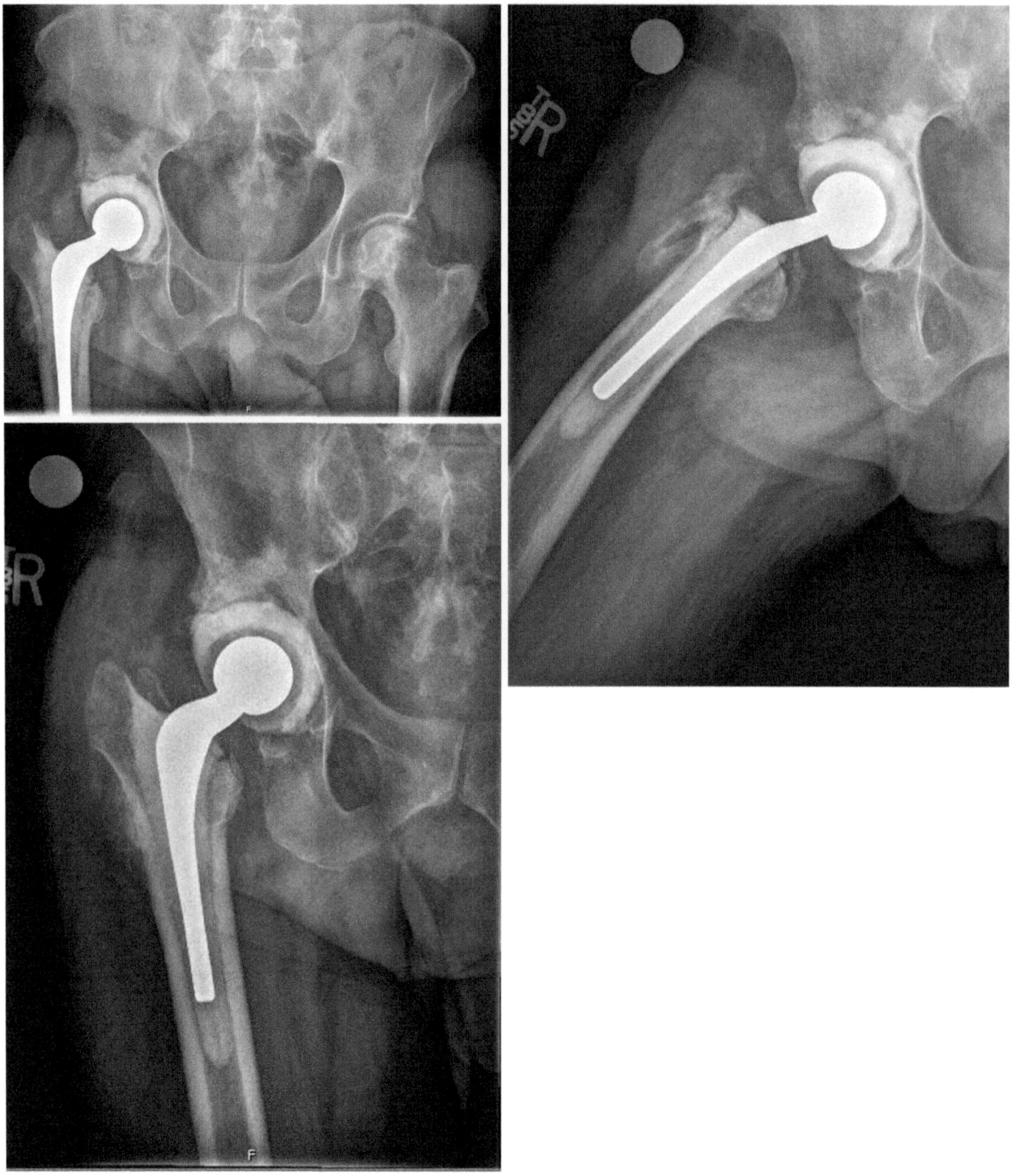

Figs. 8.33–8.35 Initial radiographs after transfer to our facility with a prostalac spacer in place

aling. Despite being cognoscente of his osteopenia and using caution with reduction and dislocation maneuvers, an intraoperative fracture still occurred. This not only added operative time and morbidity to the patient, but also limits the ability to weight bear postoperatively.

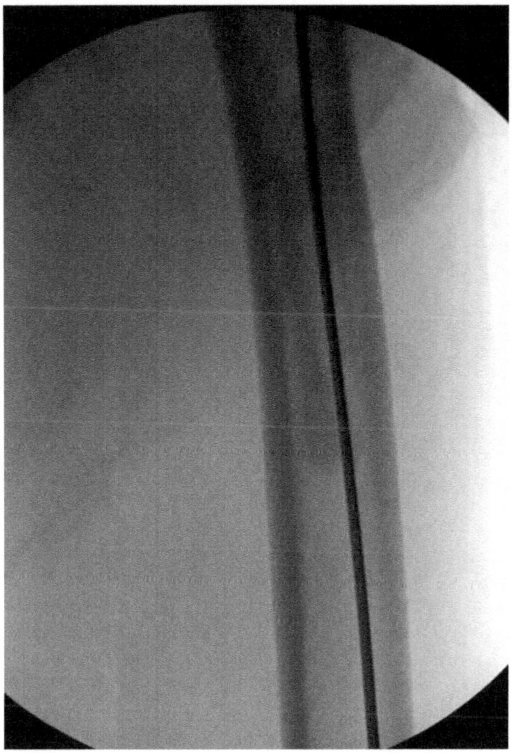

Fig. 8.36 Intraoperative C-arm image confirming guide wire placement to allow reaming through distal cement plug

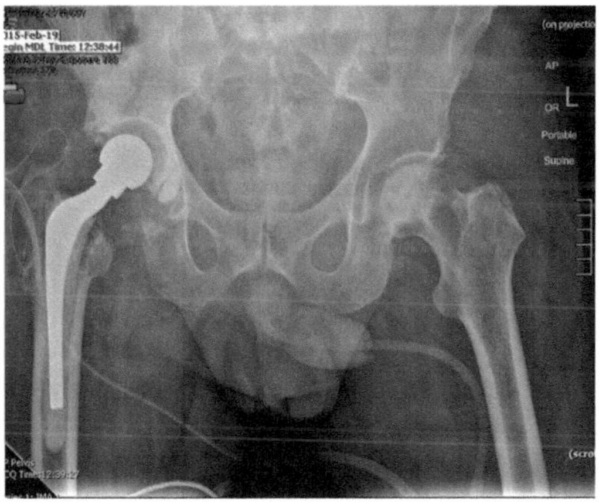

Fig. 8.37 AP pelvis after spacer exchange

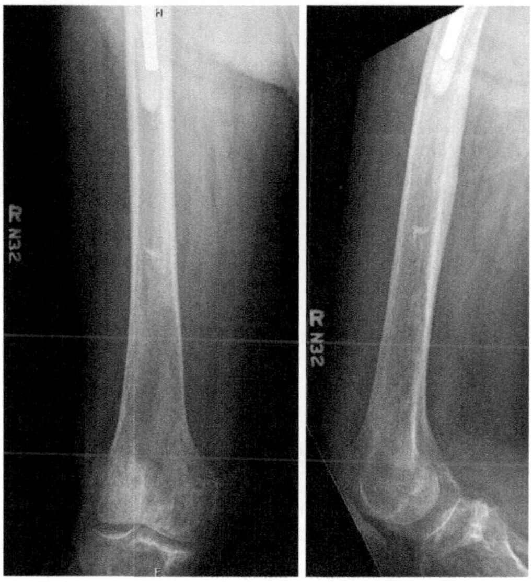

Figs. 8.38–8.39 AP and lateral of the distal femur showing significant osteopenia

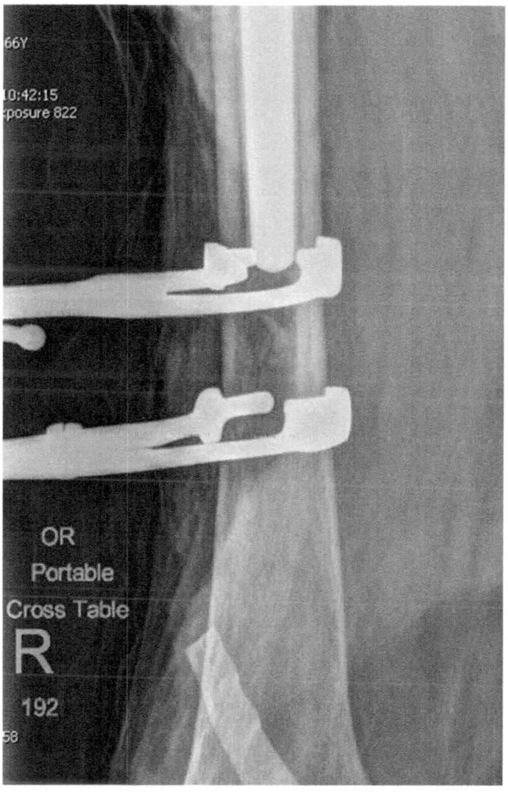

Fig. 8.40 C-arm image taken after open reduction and provisional bone clamp fixation of the intraoperative fracture. The radiolucent fracture line is still faintly visible running obliquely in between the two clamps

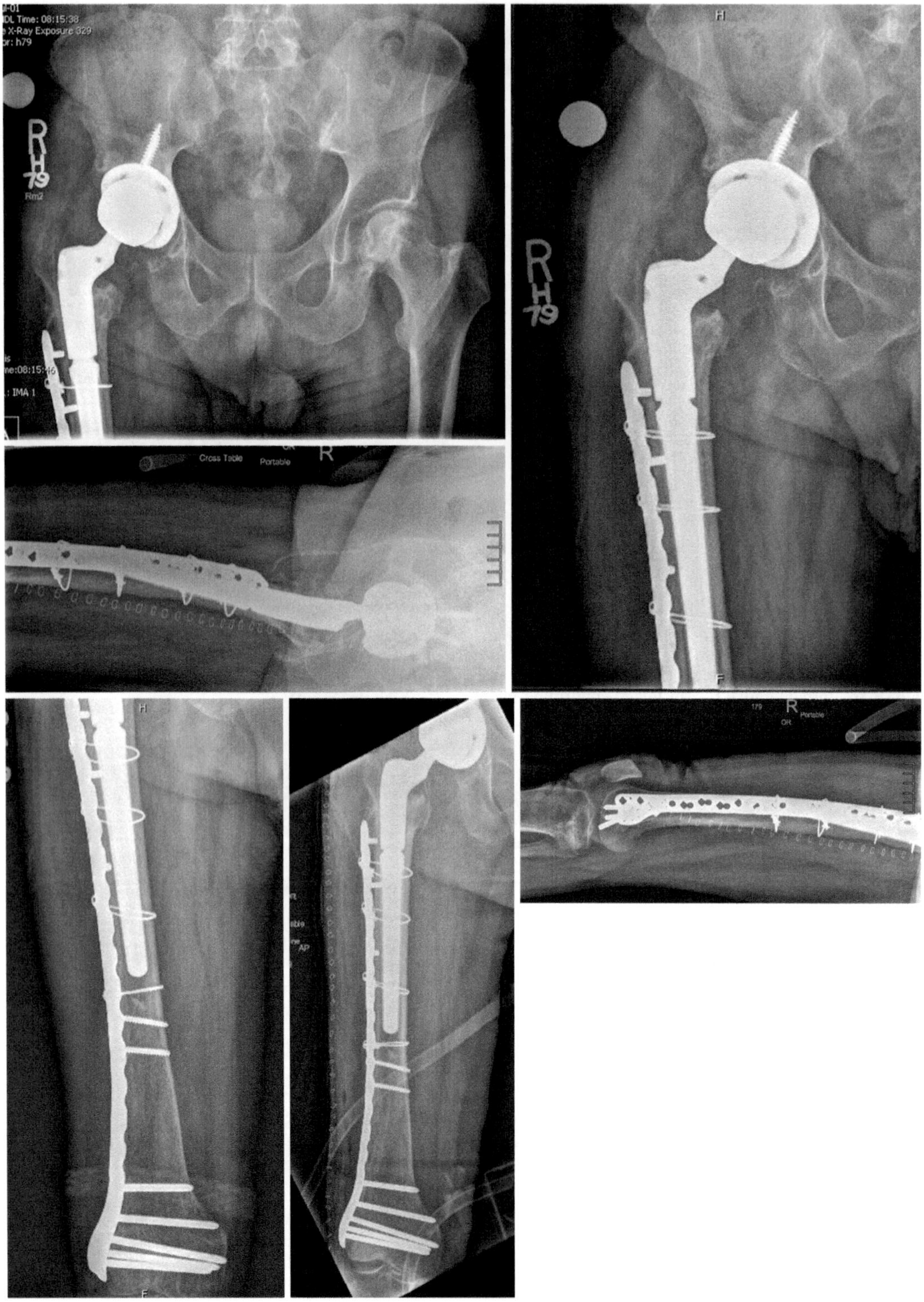

Figs. 8.41–8.46 Immediate postoperative radiographs after re-implantation and lateral locking plate fixation for intraoperative periprosthetic fracture of the femur at the distal stem tip. Locking screws were used distally at the knee and three unicortical locking screws along with cerclage cables were used more proximally where the stem was. Two interfragmentary lag screws were placed through the plate to cross the fracture line

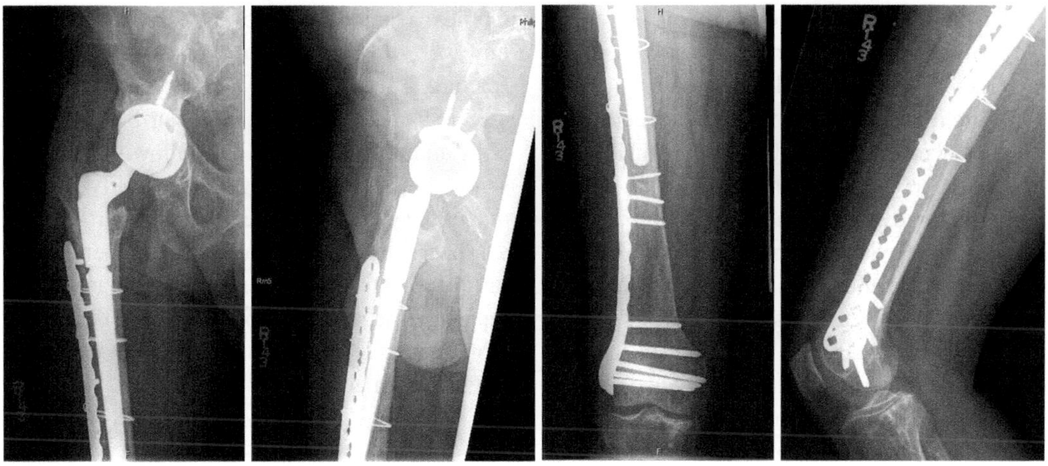

Figs. 8.47–8.50 Radiographs taken 4 months after surgery. The patient was ambulating with a cane and bearing full weight at the time of these radiographs

Issues/Controversies/Problems

Diagnosing a prosthetic joint infection can be difficult. Fortunately, the Musculoskeletal Infection Society definition of PJI has provided a standardized means for diagnosis [10]. If there is any suspicion for infection, aspiration should be performed and repeated if clinical suspicion remains high despite a negative aspiration. Once diagnosed, PJI can be classified into acute or chronic although the exact distinction between these two is of debate. A staged procedure is the gold standard although high rates of success have been reported with direct exchange arthroplasty [11]. With a two-stage procedure, antibiotic spacers are often used after extraction of the implants and radical debridement. These can be either articulating or non-articulating. The benefit of articulating spacers is the preservation of length and prevention of soft tissue contractures. Subsequent exposures can be easier and weight bearing may be allowed thus improving patient function [12]. It is important, however, to confirm that the hip is stable with the articulating spacer. An unstable articulating spacer will only lead to bony resorption as the head subluxates or even dislocates out of the acetabulum and cause discomfort for the patient. In this situation, non-articulating spacers should be used as highlighted in the case examples.

Several criteria must be met in order to incorporate antibiotic into methyl-methacrylate. The antibiotic must be thermally stable to withstand the heat created during polymerization. It must be water soluble to diffuse into local tissues and be effective at the concentration achieved. Lastly, it should elude into the local tissues gradually over time. Commonly used antibiotics include vancomycin and aminoglycosides such as tobramycin or gentamycin. High doses of antibiotic can be safely used in patients with normal kidney function [13].

Tips/Tricks/Avoiding Pitfalls

As mentioned previously, prevention is paramount. Every possible measure to prevent infection should be taken. Despite a correlation between operating room door openings and increased colony forming unit counts, there's no proof in the current literature that this increases surgical site infection [14]. Common sense should still be used and an attitude that embraces the idea that each individual step, no matter how negligible it may seem, contributes to the whole. Unnecessary OR traffic and personnel in the operating room should be minimized. Skin preparation and draping should be done by experienced OR personnel. The surgical approach should be chosen based on surgeon preference but keeping in mind the prior approach used. The approach chosen should allow for expansile exposure if necessary. Prior operative reports and implant labels should be obtained well in advance of the case to assist in planning.

When removing prostheses or antibiotic spacers, complete visualization and circumferential exposure of the entire implant are necessary prior to attempting extraction as even soft tissue will hinder removal and only increase risk for fracture. Radical debridement of all infected or questionable tissue until bleeding tissue is encountered is absolutely necessary for eradication of sepsis. This also enhances the delivery of systemic antibiotics to the area.

Proper cement technique dictates the efficacy of the antibiotic spacer. Elution of antibiotic is dependent on the surface area of the cement. Cement should not be mixed in a vacuum as typically done. This allows the cement to be more porous, therefore allowing greater elution of antibiotic from the cement. Palacos cement also has better elution properties as shown in prior studies [15, 16].

The use of locally administered antibiotics into the surgical wound has been used since the mid-1900s [17]. Benefits include direct action at the surgical site without the need for diffusion into the wound which is required with systemic antibiotics. Furthermore, with such high concentrations attained locally, the antibiotic can become bactericidal even to resistant bacteria [18]. Intra-wound antibiotic powder has been extensively studied in the spine literature with results showing its safety and efficacy with lower rates of postoperative infections [19–23].

Removing cement from the femoral canal can prove difficult even for an experienced surgeon. Reverse hooks or curettes can be used to remove loose pieces of cement along with a pituitary rongeur. In cases where cement is very distal in the canal, a drill bit can be used with C-arm guidance to create a path down the center of the cement. A guide wire is then placed, and flexible reamers can be used. An example of such is seen in Figs. 8.51–8.53.. Extra long pituitary rongeurs can be found in the obstetrical instruments and can aid with removal of cement fragments. Cortical windows can be made as a last resort; however, this carries morbidity and risk of fracture.

Small medial wall defects can be addressed with multi-hole revision cups allowing multiple screw trajectories to augment stability. Larger defects can be filled by denuding the cartilage off a frozen allograft femoral head and then boring out the center with a small sized acetabular reamer. This can then be placed in the defect along with allograft croutons and reverse reamed to impact the graft.

Authors Preferred Method/Take Home Points

Aggressive debridement of all affected tissues is performed to reduce bacterial burden and allow delivery of systemic antibiotics to the living tissue. A minimum of three cultures are taken including superficial and deep cultures depending on what is encountered during the exposure. An odd number of cultures is always chosen to aid in decision-making whenever there is suspicion of a false positive culture. Prior to attempting extraction of any implant, the bone–implant interface is circumferentially exposed and all soft tissue is excised as this may prevent successful extraction. Further debridement of the femoral canal and the acetabulum is performed followed by irrigation. Pseudomembranes are removed from the acetabulum, and reverse curettes are used to remove all membranes and remaining cement from the femoral canal. Flexible reamers are often used to ream the canal over a guide wire which is confirmed to be intramedullary with intraoperative C-arm imaging. Dilute betadine is routinely used and often repeated if operative time is prolonged. After all infected implants have been removed and debridement and irrigation are complete, a second sterile setup with clean sterile instruments is used and new draping is placed over the initial drapes to reduce bacterial load. All members scrubbed change their outer gloves. The “dirty” setup with all prior instruments and the extracted implants are no longer be used.

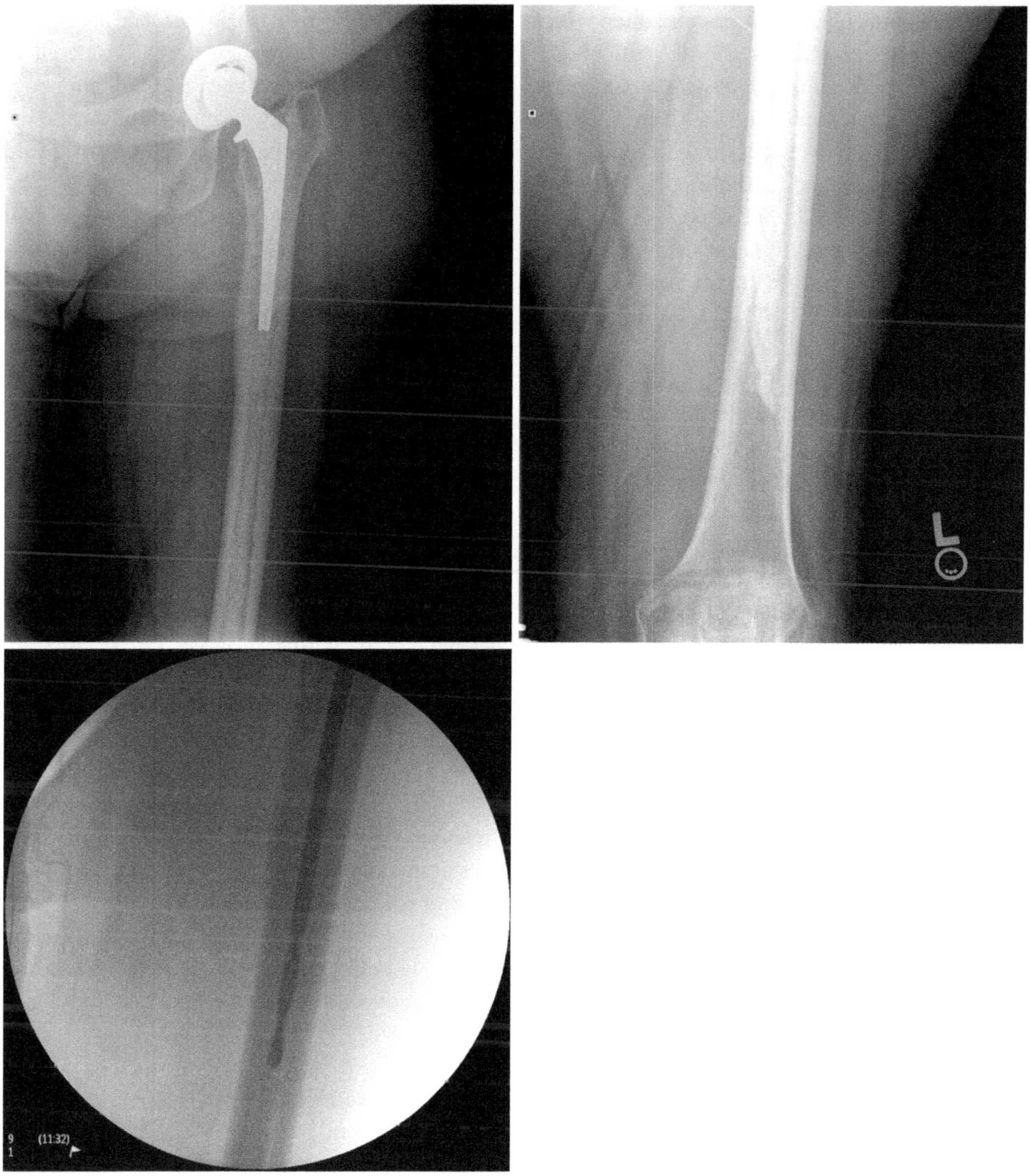

Figs. 8.51–8.53 Radiographs of the left femur in a patient who had undergone a cemented THA at another facility. Intramedullary bone cement is seen throughout the entire diaphysis of the femur. This patient required revision for aseptic loosening. A long drill bit was used to create a path in the center of the cement mantle. Flexible reamers were then used over a guide wire to remove the cement

The authors routinely use antibiotic cement spacers, either articulating or non-articulating depending on the sufficiency of the acetabular cavity and the ability to contain the head component of the spacer. Four grams of vancomycin and 4.6 g of tobramycin are mixed in 40 g of cement. The spacer is inserted after the doughy stage of the methyl-methacrylate to allow insertion of the spacer without interdigitation of the cement with bone. This facilitates easy removal and preservation of bone stock for the second stage. Non-articulating spacers are made using a hemispherical ball of cement that sits in the acetabulum. An antibiotic cement nail is made using a steinmann pin coated with cement, often with a proximal bend to ease retrieval. Articulating spacers are made again by using a steinmann pin with a gentle bend to recreate the shape of a typical femoral stem. This is coated with cement and a cement sphere is made and placed on the top of the steinmann pin for the head portion. An alternative is to use a small femoral stem of any kind and coat the stem with cement. See Figs. 8.54, 8.55–8.59, 8.60, and 8.61–8.62 for a step-by-step illustration of spacer fabrication.

A deep drain is routinely used, and lavage is performed with each layer of closure. A small amount of tobramycin powder is routinely used in the deep aspect of the wound as well as after fascial closure if the patient has normal renal function. Tobramycin is used over vancomycin as it does not have the risk of hypotension that can be observed with vancomycin although this is more of a risk with intravenous use. If there is any concern about drainage or if the patient is obese an incisional vacuum-assisted closure device is used and left in place for 3 days. The patient is closely monitored with inflammatory markers and kept on appropriate antibiotics with the help of the infectious disease service. Occasionally, the patient will require more than 6 weeks of antibiotic coverage depending on the organism and response to treatment. Repeat irrigation or spacer exchange may be required and is decided on a case-by-case basis. Once antibiotics are discontinued, the patients are considered to be on an antibiotic holiday and inflammatory markers are monitored during this period. This can take up to 1–2 months in some cases to ensure complete resolution of infection.

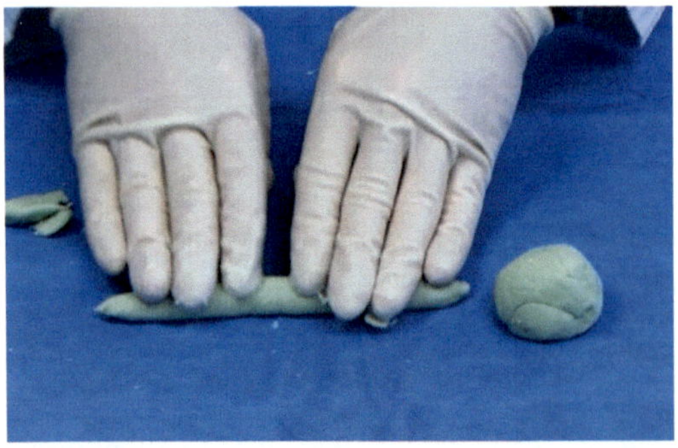

Fig. 8.54 Lab demonstration showing fabrication of a non-articulating spacer consisting of an antibiotic cement coated steinmann pin which is placed in the femoral canal and a smooth sphere of cement which is placed in the acetabulum

Preoperative templating is always performed prior to re-implantation. The second stage begins again with cultures and deep tissue sent for frozen section to evaluate the number of white blood cells per high power field. If there is doubt, spacers are exchanged and cultures are followed. If however, an aseptic environment is determined, re-implantation ensues. Previous spacers are removed, again circumferentially exposing the implants prior to attempting extraction. Again, pseudomembranes are removed from the acetabulum and the femoral canal. With adequate acetabular bone stock, reaming and cup insertion are carried out in normal fashion. Large cups are used for medial wall defects and femoral head allograft, and cancellous bone graft can be placed prior to cup insertion. A modular, fully coated tapered femoral stem is used being cautious during trialing to prevent periprosthetic fracture. Reaming of the femur is routinely done under C-arm imaging to confirm intramedullary placement of reamers and the stem. Again, dilute betadine is used as well as tobramycin powder. Lavage is performed with each layer of closure. Postoperative antibiotics are continued until cultures finalize.

Author's Take Home Points

- Radical debridement of infected tissue
- Send multiple cultures
- Consider local antibiotics
- Use antibiotic cement spacers, either articulating or non-articulating
- Some infections may require more than 6 weeks of antibiotic treatment
- Repeat debridement and antibiotic spacer exchange may be required
- Perform circumferential exposure of implant prior to attempting extraction
- Use fully porous modular revision systems

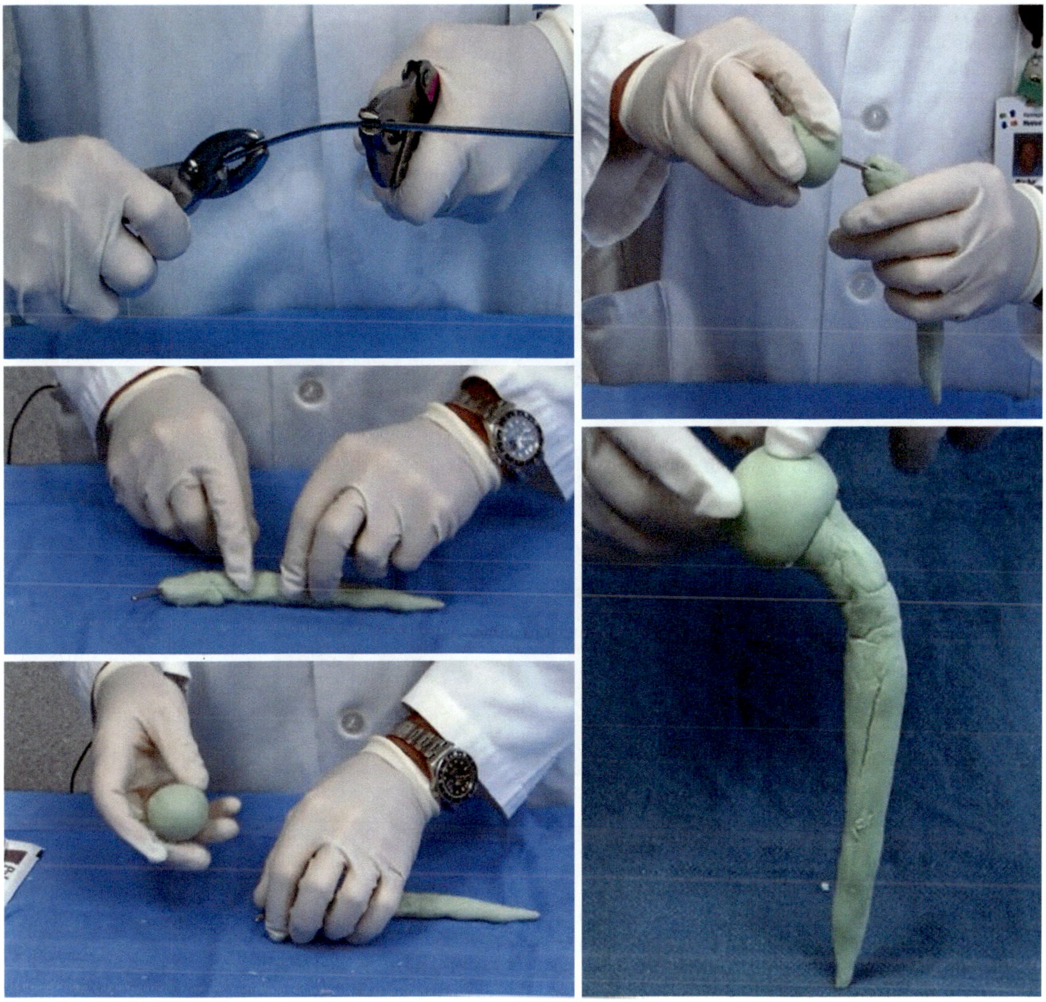

Figs. 8.55–8.59 Fabrication of an articulating antibiotic spacer. First a Steinmann pin is gently bent. Antibiotic cement is then placed around the pin which will be the stem portion inside the femur. A smooth sphere of cement is then placed on the top of the pin for the head portion. This creates a very highly concentrated antibiotic cement spacer which mimics a normal femoral stem and articulates in the acetabulum

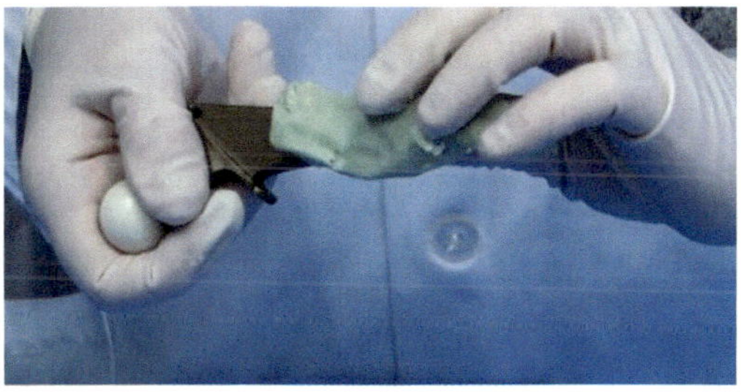

Fig. 8.60 Articulating antibiotic cement spacer fabricated using an actual femoral stem. After picking out the smallest size stem available, an antibiotic cement mantle is then formed around the stem. If the stem ends up too large to fit in the femur after the cement is hard, a burr can be used to shave the cement so it fits into the femur

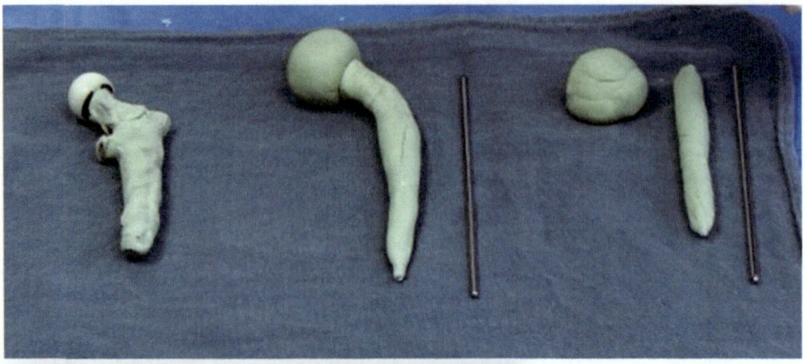

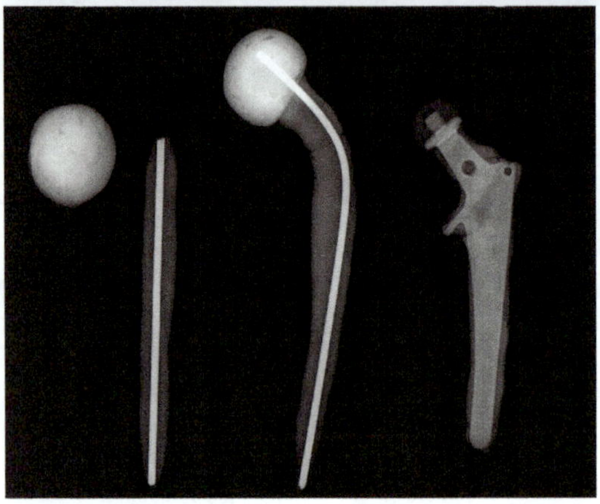

Figs. 8.61–8.62 Photograph and radiograph of the three different spacers

References

1. Charnley J. Postoperative infection after total hip replacement with special reference to air contamination in the operating room. Clin Orthop Relat Res. 1972;87:167–87.
2. Charnley J, Eftekhar N. Postoperative infection in total prosthetic replacement arthroplasty of the hip-joint. With special reference to the bacterial content of the air of the operating room. Bone Joint J. 1969;56:641–9.
3. Kurtz SM, Lau E, Watson H, Schmier JK, Parvizi J. Economic burden of periprosthetic joint infection in the United States. J Arthroplasty. 2012;27(8):61–5.
4. Kurtz S, Ong K, Lau E, Mowat F, Halpern M. Projections of primary and revision hip and knee arthroplasty in the United States from 2005 to 2030. J Bone Joint Surg. 2007;89:780–5.
5. Bozic KJ, Ries MD. The impact of infection after total hip arthroplasty on hospital and surgeon resource utilization. J Bone Joint Surg. 2005;87:1746–51.
6. Hill C, Flamant R, Mazas F, Evrard J. Prophylactic cefazolin versus placebo in total hip replacement: report of a multicentre double-blind randomised trial. Lancet. 1981;1:795–6.
7. Rao N, Cannella BA, Crossett LS, et al. Prospective screening/decolonization for *Staphylococcus aureus* to prevent orthopedic surgical site infection: prospective cohort study with 2-year follow-up. J Arthroplasty. 2011;26(8):1501–7.
8. Brown NM, Cipriano CA, Moric M, Sporer SM, Della Valle CJ. Dilute Betadine lavage before closure for the prevention of acute postoperative deep periprosthetic joint infection. J Arthroplasty. 2012;27(1):27–30.
9. Cai J, Karam JA, Parvizi J, et al. Aquacel surgical dressing reduces the rate of acute PJI following total joint arthroplasty: a case-control study. J Arthroplasty. 2014;29:1098–100.
10. Parvizi J, Gehrke T. Definition of periprosthetic joint infection. J Arthroplasty. 2014;29(7):1331.
11. Garvin KL, Hanssen A. Current concepts review. Infection after total hip arthroplasty. Past, present, and future. J Bone Joint Surg. 1995;77:1576–88.
12. Hofmann AA, Goldberg TD, Tanner AM, Cook TM. Ten-year experience using an articulating antibiotic cement hip spacer for the treatment of chronically infected total hip. J Arthroplasty. 2005;20(7):874–9.
13. Springer BD, Lee GC, Osmon D, Haidukewych GJ, Hanssen AD, Jacofsky DJ. Systemic safety of high-dose antibiotic-loaded cement spacers after resection of an infected total knee arthroplasty. Clin Orthop Relat Res. 2004;427:47–51.
14. Salassa T, Swiontkowski M. Surgical attire and the operating room: role in infection prevention. J Bone Joint Surg. 2014;96:1485–92.
15. Greene N, Holtom PD, Warren CA, et al. In vitro elution of tobramycin and vancomycin polymethylmeth-

acrylate beads and spacers from Simplex and Palacos. Am J Orthop. 1998;27:201–5.

16. Penner MJ, Duncan CP, Masri BA. The in vitro elution characteristics of antibiotic-loaded CMW and Palacos-R bone cements. J Arthroplasty. 1999;14(2):209–14.
17. Bingham R, Fleenor WH, Church S. The local use of antibiotics to prevent wound infection. Clin Orthop Relat Res. 1974;99:194–200.
18. Burdon DW. Principles of antimicrobial prophylaxis. World J Surg. 1982;6:262–7.
19. Bakhsheshian J, Dahdaleh NS, Lam SK, Savage JW, Smith ZA. The use of vancomycin powder in modern spine surgery: systematic review and meta-analysis of the clinical evidence. World Neurosurg. 2015;83:816 23.
20. Molinari RW, Khera OA, Molinari WJ III. Prophylactic intraoperative powdered vancomycin and postoperative deep spinal wound infection: 1,512 consecutive surgical cases over a 6-year period. Eur Spine J. 2012;21:S476–82.
21. O'Neill KR, Smith JG, Abtahi AM, Archer KR, Spengler DM, McGirt MJ, Devin CJ. Reduced surgical site infections in patients undergoing posterior spinal stabilization of traumatic injuries using vancomycin powder. Spine J. 2011;11:641–6.
22. Pahys J, Pahys JR, Cho SKW, Kang MM, Zebala LP, Hawasli AH, Sweet FA, Lee DH, Riew KD. Methods to decrease postoperative infections following posterior cervical spine surgery. J Bone Joint Surg. 2013;95:549–54.
23. Sweet FA, Roh M, Sliva C. Intrawound application of vancomycin for prophylaxis in instrumented thoracolumbar fusions: efficacy, drug levels, and patient outcomes. Spine J. 2011;36:2084–8.

Revision Total Knee Arthroplasty: From Minimal to Severe Bone Loss

9

Aldo M. Riesgo, Richard S. Yoon, and Frank A. Liporace

Introduction

With increasing numbers of younger and more active patients undergoing total knee arthroplasty (TKA) [1], the number of patients requiring revision surgery is expected to increase [2, 3]. While revision TKA can be complicated, bone loss encountered during the revision setting can present a significant challenge for even an experienced arthroplasty surgeon. Bony deficiencies are common in the revision setting and can affect implant choice, ligament stability, and achieving initial and long-term fixation. The purpose of this chapter is to present different strategies and treatment options for management of minimal to severe bony deficiencies in revision TKAs.

Background

Management of osseous defects begins with a thorough preoperative assessment and classification of bone loss. The etiology of bone loss can be multifactorial, including stress shielding, wear debris, infection, fracture, implant loosening, and iatrogenic [4]. These can be present simultaneously, so understanding the underlying issues and mitigating the risk of further damage are paramount. Preoperative planning with appropriate radiographic imaging allows for appropriate implant selection, adequate back-up equipment, and a systematic intraoperative surgical plan.

The Anderson Orthopaedic Research Institute (AORI) is the most widely used classification system for osseous defects about the knee [5]. Briefly, type I defects involve an intact cortical rim near the original joint line with defects less than 1 cm. Type II defects are further subclassified into IIa (loss of one femoral condyle or tibial plateau) or IIb (loss of both femoral condyles and tibial plateaus). Type III defects are the most substantial and involve almost complete loss of metaphyseal bone, commonly with collateral ligament insufficiency. The tibial tubercle and extensor mechanism insertion can also be affected and must be addressed cautiously.

Depending on the size of the defect, bone defects can be managed with cement, morselized allograft, structural allograft, adjusting component positioning, or metal augmentation(stems, sleeves, cones, megaprosthesis, etc.) depending on their size and location. Several studies have reported on the short-, mid-, and long-term follow-up of the aforementioned reconstructive options with overall good results.

A. M. Riesgo (✉)
Division of Adult Reconstruction, Department of Orthopaedic Surgery, Baptist Health, Miami, FL, USA

R. S. Yoon · F. A. Liporace
Division of Orthopaedic Trauma and Adult Reconstruction, Department of Orthopedic Surgery, Cooperman Barnabas/Jersey City Medical Center - RWJBH, Livingston/Jersey City, NJ, USA

R. S. Yoon et al. (eds.), *Trauma and Infection Control in Revision Hip and Knee Arthroplasty*,
https://doi.org/10.1007/978-3-031-71971-4_9

Regardless of the reconstructive method, an anatomic joint line must be restored to optimize joint stability. This will affect options for constraint. With moderate bone loss and possible collateral ligament insufficiency, a constrained condylar knee (CCK)-type of prosthesis will be sufficient [6]. With more substantial bone loss, medial collateral insufficiency, or gross flexion-extension gap mismatch, a hinged-type revision TKA is warranted [7]. In general, the lowest degree of constraint should be used to minimize the stress experienced at the bone–implant interface.

Cement

For AORI type I defects less than 5 mm, polymethylmethacrylate (PMMA) cement is usually sufficient. Primary knee arthroplasty components can be used in small Type I AORI defects, but use of stems is recommended in larger defects [8, 9]. For type II defects, cement alone is inadequate but may be reinforced with 6.5 mm cancellous screws. While some authors have reported poor results with this technique [10], other have reported good short- and medium-term results [11]. Despite the good results, radiolucent lines are very common. It is unclear if screw augmentation actually improves the mechanical properties of PMMA in setting of larger defects [12]. As such, PMMA augmentation should only be used in elderly or low-demand patients with peripheral defects less than 5 mm in depth.

Additionally, adjusting component positioning away from the bony defect can be effective, especially on the tibia. Commonly, the surgeon can adjust the tibial baseplate laterally to avoid an uncontained medial defect. This technique has been used effectively in setting of large varus deformity [13, 14], but care must be taken as significant downsizing of tibial baseplates can concentrate forces onto a smaller surface area with less cortical support.

Impaction Grafting

For larger bone defects, impaction grafting represents an attractive reconstructive option. Proponents of impaction grafting cite its cost-effectiveness and the ability to reconstruct bone stock, advantageous in younger patients who may require further revisions in the future. However, it is technically demanding, time-consuming, and significant risk of graft collapse or resorption [15]. Morselized allograft is impacted into contained defects, but uncontained defects require use of a wire mesh. The use of allograft also carries with it a small risk of disease transmission.

While mid-term results demonstrate good outcomes with impaction grafting in the revision TKA setting, the durability of these outcomes with long-term follow-up is questionable. One study with average 4-year follow-up prospectively reported on 48 revision TKA cases with substantial bone loss treated with impaction allograft. All radiographs demonstrated incorporation and remodeling of the bone graft with no mechanical failures [16]. Hanna et al. also reported on impaction grafting for moderate to severe bone loss. At 10-year follow-up, cumulative prosthesis survival was 98%. Five patients (9%) had reoperations for complications unrelated to the bone graft [17]. Lonner et al. reported on 17 revision TKA cases in 14 patients with large uncontained defects treated with impaction allograft and molded wire mesh for containment. No patients required further revision surgery, although non-progressive tibial radiolucency was observed in three patients [18].

While the above-mentioned studies present satisfactory to good results with impaction grafting at mid- to long-term follow-up, there is some controversy if the long-term results of impaction grafting are durable. A recent study evaluated the 10-year outcomes following impaction grafting in revision of rotational and hinged knee arthroplasty [19]. At final follow-up, only 50% survival rate was noted. Twelve knees required re-revision surgery at a mean 5 years after the first revision due to mechanical failure and aseptic loosening of the components. In all failed cases, a lack of incorporation with graft resorption was noted during the re-revision procedure.

Bulk Allograft

Bulk structural allografts represent an alternative option for reconstruction of type II and III defects without the need for wire mesh. Structural bone allograft offers numerous advantages, including biocompatibility, bone stock restoration, potential for ligament reattachment, and can be relatively cost effective compared to large custom endoprostheses. Disadvantages include technical difficulty and prolonged operative times required to fashion the grafts, limited availability of adequate graft, nonunion, delayed union, collapse, graft resorption, graft infection, and the possibility of disease transmission. The goals of structural allograft reconstruction are to maximize the stability of the graft-bone contact and provide a stable platform for fixation of the implant. Despite meticulous technique, the early-to-mid-term results of bulk structural allografts in the revision setting are variable.

Several studies have reported the long-term outcomes of structural allografts in revision TKA with an average 74% graft survivorship at 10 years [20]. In their study of revision TKA with severe bone loss, Engh and Ammeen reported an 87% good-to-excellent outcome at a mean follow-up of 4.2 years and no collapse or aseptic loosening at a mean of 7.9 years [21]. Another larger study by Backstein et al. reported on 68 revision TKAs that required a structural allograft for the treatment of uncontained defects. They reported 85.2% of success rate at an average follow-up of 5.4 years. Thirteen revision TKAs failed due to graft related complications including one graft nonunion, three cases of aseptic loosening, three periprosthetic fractures, four infections, and two cases of instability. There were three cases of graft resorption, two graded as severe and one as moderate [22]. The Mayo Clinic also reported on 70 revision TKA cases with bulk structural allograft reconstruction with 5-year follow-up. Sixteen patients required additional revision surgery with half of them due to allograft failure and three due to failure of a component not supported by the allograft. Overall, they reported a revision-free survival rate of 75.9% at 10 years [23]. While most authors support the use of bulk structural allograft for reconstruction of severe tibial or femoral bone defects in revision TKA, the rate of complications and reoperations suggests a need for more durable alternative methods for these challenging reconstructions.

Modular Augments

In the setting of type II defects, modular augments can help to fill bony defects, ensure implant contact with host bone, and restore joint line and balance flexion and extension gaps. Augments are available in many shapes and forms, can be applied quickly, and can be attached with the use of cement or screws. They allow intraoperative customization, supply excellent biomechanical properties, and require minimal bone resection as the augments attach on the residual bone. Biomechanical testing has demonstrated that modular augments provide equivalent stability to custom-fabricated implants [10]. In addition, block augments are more stable than wedge augments which have a higher shear force [24]. Distal and posterior femoral defects managed with modular augments allow for the placement of a well-positioned and correctly sized femoral component in contact with host bone. The clinical results using small metal augments to treat these types of bone defects have been excellent. Patel et al. reported a 92% survival rate at 11 years in 79 revision TKAs treated with metal augments. Non-progressive radiolucent lines were evident in 14% but this had no effect on the clinical outcome at final follow-up [25].

In the revision setting where gap mismatch is common, our preference is to liberally use femoral augments, particularly distal and posterolateral, to recreate the joint line and assist with femoral component rotation. Tibial baseplate augments are best used to minimize polyethylene size. Unfortunately, several hemi tibial augments remove significant amounts of native bone during preparation. Our goal is usually to preserve bone whenever possible and use metaphyseal cones and sleeve with nonaugmented baseplates, if possible.

Metaphyseal Cones and Sleeves

The use of metaphyseal cones and sleeves allows for treatment of bone loss and provides additional fixation near the joint line. Both cones and sleeves can be used in direct contact with the bone in a press-fit fashion or as part of a fully cemented construct. When used in press-fit fashion, cones and sleeves can achieve peripheral osseous ingrowth and offer the potential for long-term structural support. Cones and sleeves offer potential advantages over traditional reconstructive techniques like bulk allograft or impaction grafting. Advantages include the ability to provide mechanical support and the potential for long-term biologic fixation, decrease the complexity of the reconstruction, enable immediate weight-bearing, and avoid the issues of disease transmission, graft resorption, and collapse associated with bone graft. Disadvantages include expense, native host bone removal during preparation, and difficulty with extraction if necessary.

Sleeves are typically made of titanium and stepped in shape. They are typically prepared via broach technique and fashioned directly to the implant via a Morse taper. When coated with titanium beads, they provide a porous ingrowth surface for osseous integration. If sufficient rotational stability is achieved after host bone preparation, they can be used in uncemented fashion. If inadequate rotational control is achieved, they can be used in a cemented fashion with the host bone, akin to a very large keel. Whether used in a cemented or uncemented fashion, there is currently no consensus on the superiority of one technique over the other for type 2 defects. Our preference is to use titanium sleeves in an uncemented technique whenever possible.

The use of sleeves in revision total knee arthroplasty is primarily supported by short- and mid-term results. Alexander et al. reported on the use of 30 tibial metaphyseal sleeves for type 2B and type 3 AORI defects with minimum 2-year follow-up. All radiographs at final follow-up showed well-fixed components with osseous ingrowth [26]. Agarwal et al. reported on 104 revision TKAs treated with metaphyseal sleeves with a mean follow-up of 43 months. At final follow-up, 102 knees had achieved osseointegration with only two tibial sleeves revised for loosening. The authors noted that both loose sleeves did not have stems and recommended the use of stems in all patients [27]. Huang et al. prospectively reported the short-term results of revision TKA in 83 knees with both femoral and tibial metaphyseal sleeves using both nonhinged and hinged designs over a minimum 2-year follow-up. None of the cases demonstrated progressive radiolucent lines around the metaphyseal sleeves. At final follow-up, two (2.7%) tibial components required revision for aseptic loosening [28]. Barnett et al. retrospectively reviewed data on 40 patients who underwent revision TKA utilizing a metaphyseal sleeve for AORI type 2 and 3 tibial defects. At a mean of 38 months, no patients demonstrated aseptic loosening. Radiographic review at final follow-up revealed stable, osseointegrated components in all cases [29]. As for mid-term follow-up, there are fewer studies available that report on the outcomes of metaphyseal sleeves. Jones et al. reported on 30 hinged revision TKAs at a mean of 4 years with no mechanical failures, and all sleeves showed radiographic apposition and positive remodeling of bone [30]. A more recent study reported on 134 revision TKAs with titanium sleeves with median follow-up 72 months. Radiological evaluation showed osseous integration in all patients without implant migration nor radiolucent lines. Two patients were revised in the first year for septic failure, but no aseptic revisions were reported at final follow-up [31].

Overall, the above-mentioned studies only included type 2 defects with the exception of Alexander et al. (2013) that also reported on some type 3 defects. As such, the use of metaphyseal sleeves has mainly been reserved for less severe defects and should be used cautiously when treating massive bone loss. This is particularly important if initial axial and rotational stability cannot be achieved. In these cases, our preference would be to use cones or segmental replacements. Overall, short-term results demonstrate 2.6% revision rate for aseptic loosening.

Cones, most commonly made of tantalum, are prepared independently of the final implant using broaches, burrs, or reamers. Cones must be cemented to unitize to the final implant construct. The high porosity of tantalum enables bone ingrowth. Upon osseous integration, the cone shares the intramedullary axial loading forces, effectively protecting the epiphyseal fixation and improving the rotational stability of the construct. With significant scratch fit and proper preparation, however, early postoperative restrictions are not necessary. Clinical loosening of the cement interface between implant and cone has not been reported.

Several studies have reported on the excellent short-term outcomes of cones in the revision TKA setting. Long and Scuderi described 16 patients who were treated with tibial metaphyseal cones with 31-month follow-up. There were no revisions for aseptic loosening, and all patients showed radiographic evidence of osseointegration. Two cones required removal for septic revision but were well-fixed at the time of surgery [32]. The other series reported on 15 patients who underwent revision TKA with tibial cones and were followed for a minimum of 2 years. All of the cones demonstrated radiographic evidence of ingrowth without failures [33]. Lachiewicz et al. retrospectively reviewed 27 patients followed for a minimum of 2 years (mean 3.3 years) after implantation of 33 tantalum cones (9 femoral, 24 tibial). All but one cone showed osseointegration, which required revision for femoral cone and component loosening [34].

The encouraging short-term results of metaphyseal cones have proved to be durable at mid-term follow-up. Kamath et al. reported on 66 tibial cones for type 2 or 3 defects were assessed at a mean follow-up of 5.8 years (range, 60 to 106 months). One patient had progressive radiolucency about the tibial stem and cone. One patient had complete radiolucency about the tibial cone, concerning for fibrous ingrowth. Three cones were revised: one for infection, one for aseptic loosening, and one for periprosthetic fracture. Revision-free survival of the tibial metaphyseal cone was >95% at the time of the latest follow-up. Overall, the published studies of short- and mid-term results of metaphyseal cones have demonstrated a cumulative mean revision rate for aseptic cone loosening of 1.1% [35].

Patellar Bone Loss

In the revision knee setting, patellar bone stock can be severely compromised. Most commonly, bone loss is secondary to patellar button loosening and osteolysis. Trabecular metal patella represents a viable therapeutic option for severe damaged patella [36]. In our practice, we limit use of trabecular metal patellar components to revision cases with more than 50% amount of residual bone, with care in obtaining reliable bony fixation despite usual poor quality of residual bone. In cases of previous patellectomy, we caution the use of trabecular metal patella relying only on soft tissue fixation due to reports of migrations and loosening [37].

Case Presentations

Case #1 (Figs. 9.1, 9.2, and 9.3–9.4)

A 72-year-old female presented with acute onset of left knee pain status-post mechanical fall. She had undergone left total knee arthroplasty 34 years ago. She states that she had developed progressive bowing of her legs over the last several years but had not sought orthopedic follow-up in over a decade. For the last 6 months, she had required the use of a walker at all times for ambulation. Workup demonstrated an acute distal

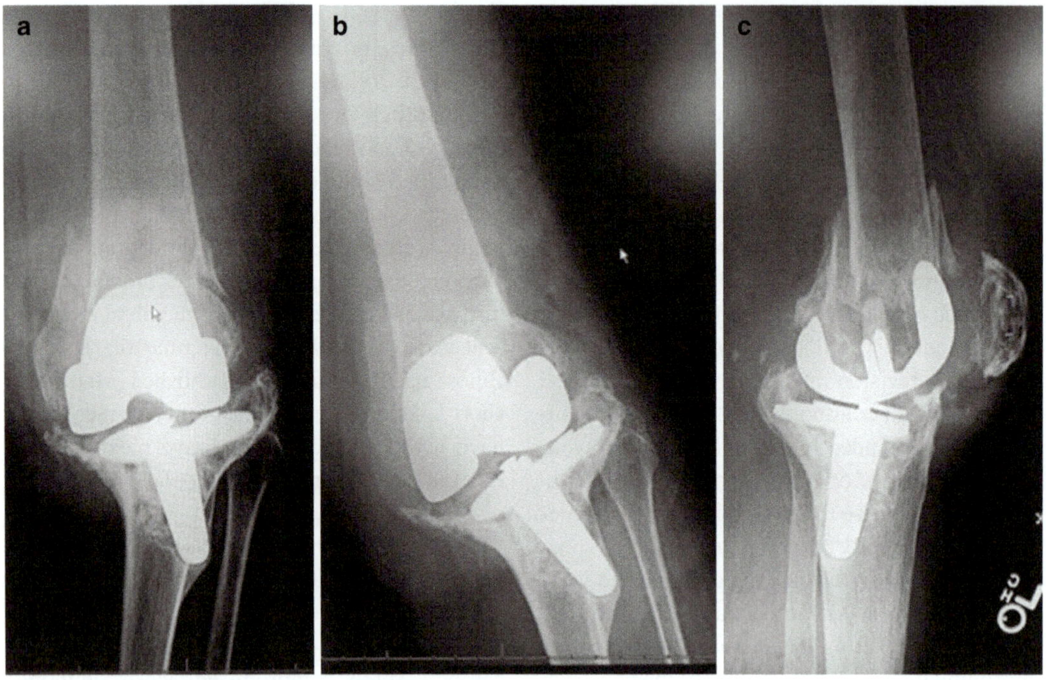

Fig. 9.1 (a–c) AP oblique and lateral radiographs exhibiting a periprosthetic fracture about the femoral component of a TKA. Of note, there is severe lysis and deformity of the tibial component, with radiographic periosteal changes that can be consistent with comcomitant a loose tibial component

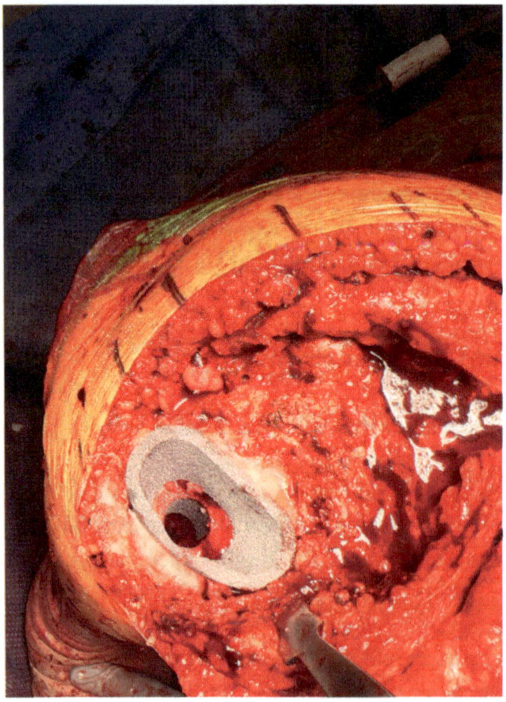

Fig. 9.2 Intraoperative clinical photograph exhibiting the use of a cementless, trabecular metal cone

femur periprosthetic fracture in the setting of a failed total knee arthroplasty. The femoral component was well-fixed but there was extensive osteolysis noted in the entire distal femur. The tibial component demonstrated chronic varus collapse with obvious loosening and extensive remodeling of the proximal tibia.

Intraoperatively, the polyethylene liner was partially fractured and worn due to baseplate on the medial side. Due to the unreconstructible nature of the distal femur in the setting of periprosthetic fracture, decision was made to proceed with distal femoral replacement with a hinged construct. On the tibia, bone loss was assessed after removal of the grossly loose baseplate as AORI Type III with only a partial rim of cortical bone. This bone was deemed unsupportive for baseplate. Decision was made to obtain fixation in the diaphysis with a femoral diaphyseal trabecular metal cone (Zimmer-Biomet, Warsaw, IN) and stack a tibial metaphyseal cone on top. The cones were inserted in a press-fit fashion and demineralized bone matrix putty was used to fill

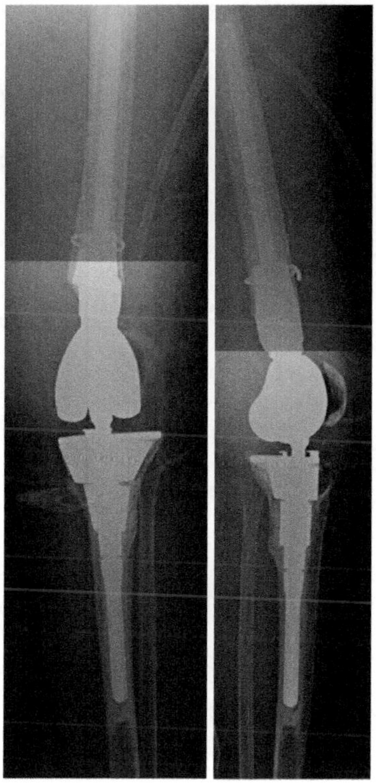

Figs. 9.3–9.4 AP and lateral post-operative radiograph with DFR and tibial reconstruction with cones and cemented stems

gaps between cones and bone. To complete the reconstruction, a long cemented stem with restrictor was used for immediate fixation.

Case #2 (Figs. 9.5, 9.6, 9.7–9.8, and 9.9)

An 80-year-old female presented with over 15-year history of bilateral knee pain and end-stage osteoarthritis. On examination, she is an obese woman (BMI 36) of average height with bilateral uncorrectable varus alignment. She underwent uncomplicated left total knee arthroplasty and was discharged to home on postoperative day #2. She was pleased with her postoperative correction in her alignment and ROM. While working with home physiotherapy 1 week after surgery, she noted atraumatic onset of increasing pain with progressive bowing of her operative leg. She presented to her surgeon's office where radiographs demonstrated a displaced medial femoral condyle periprosthetic fracture in significant varus alignment. Based on prior experience with similar periprosthetic insufficiency fractures, decision was made to pursue with revision surgery in a delayed manner. She was made non-weightbearing on the left lower extremity for approximately 6 weeks. Repeat radiographs prior to surgery revealed partial fracture healing without further displacement. She underwent revision total knee arthroplasty in an uncomplicated manner. Her medial femoral condyle had healed in a proximal and posteromedial position. This created a severe mismatch with the flexion and extension gaps. Several distal femoral and posterior augments were used to recreate the joint line and extensive soft tissue releases were used to balance the gaps. Large medial augments were used to reestablish the medial malunion. Given the partially united fracture, decision to use metaphyseal titanium cone (Stryker, Mahwah, NJ) fixation in addition to an intermediate length fully cemented stem for diaphyseal fixation. The metaphyseal cone was used to build a solid base upon which the distal augments were built-up and used to establish the joint line. The final construct used was large distal and posterior augments with porous uncemented metaphyseal cones and fully cemented stems for diaphyseal fixation.

With poor bone quality as in this patient, the author's experience has shown that removal of well-fixed total knee arthroplasty components in the setting of acute fracture commonly results in massive and unexpected bone loss. The end result is usually distal femoral or proximal tibia replacement. In our practice, we have recently started moving to delayed or subacute management of these periprosthetic fractures. The rationale is that with partial or full consolidation of the fracture, even in a mal-united position, is preferable to bone loss associated with acute revision and de-vascularization associated with surgical insult.

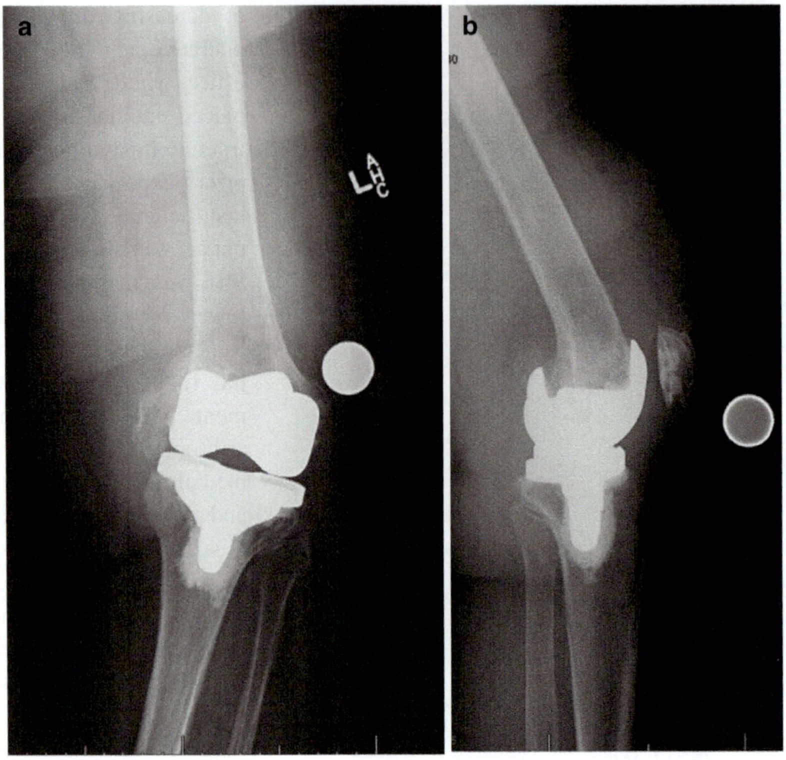

Fig. 9.5 (**a, b**) AP and lateral radiographs exhibiting periprosthetic medial condyle fracture

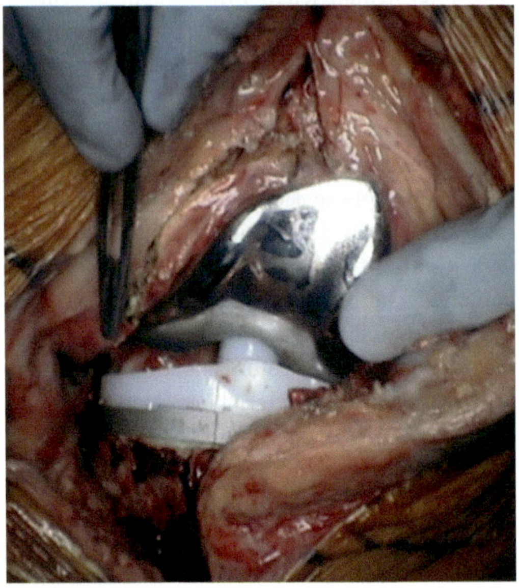

Fig. 9.6 Intraoperative clinical photo exhibiting healed fracture with deformity

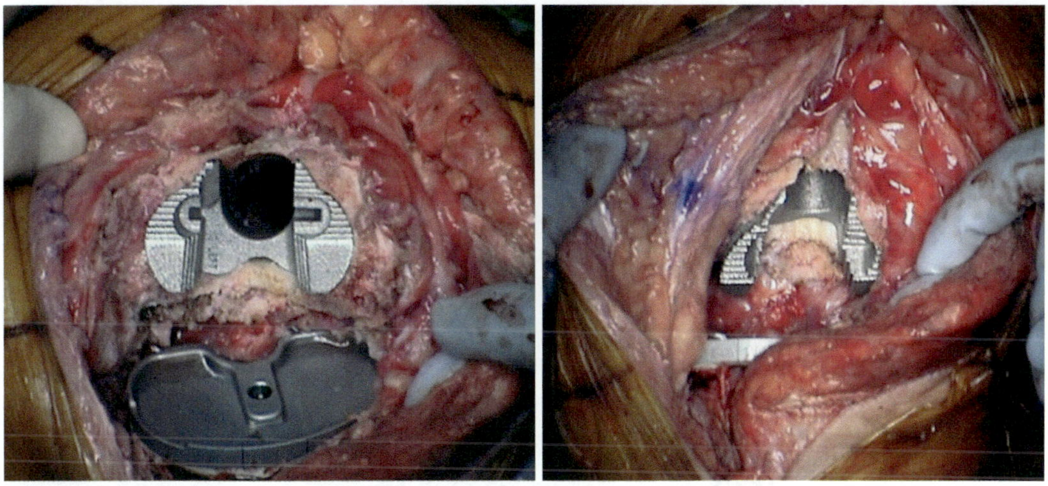

Figs. 9.7–9.8 Intraoperative clinical photo exhibiting use of metaphyseal cones to comat bone loss

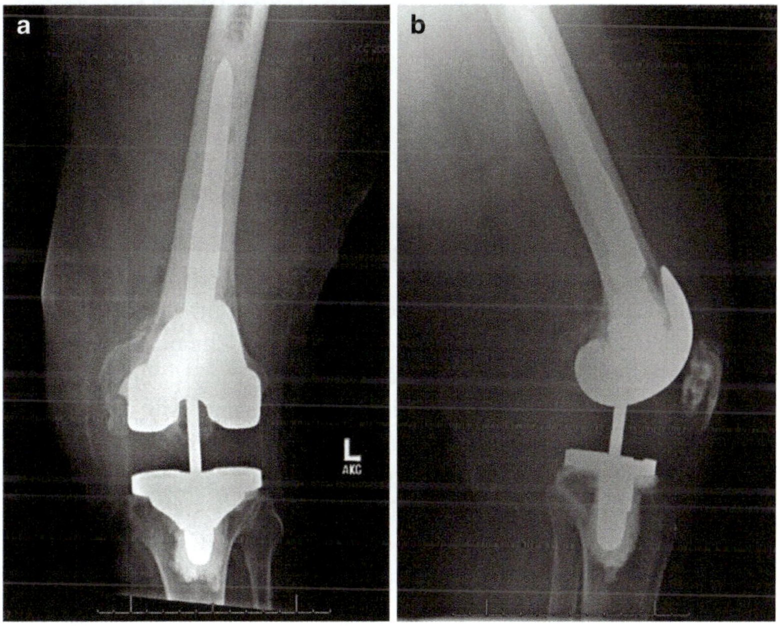

Fig. 9.9 (**a, b**) Post-op radiographs following complete femoral component revision

Case #3 (Figs. 9.10–9.11, and 9.12–9.13)

A 70-year-old female with history of multiple operations and two prior revisions of left total knee arthroplasty including patellectomy presented to our center for management of acute hematogenous periprosthetic joint infection. She initially underwent irrigation and debridement with modular component exchange but subsequently required explantation with placement of static antibiotic spacer. After an additional debridement, static spacer exchange, and antibiotic course, she was a candidate for reimplantation. After appropriate antibiotic treatment, she underwent reimplantation. Meticulous exposure of her remaining extensor mechanism was performed, including quadriceps snip, recreation of

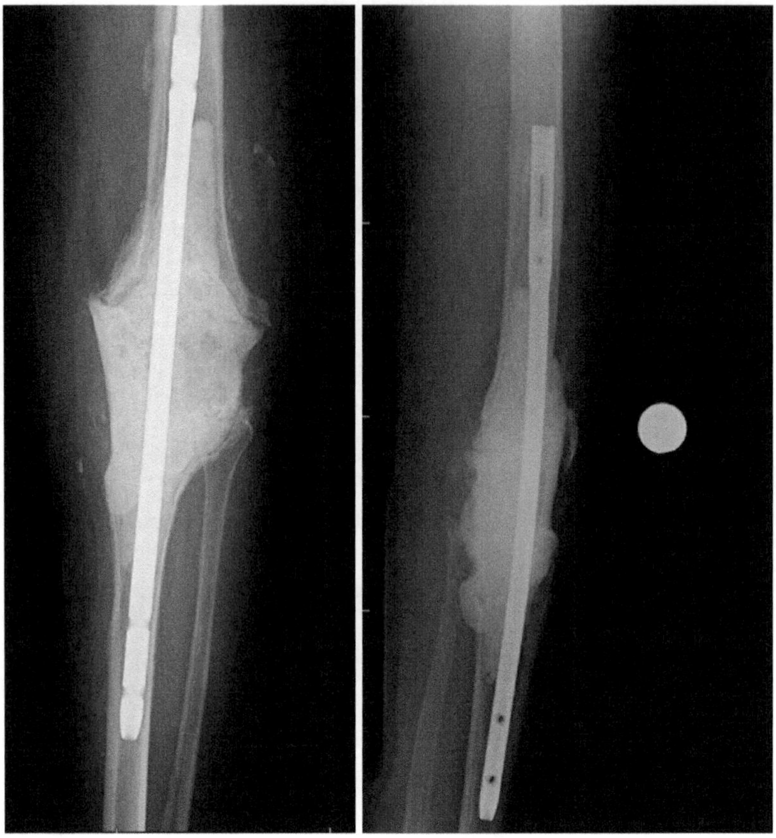

Figs. 9.10–9.11 AP and lateral radiographs following static cement spacer placement after irrigation and debridement

gutters, and posteromedial tibial release. Her prior patellectomy somewhat facilitated exposure but extreme was taken when retracting against the extensor mechanism. Using a series of osteotomes, the cement block spacer was removed. The intramedullary nail was not mobile due to retained cement in the intramedullary canal. Using a metal cutting wheel, the nail was cut and removed prior to flexing the knee. Care must be taken to avoid flexing the knee unless the IM nail can be mobilized proximal or distal. This can be a source of iatrogenic fracture that can be easily avoided with patience. After complete exposure, patient was noted to have an approximate 8 cm gap between her distal femur and tibia, with significant asymmetric bone loss of her medial tibial plateau and no remaining distal femur or epicondyles. Decision was made to manage her bone loss with fully cemented stems and stepped asymmetric trabecular metal augments on the tibia and distal femoral segmental replacement (Zimmer-Biomet, Warsaw, IN). The trabecular metal augments were fashioned for porous ingrowth against host bone and cemented on inner surface against stem. Fully cemented stems were used for diaphyseal fixation.

Additionally, setting appropriate external rotation is difficult whenever the epicondyles and collateral ligaments are absent. If an appropriately rotated implant is present, scoring the anterior cortex helps to maintain rotation when implanting the TFMT. In this case, the revision followed a static antibiotic spacer. We placed a mark on the anterior cortex prior to completely removing the antibiotic spacer. When implanting the final implant, we provided an additional five to seven degrees of external rotation. In our experience, there is little downside to additional external implant rotation in a hinged device, but significant downside to poor patellofemoral tracking.

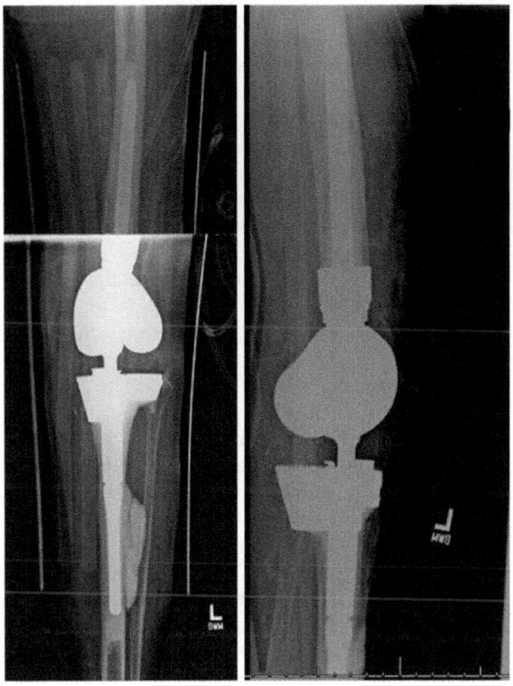

Figs. 9.12–9.13 AP and lateral radiograph exhibiting final reconstruction with DFR. Additional femoral external rotation can help assist in proper patellar tracking

Conclusion

As the number of revision TKAs continues to rise, the appropriate management of bone loss will continue to be of paramount importance for the reconstructive surgeon. While numerous reconstructive options are available to manage bone loss, the optimal method is specific to the degree of bone loss, surgeon familiarity, and the unique characteristics of the patient. In general, the larger the defect, the more robust the reconstruction should be. We recommend using stem fixation whenever a femoral or tibial component is revised. In smaller defects, knowing when to use cement or nonstructural bone graft can provide excellent results in a cost-effective manner. When dealing with larger defects, cones and sleeves represent the most recent advances in the treatment of metaphyseal bone loss during revision TKA. These implants have revolutionized how we address bone loss, offering the potential for biologic ingrowth and a mechanically stable revision construct while avoiding many of the issues associated with bone grafting. While cost may be a concern, the excellent results of metaphyseal cones and sleeves, in the authors' opinion, make the use of other less reliable techniques like impaction bone grafting and structural allografts obsolete in our practice.

Authors' Preferred Method and Take-Home Points

- Use stems whenever a femoral or tibial component is revised.
- Short cemented stems demonstrate equivalent outcomes to longer cementless stems—use the technique familiar to the surgeon.
- In small defects, cement or cement with screws is quick, cost-effective, and is likely all that is needed.
- In larger defects, avoid use of impaction bone grafting or structural allograft.
- Metaphyseal fixation, whether in the form of cones or sleeves, should be used in the vast majority of revision TKAs to offload the implant near the joint line.
- Avoid sleeves in type 3 defects. Use cones in these settings.
- Bigger is usually better—err on the side of stability in major reconstructions.

References

1. Harrysson OL, Robertsson O, Nayfeh JF. Higher cumulative revision rate of knee arthroplasties in younger patients with osteoarthritis. Clin Orthop Relat Res. 2004;421:162–8.
2. Iorio R, Robb WJ, Healy WL, Berry DJ, Hozack WJ, Kyle RF, et al. Orthopaedic surgeon workforce and volume assessment for total hip and knee replacement in the United States: preparing for an epidemic. J Bone Joint Surg Am. 2008;90(7):1598–605. https://doi.org/10.2106/JBJS.H.00067.
3. Kurtz S, Mowat F, Ong K, Chan N, Lau E, Halpern M. Prevalence of primary and revision total hip and knee arthroplasty in the United States from 1990 through 2002. J Bone Joint Surg Am. 2005;87(7):1487–97. https://doi.org/10.2106/JBJS.D.02441.
4. Lombardi AV, Berend KR, Adams JB. Management of bone loss in revision TKA: it's a changing world. Orthopedics. 2010;33(9):662. https://doi.org/10.3928/01477447-20100722-37.

5. Engh GA, Ammeen DJ. Bone loss with revision total knee arthroplasty: defect classification and alternatives for reconstruction. Instr Course Lect. 1999;48:167–75.
6. Vasso M, Beaufils P, Schiavone Panni A. Constraint choice in revision knee arthroplasty. Int Orthop. 2013;37(7):1279–84. https://doi.org/10.1007/s00264-013-1929-y.
7. Daines BK, Dennis DA. Management of bone defects in revision total knee arthroplasty. Instr Course Lect. 2013;62:341–8.
8. Lachiewicz PF, Soileau ES. A 30-mm cemented stem extension provides adequate fixation of the tibial component in revision knee arthroplasty. Clin Orthop Relat Res. 2015;473(1):185–9. https://doi.org/10.1007/s11999-014-3529-6.
9. Nelson CL, Vanushkina M, Irgit K, Strohecker K, Bowen TR. Stemmed femoral implants show lower failure rates in revision total knee arthroplasty. Knee. 2015;22(5):429–34. https://doi.org/10.1016/j.knee.2015.02.013.
10. Brooks PJ, Walker PS, Scott RD. Tibial component fixation in deficient tibial bone stock. Clin Orthop Relat Res. 1984;184:302–8.
11. Lotke PA, Wong RY, Ecker ML. The use of methylmethacrylate in primary total knee replacements with large tibial defects. Clin Orthop Relat Res. 1991;270:288–94.
12. Ritter MA. Screw and cement fixation of large defects in total knee arthroplasty. J Arthroplast. 1986;1(2):125–9.
13. Krackow KA, Raju S, Puttaswamy MK. Medial over-resection of the tibia in total knee arthroplasty for varus deformity using computer navigation. J Arthroplast. 2015;30(5):766–9. https://doi.org/10.1016/j.arth.2014.11.034.
14. Mullaji AB, Shetty GM. Correction of varus deformity during TKA with reduction osteotomy. Clin Orthop Relat Res. 2014;472(1):126–32. https://doi.org/10.1007/s11999-013-3077-5.
15. Mabry TM, Hanssen AD. The role of stems and augments for bone loss in revision knee arthroplasty. J Arthroplast. 2007;22(4 Suppl 1):56–60. https://doi.org/10.1016/j.arth.2007.02.008.
16. Lotke PA, Carolan GF, Puri N. Impaction grafting for bone defects in revision total knee arthroplasty. Clin Orthop Relat Res. 2006;446:99–103. https://doi.org/10.1097/01.blo.0000214414.06464.00.
17. Hanna SA, Aston WJ, de Roeck NJ, Gough-Palmer A, Powles DP. Cementless revision TKA with bone grafting of osseous defects restores bone stock with a low revision rate at 4 to 10 years. Clin Orthop Relat Res. 2011;469(11):3164–71. https://doi.org/10.1007/s11999-011-1938-3.
18. Lonner JH, Lotke PA, Kim J, Nelson C. Impaction grafting and wire mesh for uncontained defects in revision knee arthroplasty. Clin Orthop Relat Res. 2002;404:145–51.
19. Hilgen V, Citak M, Vettorazzi E, Haasper C, Day K, Amling M, et al. 10-year results following impaction bone grafting of major bone defects in 29 rotational and hinged knee revision arthroplasties: a follow-up of a previous report. Acta Orthop. 2013;84(4):387–91. https://doi.org/10.3109/17453674.2013.814012.
20. Clatworthy MG, Ballance J, Brick GW, Chandler HP, Gross AE. The use of structural allograft for uncontained defects in revision total knee arthroplasty. A minimum 5-year review. J Bone Joint Surg Am. 2001;83-A(3):404–11.
21. Engh GA, Ammeen DJ. Use of structural allograft in revision total knee arthroplasty in knees with severe tibial bone loss. J Bone Joint Surg Am. 2007;89(12):2640–7. https://doi.org/10.2106/JBJS.F.00865.
22. Backstein D, Safir O, Gross A. Management of bone loss: structural grafts in revision total knee arthroplasty. Clin Orthop Relat Res. 2006;446:104–12. https://doi.org/10.1097/01.blo.0000214426.52206.2c.
23. Bauman RD, Lewallen DG, Hanssen AD. Limitations of structural allograft in revision total knee arthroplasty. Clin Orthop Relat Res. 2009;467(3):818–24. https://doi.org/10.1007/s11999-008-0679-4.
24. Chen F, Krackow KA. Management of tibial defects in total knee arthroplasty. A biomechanical study. Clin Orthop Relat Res. 1994;305:249–57.
25. Patel JV, Masonis JL, Guerin J, Bourne RB, Rorabeck CH. The fate of augments to treat type-2 bone defects in revision knee arthroplasty. J Bone Joint Surg Br. 2004;86(2):195–9.
26. Alexander GE, Bernasek TL, Crank RL, Haidukewych GJ. Cementless metaphyseal sleeves used for large tibial defects in revision total knee arthroplasty. J Arthroplast. 2013;28(4):604–7. https://doi.org/10.1016/j.arth.2012.08.006.
27. Agarwal S, Azam A, Morgan-Jones R. Metal metaphyseal sleeves in revision total knee replacement. Bone Joint J. 2013;95-B(12):1640–4. https://doi.org/10.1302/0301-620X.95B12.31190.
28. Huang R, Barrazueta G, Ong A, Orozco F, Jafari M, Coyle C, Austin M. Revision total knee arthroplasty using metaphyseal sleeves at short-term follow-up. Orthopedics. 2014;37(9):e804–9. https://doi.org/10.3928/01477447-20140825-57.
29. Barnett SL, Mayer RR, Gondusky JS, Choi L, Patel JJ, Gorab RS. Use of stepped porous titanium metaphyseal sleeves for tibial defects in revision total knee arthroplasty: short term results. J Arthroplast. 2014;29(6):1219–24. https://doi.org/10.1016/j.arth.2013.12.026.
30. Jones RE, Barrack RL, Skedros J. Modular, mobile-bearing hinge total knee arthroplasty. Clin Orthop Relat Res. 2001;392:306–14.
31. Martin-Hernandez C, Floria-Arnal LJ, Muniesa-Herrero MP, Espallargas-Donate T, Blanco-Llorca JA, Guillen-Soriano M, Ranera-Garcia M. Mid-term results for metaphyseal sleeves in revision knee surgery. Knee Surg Sports Traumatol Arthrosc. 2017;25(12):3779–85. https://doi.org/10.1007/s00167-016-4298-4.

32. Long WJ, Scuderi GR. Porous tantalum cones for large metaphyseal tibial defects in revision total knee arthroplasty: a minimum 2-year follow-up. J Arthroplast. 2009;24(7):1086–92. https://doi.org/10.1016/j.arth.2008.08.011.
33. Meneghini RM, Lewallen DG, Hanssen AD. Use of porous tantalum metaphyseal cones for severe tibial bone loss during revision total knee replacement. J Bone Joint Surg Am. 2008;90(1):78–84. https://doi.org/10.2106/JBJS.F.01495.
34. Lachiewicz PF, Bolognesi MP, Henderson RA, Soileau ES, Vail TP. Can tantalum cones provide fixation in complex revision knee arthroplasty? Clin Orthop Relat Res. 2012;470(1):199–204. https://doi.org/10.1007/s11999-011-1888-9.
35. Sculco PK, Abdel MP, Hanssen AD, Lewallen DG. The management of bone loss in revision total knee arthroplasty: rebuild, reinforce, and augment. Bone Joint J. 2016;98-B(1 Suppl A):120–4. https://doi.org/10.1302/0301-620X.98B1.36345.
36. Tigani D, Trentani P, Trentani F, Andreoli I, Sabbioni G, Del Piccolo N. Trabecular metal patella in total knee arthroplasty with patella bone deficiency. Knee. 2009;16(1):46–9. https://doi.org/10.1016/j.knee.2008.08.005.
37. Ries MD, Cabalo A, Bozic KJ, Anderson M. Porous tantalum patellar augmentation: the importance of residual bone stock. Clin Orthop Relat Res. 2006;452:166–70. https://doi.org/10.1097/01.blo.0000229359.27491.9f.

10 Revision Knee Arthroplasty in the Setting of a Deficient Extensor Mechanism

George J. Haidukewych and Obinna O. Adigweme

Background

Quadriceps Rupture

Quadriceps tendon rupture after TKA is very uncommon with an incidence around 0.1–1.1% [2, 3]. The incidence increases in the setting of revision knee arthroplasty [3]. Quadriceps rupture is the least common form of extensor mechanism disruption after TKA. Systemic risk factors for this include diabetes mellitus, chronic renal failure, rheumatoid arthritis, obesity, and hyperthyroidism [3, 4]. Surgical risk factors include an aberrant parapatellar approach or lateral release, decreased vascularity after lateral release, previous patellectomy, and over-resection of the patella [2]. The friability of the tissues and need for better exposure in the case of revision surgery also places the quadriceps tendon at risk. Additionally, when performing a quadriceps snip for exposure, the surgeon must ensure not to transect the tendon.

Due to the rarity of this complication, there is a paucity of literature addressing its management. Partial tears may be treated nonoperatively with the knee immobilized in full extension for 6 weeks. Complete ruptures generally require operative treatment. Options for operative treatment include direct repair, allograft reconstruction, or autograft reconstruction.

Direct repair is historically unsuccessful with high failure rates. Dobbs et al. reviewed ten patients with complete quadriceps tears after TKA treated with direct repair. Six patients had unsatisfactory results, including four re-ruptures. They concluded that primary repair resulted in poor outcomes and an unacceptably high complication rate [3].

More recently, however, Chhappan et al. reported successful results with direct repair of acute quadriceps ruptures after TKA. Ten postoperative quadriceps ruptures within 3 months of TKA were treated with direct repair. Within 6 months, all patients exhibited no extension lag and good range of motion. Thus, prompt repair of acute quadriceps rupture after recent TKA was shown to be a viable option.

Extensor mechanism reconstruction is considered the gold standard for operative treatment. Reconstruction options include autograft, allograft, and synthetic mesh.

Shi et al. reported results of autogenous reconstruction for quadriceps tendon ruptures after TKA. In this technique, a direct repair was performed followed by a full-thickness triangular V-Y turndown flap of quadriceps tendon for augmentation of the repair. At average 2-year follow-up, only one failure was observed, the majority achieved successful outcomes [5].

G. J. Haidukewych (✉)
Department of Orthopedic Surgery, Orlando Health, Orlando, FL, USA

O. O. Adigweme
Rothman Orthopedic Institute, Orlando, FL, USA

R. S. Yoon et al. (eds.), *Trauma and Infection Control in Revision Hip and Knee Arthroplasty*,
https://doi.org/10.1007/978-3-031-71971-4_10

Rust et al. reported on the use of the Leeds-Keio artificial ligament to reconstruct a quadriceps tendon rupture after revision knee arthroplasty [6]. The ligament is made of polyester and has a mesh structure. The technique involves insertion of the ligament in a figure of eight fashion, and weaving through the retracted quadriceps muscle and tendon proximally and the patellar tendon distally. The graft is then passed anterior to the patella and sutured anteriorly to the periosteum. At 2-year follow-up, the patient had an intact straight leg raise, minimal extensor lag, and 100 degrees of flexion. Larger series are needed to evaluate this technique.

Achilles tendon allograft and synthetic mesh reconstruction techniques will be discussed later in this chapter.

Patellar Fractures

Periprosthetic patellar fractures represent a rare and potentially debilitating injury. The prevalence of this injury is 0.1–0.68% and is notably higher after revision arthroplasty [7, 8]. Patient-related risk factors include obesity, osteoporosis, increased activity level, inflammatory arthritis, and excessive knee flexion. Surgical factors that may increase risk include a lateral release, decreased patellar thickness, limb or component malalignment, and metal-backed patellar component designs [9–13].

Historically, operative treatment for these injuries is wrought with complications. Nonoperative treatment is preferred in the setting of an intact extensor mechanism and a stable patellar component. Loose patellar components should be removed only if symptomatic, and loss of extension may be addressed surgically. Patellar bone stock must be considered in treatment decisions. If the patient has loss of extension and adequate bone stock, open reduction and internal fixation can be considered. Allograft augmentation is often required for an extensor repair in the setting of poor patellar bone stock. Extensor allograft reconstruction with patellectomy should be considered in failed repairs as a salvage procedure. However, even in the setting of extensor disruption after patellar fracture, nonoperative treatment should be considered with immobilization for 6–8 weeks. Again, this is due to high complication rates with operative treatment. If a trial of nonoperative management fails, reconstructive techniques remain an option.

Ortiguera and Berry reviewed 85 patellar fractures following TKA [8]. A total of 38 fractures were associated with a stable component and an intact extensor mechanism. Thirty-seven were treated nonoperatively with good results in 97%. Twelve fractures were associated with extensor mechanism disruption, 11 of which were treated operatively. Patients underwent internal fixation (6 knees) or partial patellectomy with tendon repair (5 knees). Six patients (55%) undergoing surgical treatment had complications. Five required reoperation and seven had pain, patellar or extensor instability, or weakness. An additional 12 fractures in this series were associated with a loose patellar component and supportive bone stock. Four of these were treated nonoperatively, whereas eight underwent surgical intervention. All five knees treated with resection of patellar component and internal fixation had complications, with two knees requiring a reoperation. Sixteen fractures were associated with a loose patellar implant and poor bone stock, of which 12 were treated operatively. Of these, seven had persistent pain, patellar or extensor instability, or weakness, and one had an operative complication.

Keating et al. retrospectively reviewed 177 periprosthetic patellar fractures [9]. Twenty-two fractures had stable components and intact extensor mechanisms. Twenty-one of these fractures were treated nonoperatively with good results. There were an additional 22 fractures with disrupted extensor mechanisms and stable components, of which 21 were treated nonoperatively. These resulted in excellent function and no extensor lag. Of the 17 fractures noted to have both an extensor mechanism discontinuity and a loose component, 3 were treated operatively with postoperative infection occurring in 1 patient. The remaining patients possessed intact extensor mechanisms and loose components. Only six of these were treated surgically; however, 50% of these patients developed complications. The authors concluded that operative treatment should be avoided if possible due to high complication rates.

Parvizi et al. compared patients treated nonoperatively and operatively [14]. Twelve periprosthetic patellar fractures were reviewed. Seven were nondisplaced and treated nonoperatively with good-to-excellent outcomes. Operative treatment was performed in five knees with three good outcomes and two fair outcomes; however, two of the five surgically treated fractures had complications (40%) requiring reoperation.

Patellar Tendon Ruptures

Patellar tendon rupture or avulsion after total knee arthroplasty is a rare and potentially devastating problem. The incidence of patellar tendon disruption in primary TKA is reported around 0.17–2.5% [1, 2, 15]. The incidence after revision TKA has not been reported but is expected to be significantly higher due to poor tissue quality. Patient factors that increase risk include diabetes mellitus, chronic kidney disease, and rheumatoid arthritis. Surgical risk factors include difficult exposure in the revision setting, previous high tibial osteotomy, and systemic disease. Postoperative trauma, usually a fall directly onto a hyperflexed knee, may result in patellar tendon injury. Rupture may also occur postoperatively without trauma. Patients may present with a palpable defect, patella alta, and an extension lag.

The options for management include casting and bracing, primary repair, and reconstruction. Nonoperative management has yielded generally poor results, as expected, and is reserved for nonambulatory patients or those with prohibitive medical comorbidities. Primary repair has demonstrated unacceptably high failure rates [1]. Rand et al. reported only a 25% success rate with operative treatment of the patellar tendon after TKA using a variety of techniques [1]. Techniques included staple fixation, xenograft reconstruction, semitendinosus reconstruction, and direct repair. All direct repairs failed.

Reconstruction is the standard of care for the treatment of extensor mechanism disruption after TKA. Reconstruction options include autograft (e.g., gastrocnemius rotational flap, semitendinosus), allograft (Achilles tendon bone block, whole extensor mechanism allograft), or synthetic mesh.

Crossett et al. reviewed the use of Achilles tendon allograft in the treatment of patellar tendon rupture after TKA in nine patients [16]. The average extensor lag decreased from 44° preoperatively to 3° postoperatively, with six patients having full active extension. All patients reported improved functional ability. There were two graft failures and one deep infection.

Ares et al. reviewed five patients with chronic patellar tendon ruptures after TKA [17]. These patients were treated with a modified Achilles allograft reconstruction technique which involved dividing the Achilles tendon into two bundles and overcrossing these through the distal aspect of the quadriceps tendon. The mean active extension was −1.4°, and all patients were able to ambulate without crutches.

Nazarian and Booth reported on 36 knees with complete extensor mechanism disruption after TKA who underwent allograft reconstruction with whole extensor allograft [18]. At a minimum 2-year follow-up, 21 patients had full active extension. The other 13 patients had an average extension lag of 13°. There were eight re-ruptures which were treated with repeat reconstruction. Reconstruction with complete extensor mechanism has largely been abandoned.

Barrack et al. reported a series of 14 patients with chronic extensor mechanism disruption [19]. Eight patients underwent reconstruction with an Achilles tendon with calcaneal bone block and six with whole extensor mechanism allograft. Postoperatively, 10 of 14 patients had an extensor lag of <10°, and all patients were community ambulators.

Synthetic Mesh Extensor Mechanism Reconstruction

Synthetic mesh reconstruction, an alternative to allograft reconstruction has been growing in popularity. Advantages over other reconstruction techniques include availability, cost, and no risk of disease transmission. In this technique, the mesh acts as a scaffold for tissue ingrowth. Browne and Hanssen [20] described the technique (Fig. 10.1).

Browne and Hanssen reviewed 13 patients with deficient patellar tendons who underwent reconstruction with synthetic mesh [20]. All but one patient had undergone a previous revision arthroplasty procedure. Three patients had evidence of failed mesh reconstruction. The remaining patients had an extensor lag that improved from a mean of 36° preop to 10° at most recent follow-up. Furthermore, the cost of synthetic mesh was dramatically less.

Abdel et al. reported results of 77 patient who underwent extensor Marlex mesh extensor reconstruction [21]. There were 12 failures requiring mesh revision. Four mesh failures were treated nonoperatively with bracing. At mean 4-year follow-up, 84% of mesh reconstructions remained with excellent outcomes with mean 26° extensor lag improvement.

A recent multicenter, retrospective study compared allograft reconstruction with mesh reconstruction for extensor [22]. There were no

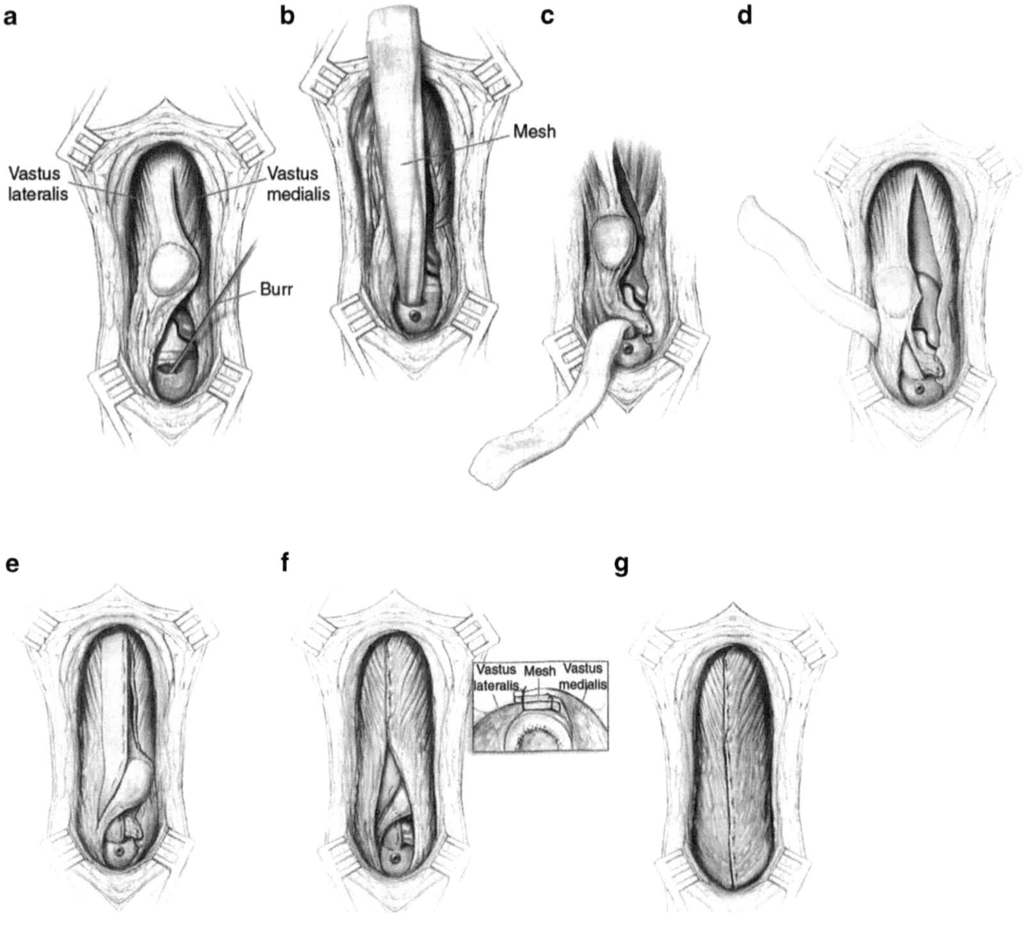

Fig. 10.1 Schematic of synthetic mesh extensor mechanism reconstruction [20]

differences in knee scores, extensor lag, graft failures, and revision rates. Allograft patients showed significant greater knee flexion. The authors concluded that both options yielded similar outcomes and acceptable survivorship.

Case Presentations

Case 1

A 55-year-old male status post left TKA after multiple revisions, presented with global knee instability. The patient underwent revision to a hinged implant. At 3-month follow-up, he presented to clinic with anterior knee pain, a 45° extensor lag, and a palpable suprapatellar defect. He had full passive extension. Radiographs in Fig. 10.2a reveal a fragmented patella along with patella baja. The decision was made to proceed with patellectomy and extensor mechanism reconstruction with Achilles allograft, shown in Fig. 10.2b.

Case 2

A 73-year-old female underwent left TKA in 1994. She subsequently required revision TKA due to aseptic loosening in early 2015. She sustained a fall causing wound dehiscence and patellar tendon rupture and presented to clinic with an extensor lag of 80° and inability to actively extend the knee fully. The radiograph in Fig. 10.3a reveals patella alta. She was initially taken to the OR for irrigation and debridement and surgical wound closure. The decision was then made to proceed with patellectomy and extensor mechanism reconstruction due to her functional deficits. Postoperative radiographs are shown in Fig. 10.3b.

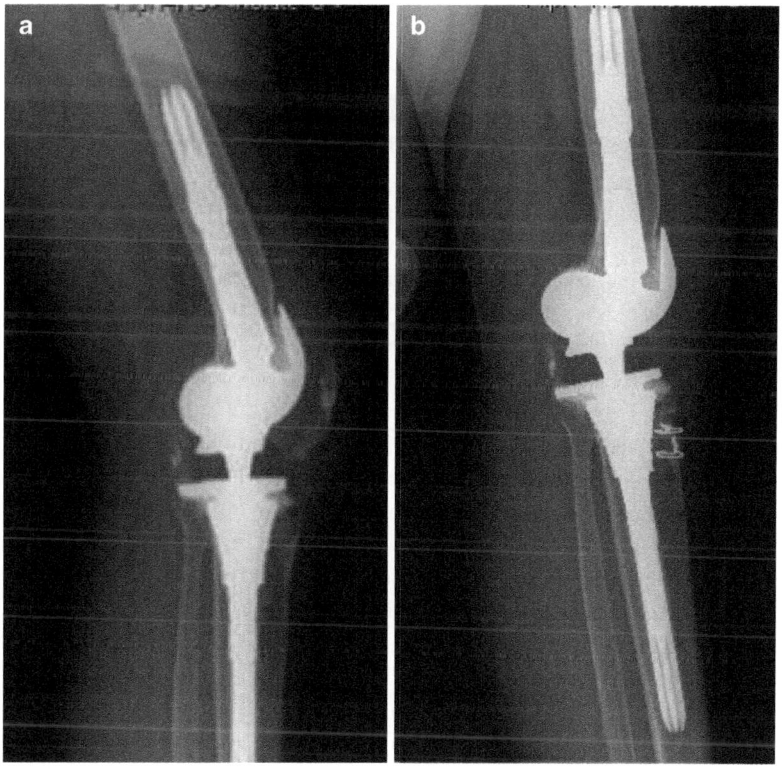

Fig. 10.2 (**a**) Fragmented patella along with patella baja; (**b**) patellectomy and extensor mechanism reconstruction with Achilles allograft

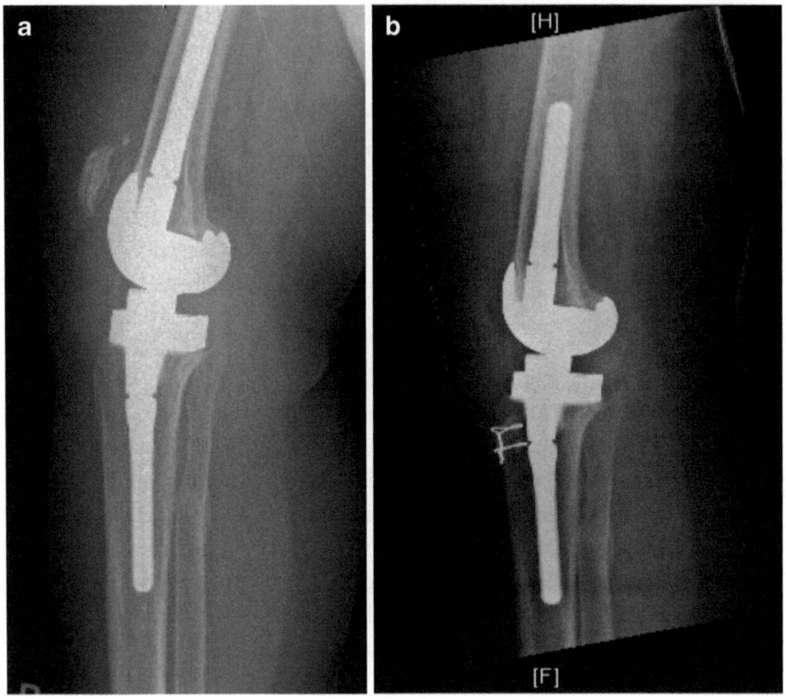

Fig. 10.3 (a) Patella alta; (b) patellectomy and extensor mechanism reconstruction due to functional deficits

Case 3

A 66-year-old female 8 years status post left TKA with subsequent complete patellectomy for AVN presented with instability and inability to perform a straight leg raise. She had full passive extension. She was treated with revision to a hinged implant and extensor reconstruction with synthetic mesh. She was placed in a cylinder cast for 10 weeks. At 6 months, she exhibited an intact straight leg raise with no extensor lag (Fig. 10.4).

Authors' Preferred Method, Take-Home Points, Tips and Tricks, and Avoiding Pitfalls

Quadriceps deficiencies are generally treated with both primary repair of the remaining tissues. The author prefers to augment the repair, typically with synthetic mesh. Achilles tendon allograft is a good alternative. The take-home point for quadriceps problems is that simple primary repair is likely to fail, especially in the chronic setting, and some form of augmentation is recommended.

Regarding patellar fractures, the authors strongly prefer nonoperative treatment, regardless of the appearance of the radiograph, if the extensor mechanism is intact and the patellar component is well fixed. Traditional methods of treating patellar fractures often fail in the setting of a periprosthetic patellar fracture. In the setting of a symptomatic loose patellar implant with intact extensor mechanism, solely removing the implant is a reasonable option. When the extensor mechanism is deficiency after fracture, a trial of conservative management with immobilization is still preferred. If extensor deficiency persists, reconstruction with Marlex mesh is the author's preference although Achilles tendon reconstruction is a reasonable option with similar results.

In the management of patellar tendon rupture, the authors prefer synthetic mesh reconstruction. Achilles tendon calcaneal bone block allograft reconstruction (Fig. 10.5) is a good alternative. In Achilles tendon allograft reconstruction, the bone block is press fit into a trough in the anterior tibia,

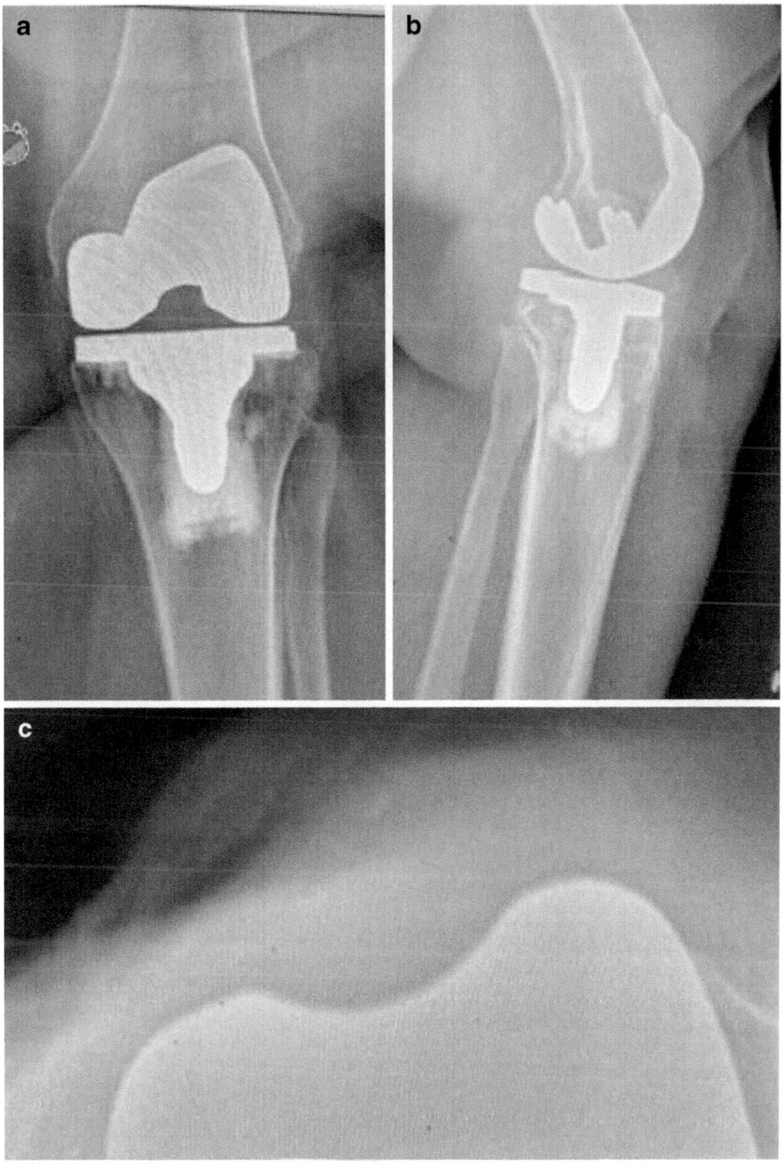

Figs. 10.4 (**a**–**c**) AP, lateral, and sunrise radiographs of a TKA after complete patellectomy, (**d**, **e**) AP and lateral radiograph after revision arthroplasty to a hinged implant along with mesh extensor mechanism reconstruction, (**f**) tubularized Marlex mesh, (**g**) 6-month postoperative visit demonstrates intact straight leg raise without extensor lag

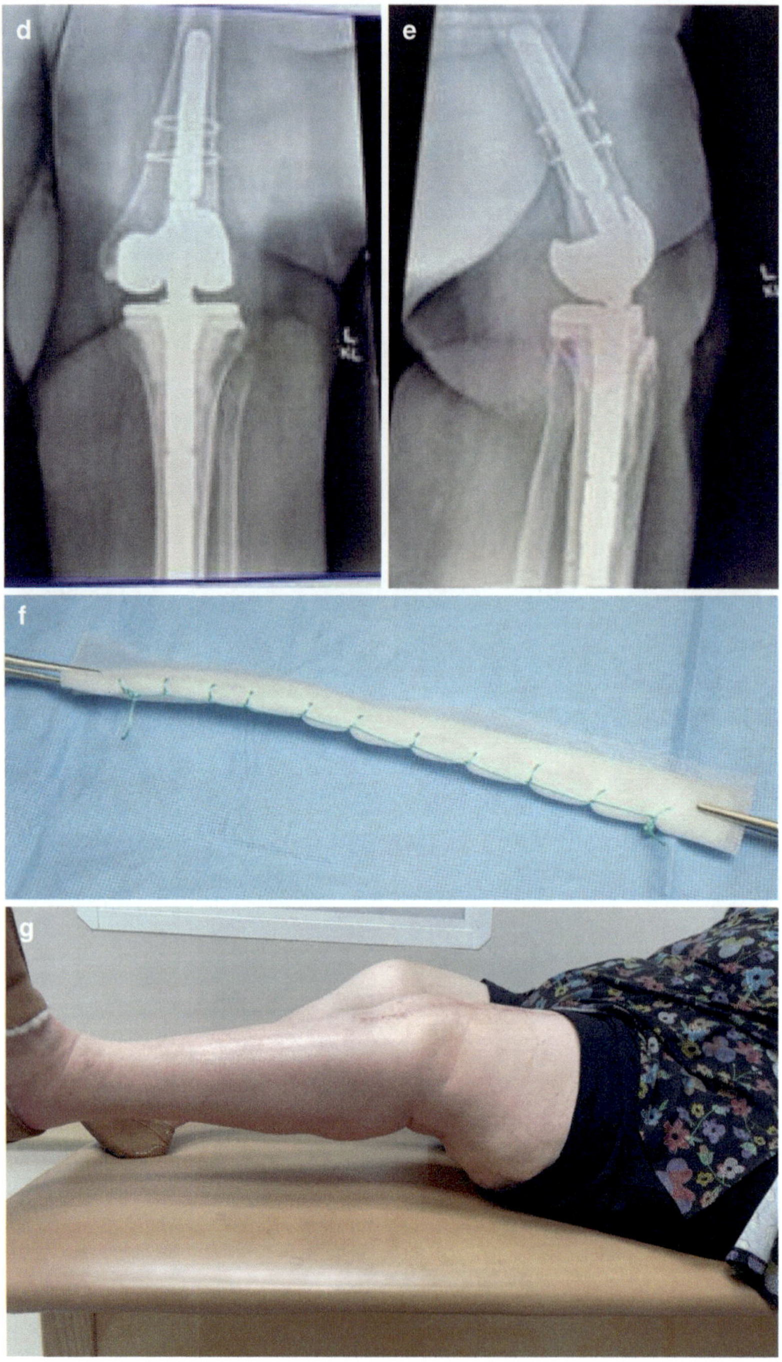

Fig. 10.4 (continued)

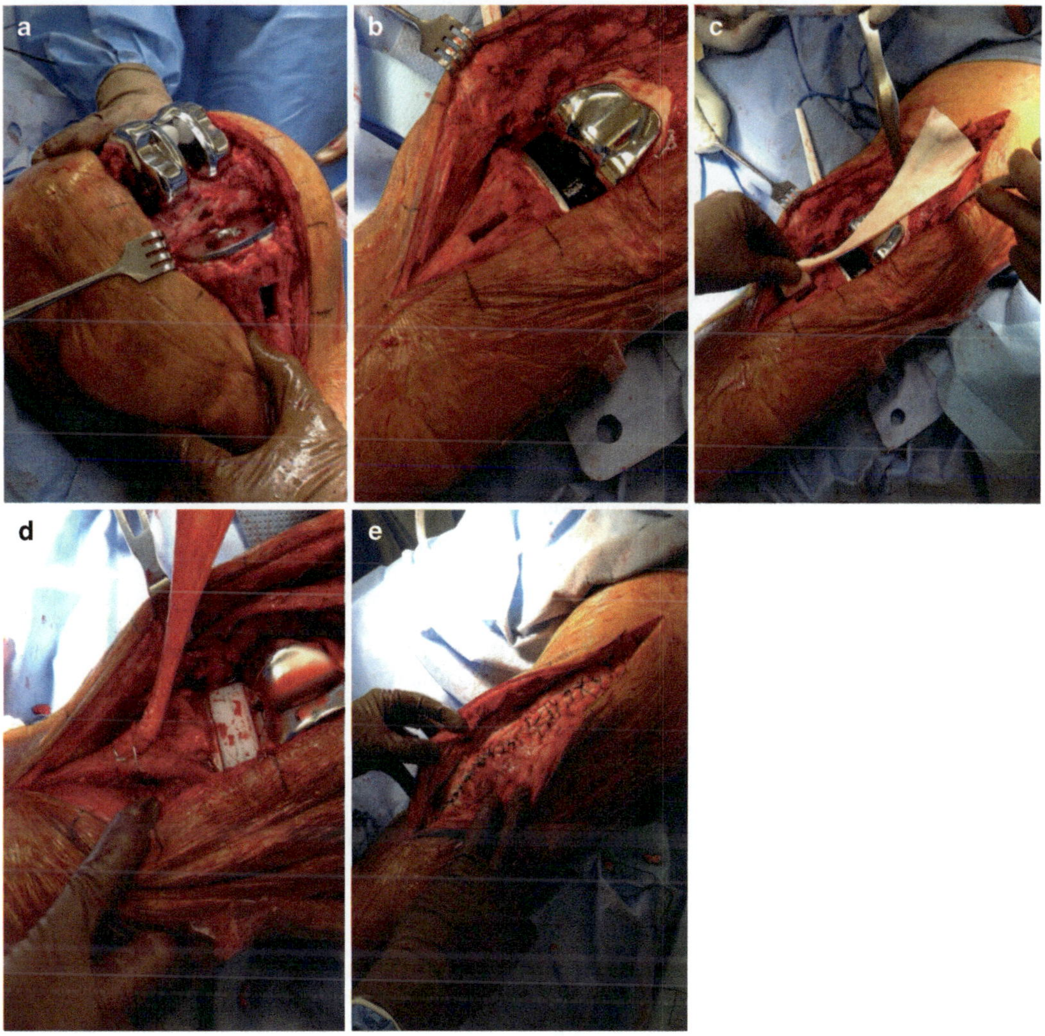

Fig. 10.5 (**a**–**e**) Achilles allograft extensor mechanism reconstruction

and fixation is supplemented with 18 gauge wires. The allograft is tensioned with the knee in full extension. Closing the native remaining extensor tissue over the allograft is preferred. Patients are immobilized in a long leg walking cast for 6 weeks. A hinge knee brace with drop locks is then used for another 6 weeks with slow progression of motion. Active extension strengthening is allowed at 12 weeks.

References

1. Rand JA, Morrey BF, Bryan RS. Patellar tendon rupture after total knee arthroplasty. Clin Orthop Relat Res. 1989;244:233–8.
2. Lynch AF, Rorabeck CH, Bourne RB. Extensor mechanism complications following total knee arthroplasty. J Arthroplasty. 1987;2:135–40.
3. Dobbs RE, Hanssen AD, Lewallen DG, Pagnano MW. Quadriceps tendon rupture after total knee arthroplasty. Prevalence, complications, and outcomes. J Bone Joint Surg Am. 2005;87(1):37–45.
4. Fernandez-Baillo N, Garay EG, Ordoñez JM. Rupture of the quadriceps tendon after total knee arthroplasty. A case report. J Arthroplasty. 1993;8(3):331–3.
5. Shi SM, Shi GG, Laurent EM, Ninomiya JT. Modified V-Y turndown flap augmentation for quadriceps tendon rupture following total knee arthroplasty: a retrospective study. J Bone Joint Surg Am. 2019;101(11):1010–5.
6. Rust PA, Tanna N, Spicer DD. Repair of ruptured quadriceps tendon with Leeds-Keio ligament following revision knee surgery. Knee Surg Sports Traumatol Arthrosc. 2008;16(4):370–2.
7. Grace JN, Sim FH. Fracture of the patella after total knee arthroplasty. Clin Orthop Relat Res. 1988;230:168–75.
8. Ortiguera CJ, Berry DJ. Patellar fracture after total knee arthroplasty. J Bone Joint Surg Am. 2002;84-A(4):532–40.
9. Keating EM, Haas G, Meding JB. Patella fracture after post total knee replacements. Clin Orthop Relat Res. 2003;416:93–7.
10. Wulff W, Incavo SJ. The effect of patella preparation for total knee arthroplasty on patellar strain: a comparison of resurfacing versus inset implants. J Arthroplasty. 2000;15(6):778–82.
11. Singerman R, Heiple KG, Davy DT, Goldberg VM. Effect of tibial component position on patellar strain following total knee arthroplasty. J Arthroplasty. 1995;10(5):651–6.
12. Singerman R, Pagan HD, Peyser AB, Goldberg VM. Effect of femoral component rotation and patellar design on patellar forces. Clin Orthop Relat Res. 1997;334:345–53.
13. Bayley JC, Scott RD, Ewald FC, Holmes GB Jr. Failure of the metal-backed patellar component after total knee replacement. J Bone Joint Surg Am. 1988;70(5):668–74.
14. Parvizi J, Kim KI, Oliashirazi A, Ong A, Sharkey PF. Periprosthetic patellar fractures. Clin Orthop Relat Res. 2006;446:161–6.
15. Schoderbek RJ Jr, Brown TE, Mulhall KJ, Mounasamy V, Iorio R, Krackow KA, Macaulay W, Saleh KJ. Extensor mechanism disruption after total knee arthroplasty. Clin Orthop Relat Res. 2006;446:176–85.
16. Crossett LS, Sinha RK, Sechriest VF, Rubash HE. Reconstruction of a ruptured patellar tendon with Achilles tendon allograft following total knee arthroplasty. J Bone Joint Surg Am. 2002;84-A(8):1354–61.
17. Ares O, Lozano LM, Medrano-Nájera C, Popescu D, Martínez-Pastor JC, Segur JM, Maculé F. New modified Achilles tendon allograft for treatment of chronic patellar tendon ruptures following total knee arthroplasty. Arch Orthop Trauma Surg. 2014;134(5):713–7.
18. Nazarian DG, Booth RE Jr. Extensor mechanism allografts in total knee arthroplasty. Clin Orthop Relat Res. 1999;367:123–9.
19. Barrack RL, Stanley T, Allen Butler R. Treating extensor mechanism disruption after total knee arthroplasty. Clin Orthop Relat Res. 2003;416:98–104.
20. Browne JA, Hanssen AD. Reconstruction of patellar tendon disruption after total knee arthroplasty: results of a new technique utilizing synthetic mesh. J Bone Joint Surg. 2011;93(12):1137–43.
21. Abdel MP, Salib CG, Mara KC, Pagnano MW, Perry KI, Hanssen AD. Extensor mechanism reconstruction with use of Marlex mesh: a series study of 77 total knee arthroplasties. J Bone Joint Surg Am. 2018;100(15):1309–18.
22. Gencarelli P Jr, Yawman JP, Tang A, Salandra J, North DD, Menken LG, Green CC, Haidukewych GJ, Liporace FA, Yoon RS. Extensor mechanism reconstruction after total knee arthroplasty with allograft versus synthetic mesh: a multicenter retrospective cohort. J Am Acad Orthop Surg. 2023;31(1):e23–34.

11 Revision Knee Arthroplasty for Periprosthetic Fractures: Loose and Well-Fixed Components

John S. Hwang and Cory A. Collinge

Introduction

Distal femur fractures are increasingly common as our population ages and more total knee arthroplasty (TKA) surgeries are used to treat arthritis. The incidence of these fractures has been reported at 0.3% to 2.5% following TKA. There is also an increasing incidence of *inter*-prosthetic fractures occurring above a TKA and below a hip arthroplasty which can necessitate treatments that are even more complex. Risk factors for periprosthetic fracture around a TKA include osteopenia, rheumatoid arthritis, prolonged corticosteroid therapy, anterior notching of the femoral cortex, and revision TKA. These scenarios present considerable challenges in treatment, and no single management method has been identified to successfully overcome all of the problems associated with these injuries.

Until the last few decades, most supracondylar femur fractures (periprosthetic or not) were treated non-operatively with or without cast bracing however angulatory deformities, knee joint incongruity, loss of knee motion, and the complications of immobility led to alternative treatments. More recently, both operative techniques and implants have seen dramatic improvements, and internal fixation is now recommended for most displaced distal femoral fractures in adults. The goals of treatment are restoration of limb alignment, length and rotation as well as stable fixation that allows for early mobilization and healing. Nevertheless, internal fixation of periprosthetic distal femur fractures may be difficult for several reasons. Thin cortices, a wide medullary canal, compromised bone stock, and fracture comminution are several contributors that render stable internal fixation difficult. Furthermore, treatment may be further complicated due to issues in the use of knee prostheses, the presence of previous surgical wounds and pre-existing knee stiffness. Over the past two decades, we have witnessed significant improvements in clinical outcomes as a result of innovative implants and improved technique, yet, the operative management of these difficult fractures has not proved uniformly successful. Patients with periprosthetic fractures have historically been treated with intramedullary nails or plate-screw constructs. As stated, both of these modalities have seen improvements in implant design and technical modifications, and yet, they still are not without limitations when applied to osteoporotic bone around a TKA.

J. S. Hwang
Department of Orthopaedic Surgery, Rutgers, The State University of New Jersey, New Jersey Medical School, Newark, NJ, USA

C. A. Collinge (✉)
Harris Methodist Hospital Fort Worth, Fort Worth, TX, USA

R. S. Yoon et al. (eds.), *Trauma and Infection Control in Revision Hip and Knee Arthroplasty*,
https://doi.org/10.1007/978-3-031-71971-4_11

The mean age of patients with periprosthetic fractures tends to be higher than that of those with non-implant-related fractures, as patients undergoing TKA tend to be older and less active than the general population. Elderly patients typically present with periprosthetic distal femur fracture cases resulting from low-energy trauma, and mortality rates are similar to that of the hip fracture population. Patients with periprosthetic distal femur fractures who also present with comorbidities such as dementia, heart failure, advanced renal disease and metastasis have shown to be independent predictors of reduced survival when compared with age-matched controls. The age-adjusted Charlson Comorbidity Index has demonstrated benefits in predicting survival for such a group of patients. In addition, a surgical delay of greater than 4 days has also been shown to increase the 6-month and 1-year mortality rates [1, 2].

The objective of this chapter is to provide useful information for the orthopedic surgeon who is treating a patient with a periprosthetic distal femur fracture. The goals of this chapter are to improve the surgeon's understanding of injury patterns, enhance his/her decision-making process, and discuss modern surgical techniques, including "tips and tricks," that may assist in obtaining a good clinical outcome.

Classification

There are multiple classifications systems for distal femur periprosthetic fracture. The most commonly used classification, developed by Rorabeck and Taylor (Table 11.1), takes into account the fracture's *displacement* and *prosthesis stability* [3]. According to this classification, type I fractures should be treated non-operatively, type II fractures should be treated with internal fixation and type III fractures should require revision surgery. While this is currently the most commonly used classification system, it falls short in its failure to consider available bone stock a key factor in surgical decision-making.

Kim et al. subsequently developed a classification system which took into consideration distal femoral bone stock, as well as component fixation and fracture displacement. Under this system, type II and type III fractures would require revision arthroplasties or distal femoral replacements (Table 11.2) [4]. Most recently, Su et al. developed a classification system based primarily on the location of the fracture. Type I fractures are proximal to the femoral component, while type II fractures originate at the femoral knee component and extend proximally. Type III fractures were defined as any fracture line distal to the upper edge of the anterior flange of the femoral knee component [5].

Table 11.1 Rorabeck and Taylor classification [3] of periprosthetic distal femur fractures

Type	Fracture displacement	Component fixation
I	Undisplaced	Well fixed
II	Displaced	Well fixed
III	Undisplaced or displaced	Loose

Table 11.2 Modified classification [4] of periprosthetic distal femur fractures

Type	Fracture displacement	Component fixation	Bone stock in distal femur
IA	Yes	Well fixed	Good
IB	No	Well fixed	Good
II	Yes/no	Loose	Good
III	Yes/no	Loose	Poor

Treatment Options

For the vast majority of patients, the ultimate goal of treatment for a periprosthetic distal femur fracture is to achieve a painless, functional, and well-aligned lower extremity that returns the patient to his/her state prior to injury. Treatment choice is typically selected based on the stability and design of TKA implants, the presence of any other implants, the quality and amount of bone stock and the physical condition and ambulatory potential of the patient. Rarely, fracture repair or surgical treatment at all is not feasible, or desirable and alternative treatments must be employed. All of these considerations are explored in greater detail below.

Non-operative Treatment

Historically, the standard non-operative management of periprosthetic distal femur fracture was skeletal traction with or without subsequent cast bracing. This changed when improved results were noted with surgical treatment. Closed methods do offer a way to avoid the risks of surgery itself; however, there are also a number of significant and potentially severe risks associated with non-operative treatment. For example, complications from prolonged bed and limb immobilization include deep vein thrombosis and pulmonary embolus, decubitus ulcer, pneumonia, urinary retention and urosepsis, and others. Furthermore, studies have shown that these patient are at high risk for malalignment/malunion and nonunion, for example, Culp et al. reported that patients treated in prolonged traction had nonunion rates of 20% and malunion rates of 23% [6]. Similar results were reported by Merkel and Johnson who additionally noted that 35% of their patients went on to revision TKA [7].

Currently, non-operative treatment is the treatment of choice for patients who present with non-displaced fractures or those who are not surgical candidates due to significant medical comorbidities such as those that are receiving palliative care. Relative indications for non-operative treatment include non-ambulatory states of patients (e.g., paraplegia), significant underlying medical disease (e.g., severe cardiopulmonary risk), lack of modern internal fixation devices or imminent death. In addition, surgeons who are unfamiliar or inexperienced with surgical techniques should avoid operative management and elect to treat the patient non-operatively until the care of a surgeon experienced in periprosthetic fractures becomes available to the patient.

Operative Treatment

Several surgical options are available to treat periprosthetic fractures of the distal femur. If the implant is stable and enough bone is still available and attached to the distal femoral component, then fracture repair with a plate or nail is recommended. Even far distal fractures that extend distal to the proximal border of the femoral TKA component can be successfully managed with internal fixation [8]. On the other hand, if the prosthesis is loose or if scant bone is available distally, then revision arthroplasty (distal femoral replacement) may be chosen for salvage of this difficult problem.

Achieving rigid internal fixation is potentially difficult—and sometimes impossible—in osteopenic bone following a comminuted periprosthetic distal femur fracture. Fixation method for distal femur fractures and periprosthetic fractures have improved greatly over the past decade or two. Techniques focusing on the preservation of biology and implants enabling improvement of stability in the short, osteoporotic condylar segment are now the standards. In addition, implant manufacturers are continuing to make improvements with each generation of products.

One of the difficulties in the treatment of periprosthetic distal femur fractures is the fixation limitation presented by the femoral component of the TKA. Fixation methods are subject to the limitations posed by the design of the femoral components. For example, retrograde nailing cannot be performed in femoral components that have narrow or closed boxes, while certain fixed-angle devices, such as a 95-degree blade plate or condylar screw, cannot be used in prostheses with deep boxes. The evaluation of the prosthesis at hand is vital to constructing an appropriate and optimal preoperative plan. Unfortunately, the information required for such an evaluation is not always readily available to the surgeon as the number of galleries displaying prostheses is very limited [9].

Open Reduction and Internal Fixation Using Conventional Plates

The use of open reduction and internal fixation (ORIF) of periprosthetic distal femur fractures with conventional plates rose in the 1970s and 1980s as techniques for periarticular fractures became more common. The goals of ORIF for periprosthetic distal femur fractures with conventional plates were anatomical reconstruction and early rehabilitation of the patient, and several authors have reported "good" clinical results. Nevertheless, it should be noted that these were small cohort studies with significant limitations.

Open anatomic reduction and internal fixation with traditional non-locked plates has been associated with relatively high rates of delayed union, nonunion, and infection (20% or higher), and historically the need for supplemental bone graft has been reported in comminuted fractures. Healy et al. treated 20 patients with periprosthetic distal femur fractures with ORIF using a variety of implants including blade plates, dynamic condylar screws, and condylar buttress plates [10]. Most of these patients required autografts with index procedure. Those grafted mostly healed, while those without graft did not, which led the authors to recommend primary bone grafting with internal fixation to increase the prospects for union.

With standard plating constructs, plating on one surface of a metaphyseal fracture (eccentric stabilization) can be particularly prone to fixation failure. Mechanically, the characteristic of the screw heads to toggle within the plate makes it difficult for these implants to maintain coronal plane alignment, particularly with opposite-cortex comminution. Additionally, because most plates are applied laterally, medial cortical comminution predisposes to loss of reduction into a varus deformity when standard implants are used [11]. Figgie et al. reported nonunions in five of ten patients with a periprosthetic distal femur fracture treated with ORIF, and eight of the ten cases subsequently fell into varus alignment despite satisfactory intraoperative alignment [12].

Locked Plating

Modern locked plating technology was proposed largely to address the difficulties with treatment of osteoporotic, metaphyseal fractures such as those discussed in this chapter. Locked plates allow the screw heads to screw into the plate, creating "fixed-angle" constructs, which are theoretically better able to resist varus displacement forces across the fracture (Fig. 11.1a–c). Most surgeons will agree that these implants have provided an excellent tool to achieve stable fixation in many osteoporotic fractures, including periprosthetic fractures. A well-fixed prosthesis is an essential prerequisite for predictably treating with locked plating systems.

Biomechanical studies using paired cadaver femurs have demonstrated that fixation with locked plates is superior to those with plates that use non-locked screws, such as blade plates and dynamic condylar screws. Various clinical studies have demonstrated union rates to be between 78–100% with locked plating systems [8, 13–18], as opposed to the poorer results seen in non-operative management or conventional plating systems. For example, Kregor et al. reported 100% union rate in 13 periprosthetic fractures using locked plating (LISS™); only one patient needed bone grafting [17]. Raab and Davis reported their results of using locked plating in 11 fractures, which included 2 nonunions: eight fractures were supplemented with non-structural allograft [18]. achieved union in all nine acute fractures and in one of two cases of nonunion with satisfactory alignment. Finally, Streubel et al. evaluated "far distal" periprosthetic supracondylar fractures of the femur and concluded they are not a contraindication to repair with lat-

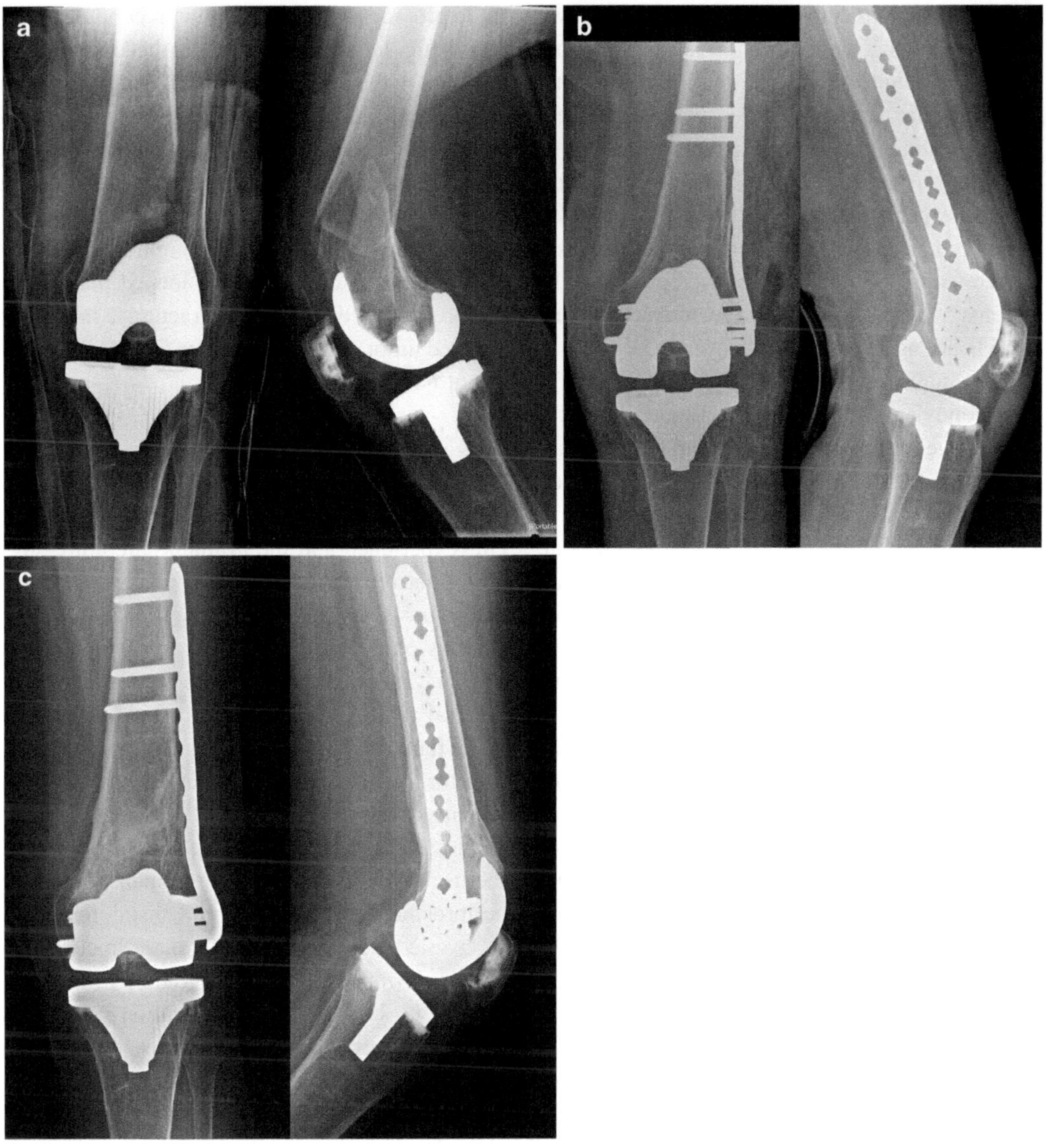

Fig. 11.1 (**a**) Periprosthetic distal femur fracture. (**b**) Repair using distal femur locking plate. (**c**) 9 month follow-up with healed fracture

eral locked plating [8]. Patients were divided into those with fractures located *proximal* to the implant (28) and those with fractures that extended *distal* to the proximal border of the femoral component (33). Delayed healing and nonunion occurred in five (18%) and three (11%) of more proximal fractures, respectively, and in two (6%) and five (15%) of the fractures with distal extension ($p = 0.23$ for delayed healing; $p = 0.72$ for nonunion), respectively. Four construct failures (14%) occurred in more proximal fractures and three (9%) in fractures with distal extension ($p = 0.51$).

The development of the LISS system™ and indirect plating systems and techniques has allowed for better management of maintaining biology and allowing for better union rates. Ricci et al. reported the results of treating 22 periprosthetic fractures by indirect reduction methods without bone graft using locked plating. Nineteen of 22 fractures (86%) healed after the index procedure. All three patients who failed to heal were insulin-dependent diabetes mellitus patients. Two of these patients developed infected nonunion. Authors concluded that fixation of periprosthetic supracondylar femur fractures with an indirect locked plating provided satisfactory results in nondiabetic patients [13]. O'Toole et al. examined nine periprosthetic fracture above a TKA and five patients with hip and knee arthroplasty treated with LISS plating. The average age of the patients were 80, and all were female, and no complications were seen in this study.

Literature has demonstrated that LISS for supracondylar distal femur fractures allows for early range of motion and more rapid bone healing [19, 20]. Falck et al. demonstrated reduction in analgesic use and accelerated mobilization in patients treated with LISS [21]. Althausen et al. reported better results using LISS to maintain alignment and return to preoperative functional status when compared with other devices for periprosthetic distal femur fractures. All patients maintained physiologic valgus and length [22]. A more recent study by Hierholzer et al. compared 115 patients with distal femur fractures that included but no limited to patients who suffered periprosthetic fracture around a total knee implant. They compared retrograde nailing with LISS plating and found no difference in fracture healing, nonunion, and infection between the two. These authors suggest precise preoperative planning and advanced surgical experience to reduce risk of revision surgery [23].

Although the mechanical basis for locked plating seemed well-suited for the osteoporotic metaphyseal fracture, it has not exactly turned out to be the panacea for which many had hoped. The vast majority of surgeons have transitioned to using locked plates for these fractures, but this appears based on anecdotal observations and lower quality studies—there remains a paucity of clear, high-level evidence proving their benefit [24]. Even though the screw heads mechanically lock to the plate, in order for the fixation to remain stable, the screw shafts must remain securely anchored in the epiphyseal, periarticular bone segment. For this to occur, there needs to be an adequate volume of bone with adequate quality to provide anchorage. The supracondylar periprosthetic femur fracture with distal extension adjacent to the prosthesis may have limited native bone stock available for placing effective locked screws. Hoffmann et al. reported a nonunion rate of 22% in 36 patients who underwent locked plating for periprosthetic distal femur fracture [16]. Ebraheim et al. found a complication rate of 37% following distal femoral locked plating for periprosthetic distal femur fractures, including delayed union (7.4%), nonunion (3.7%), and failure of fixation (26%) [25].

Intramedullary Fixation

Our experience and the available literature suggests that retrograde nailing is a safe and minimally invasive procedure that allows for early healing of this injury pattern in most patients (Fig. 11.2a–c). Implant evolution for retrograde femoral nailing has occurred just as it has with distal femur plating, and the pendulum of implant use for distal femur fractures seems to have recently swung the direction of nailing. Many studies have now shown high success rate with the use of retrograde nail in the management of periprosthetic fractures of the distal femur. A cadaveric study has reported greater fracture stability with the use of a retrograde nail as compared with less invasive stabilization systems in simulated periprosthetic fractures [26]. This technique allows for the use of the previous incision, with no soft-tissue dissection being required at the fracture site, which preserves blood supply and biology. It allows early mobilization and range-of-motion exercises of the knee joint and maintains the overall alignment at the fracture site. A recent systematic review of 415 cases of periprosthetic fracture above TKA reported that retrograde nailing is associated with relative risk reduction of 87% for developing a nonunion and 70% for requiring revision surgery when compared with traditional (non-locked) plating methods [27]. Wick et al. demonstrated that both LISS plating and retrograde nailing are useful techniques in treating periprosthetic distal femur

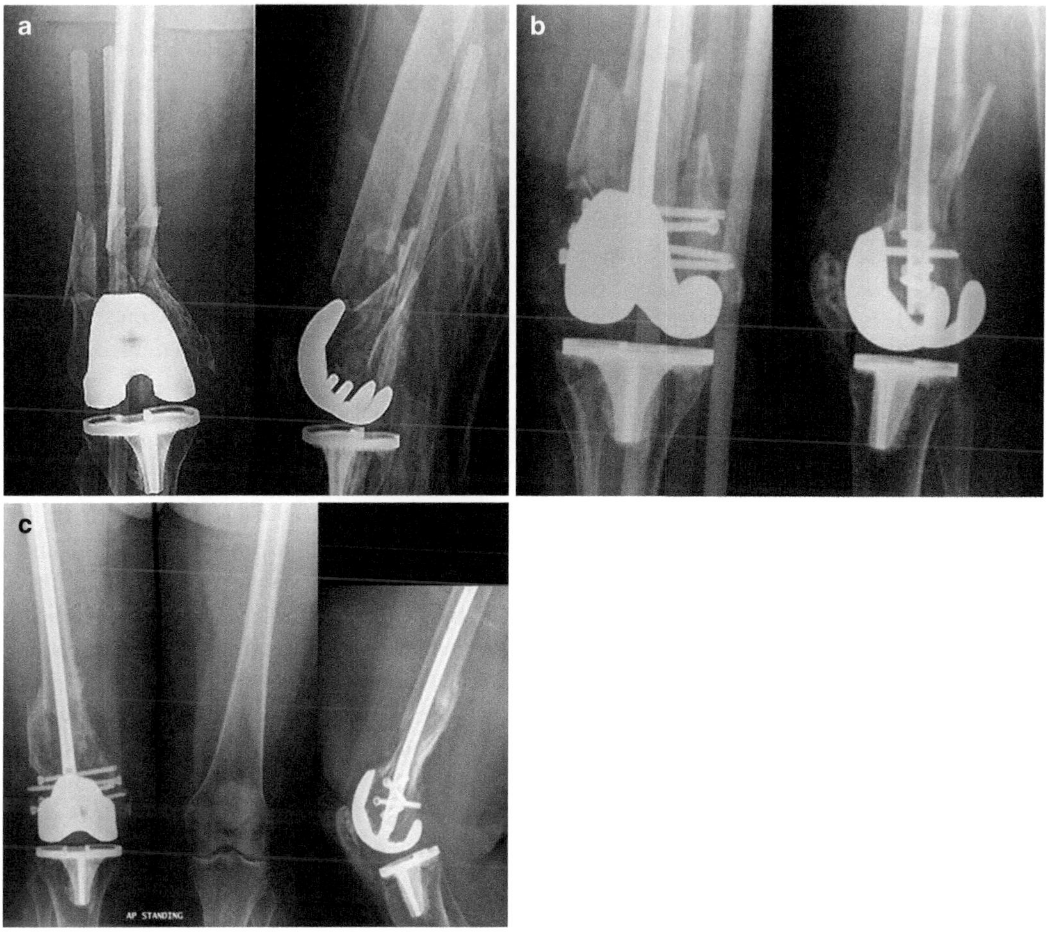

Fig. 11.2 (**a**) Periprosthetic distal femur fracture. (**b**) Repair using retrograde femoral nail. (**c**) 8.5 month follow-up with healed fracture

fracture. They did note that LISS plating was preferred in osteoporotic bone or fractures with short distal segments [28].

However, this technique also has some limitations. The reasonably common limitation of retrograde nailing for periprosthetic distal femur fracture is that the intercondylar box of the femoral component renders nailing impossible. This is more common with older implants and less problematic with newer versions. Others may have a narrow fit which may push the nail entry site posterior: this may impart an extension deformity at the fracture site (Fig. 11.2a–c). Some recent nails have been designed with a distal "kick" or exaggerated bend to move their insertion pathway more posterior (behind the available entry point of some femoral components). In addition, as previously discussed, it is not possible to use a retrograde nail in a very distal fracture, as it may not provide any fixation to the distal screws. A retrograde nail should probably not be used in the presence of a pre-existing total hip replacement, as it can create a stress riser below the femoral stem, which may, in turn, lead to a fracture between the two implants. A plate or nail-plate construct might be a good option for these cases. Although most of the modern knee prostheses would allow insertion of a retrograde nail, it is important to determine the type of the knee implant prior to surgery.

Revision Total Knee Arthroplasty (AKA Tumor Prosthesis or Distal Femoral Replacement)

Revision TKA is typically reserved for patients who have extremely distal fractures, significant comminution where secure fixation cannot be achieved, or there are loose or unstable femoral components (Fig. 11.3a, b). Typically, either long-stemmed revision components or distal femoral replacements are used. These prostheses can provide stable fixation that allows for early weight-bearing and range of motion.

Satisfactory results have been demonstrated using revision implants (i.e., distal femoral replacement [DFR]) following periprosthetic distal femur fractures in a number of limited studies. For example, Cordeiro et al. reported on nine patients with periprosthetic distal femur fractures: they found that patients who underwent DFR had better results in walking ability, range of motion, and early rehabilitation when compared to those treated non-operatively or with conventional plating [29]. Pour et al. examined 44 patients with hinged prostheses used in revision cases, including four patients with periprosthetic fracture, and found 79.6% survival rate at 1 year and 68.2% at 5 years [30]. Chen et al. in a review of 12 published reports including 195 patients, noted successful results in 10 of 11 cases who were treated with DFR as initial treatment for a periprosthetic distal femur fracture. However, there was a complication rate of 25% which included a knee dislocation [31].

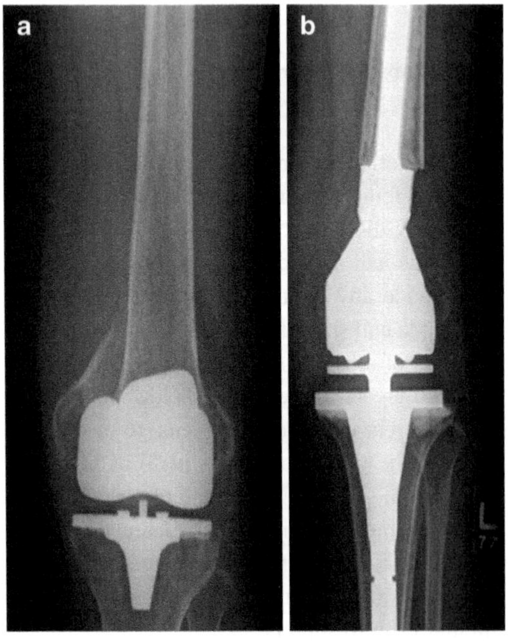

Fig. 11.3 (**a**) Far distal periprosthetic distal femur fracture in osteoporostic bone and low-demand patient (**b**) Replacement of distal femur with a "tumor" prosthesis

When significant bone loss is present, long-stemmed revision has also been used in with allografts. Kassab et al. reviewed 12 consecutive patients, two lost to follow-up, who underwent revision arthroplasty with distal femoral allograft. They found good to fair results in HSS knee score and reported the mean range of motion to be 98° (range 50°–115°). Nine patients reached full union [32]. A more recent study by Saidi et al. compared allograft prosthesis composite (APC), revisions systems and DFR. It was found that the patients with APCs had the most blood loss, longest operative time and longest hospital stay. The authors recommend the use of DFR as opposed to APC and revision systems in patients with extreme bone deficiency and advanced patient age [33].

The DFR implant should be considered as a limb-salvage option when all other surgical options are unlikely to be successful. Recently, a retrospective review by Rahman et al. examined the use of DFR of periprosthetic supracondylar fractures. They found mean final range of motion to be 2°–90.2° and moderate patient satisfaction and function. As previously discussed, Saidi et al. recommended DFRs over APC and revision systems. The disadvantage of using DFR is the early rates of aseptic loosening, and thus, it may not be suitable for younger patients. Some relative indications for DFRs are older patients, sick patients who may not tolerate more than one procedure, and patients with osteopenia with significant bone loss.

Case Presentations

Issues, Controversies, Problems

Present your perspective on the issues, controversies, problems, etc., as they relate to theme and arguments supporting your position. Utilize your own case examples (4–6 cases) with figures to illustrate how you treat and tackle these problems.

Case 1: Periprosthetic Distal Femur Fracture Treated with Plates and Screws

AP and lateral femur/knee radiographs of an 83-year-old woman fell onto her flexed knee and suffered a comminuted periprosthetic distal femur fracture above a stable TKA (Fig. 11.1a). Corresponding radiographs after she was treated with locked plating (Fig. 11.1b) using a bridge-plating technique. At 5 months follow-up, she was clinically and radiographically healed (Fig. 11.1c), and very satisfied with her outcome.

Case 2: Periprosthetic Distal Femur Fracture Treated with Retrograde Femoral Nail

An 83-year- old woman fell down a stair and suffered a comminuted distal femur fracture above a well-fixed femoral component that was compatible for nailing (Fig. 11.2a). She was treated with retrograde femoral nailing (Fig. 11.2b) using four fixed-angle distal locking screws (Phoenix®, Biomet, Parsippany, NJ). At 6 month follow-up, she was clinically and radiographically (Fig. 11.2c) healed, and ambulatory to her pre-injury level.

Case 3: Periprosthetic Distal Femur Fracture Treated with Revision Knee Arthroplasty

An 88-year- old woman with severe osteoporosis had a ground level fall causing a very far distal periprosthetic fracture (Fig. 11.3a). Predictable repair with internal fixation did not seem likely so she was treated with revision TKA (Fig. 11.3b). She was able to bear weight immediately which allowed for improved post-operative rehabilitation.

Case 4: Massively Unstable Fracture in a Young Patient Treated with Nail-Plate Construct

A 49-year-old "fluffy" woman with a TKA was involved in a car crash and suffered polytrauma. The TKA was recognized as likely to be "unstable" with standard fixation (Fig. 11.4) but distal femoral replacement appeared unsatisfactory treatment choice due the patient age and size. AP and lateral X-rays (a,b) and CT (c) reconstruction show osteopenia and limited bone stock associated with femoral component. The patient was treated with staged surgery using an external fixator and ultimately underwent ORIF with an arthrotomy and repair with a nail-plate construct (Fig. 11.4d).

Case 5: Periprosthetic Distal Femur Fracture Treated with Locked Plating Resulting in Nonunion

Radiographs of a 68-year-old woman with low-energy mechanism suffered a distal femur fracture (Fig. 11.5a) which was treated with locked plating (Fig. 11.5b). She went on to develop an atrophic nonunion (Fig. 11.5c). Hypovitaminosis D was diagnosed and she was treated. Revision surgery included compression of the nonunion with a 95 degree angled blade plate and autograft. X-rays from 6 months show that she healed reasonably quickly thereafter (Fig. 11.5e).

Case 6: Nail Causing Extension Deformity

Lateral knee X-ray of a nailed periprosthetic femur fracture where the arthroplasty implant forced the insertion point posterior. This may create and extension deformity as the nail crosses the fracture as seen in Fig. 11.6.

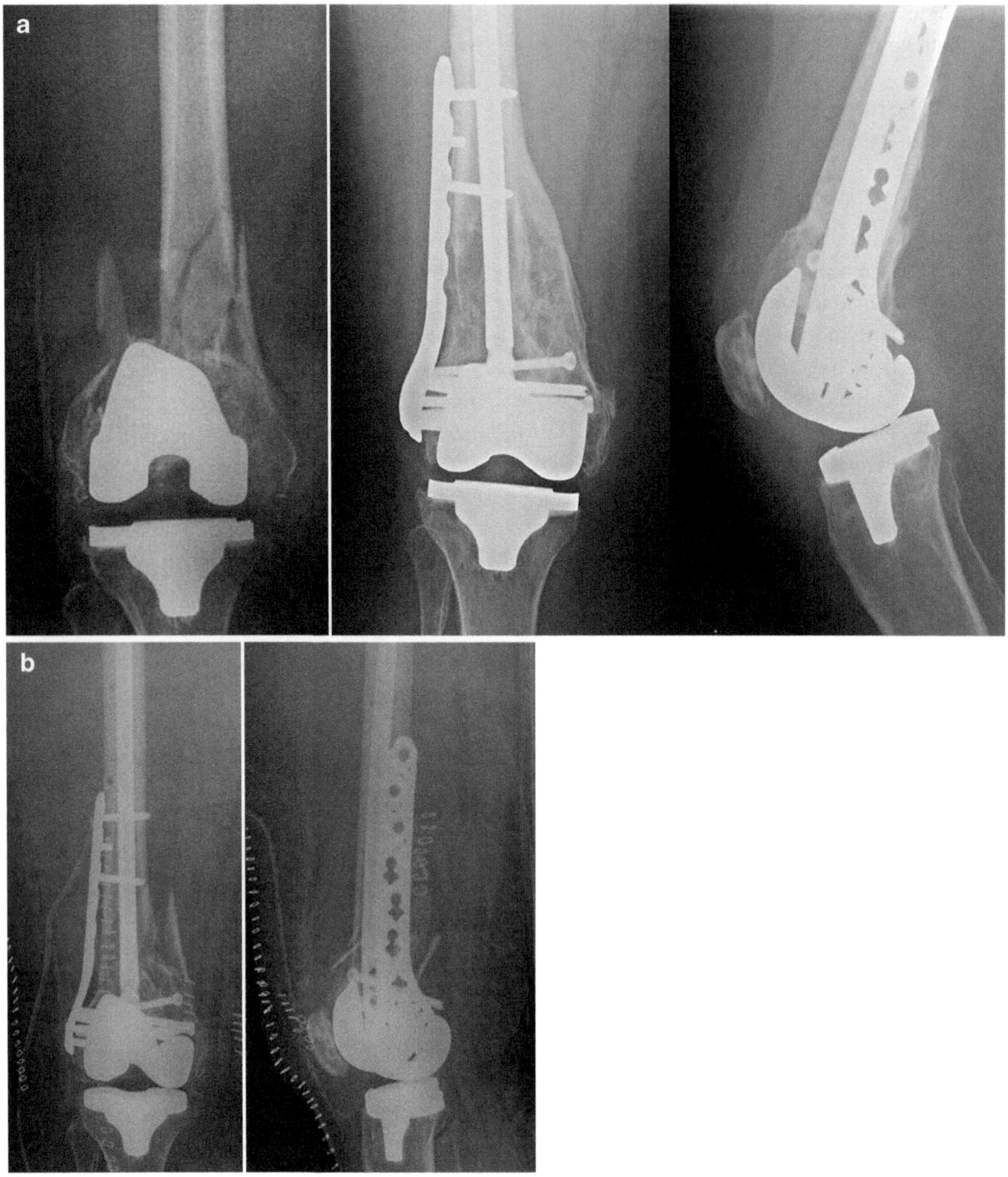

Fig. 11.4 (**a**) Comminuted distal femur fracture in a 56yo active, osteoporotic woman. (**b**) Repair of injury with a nail and plate combination

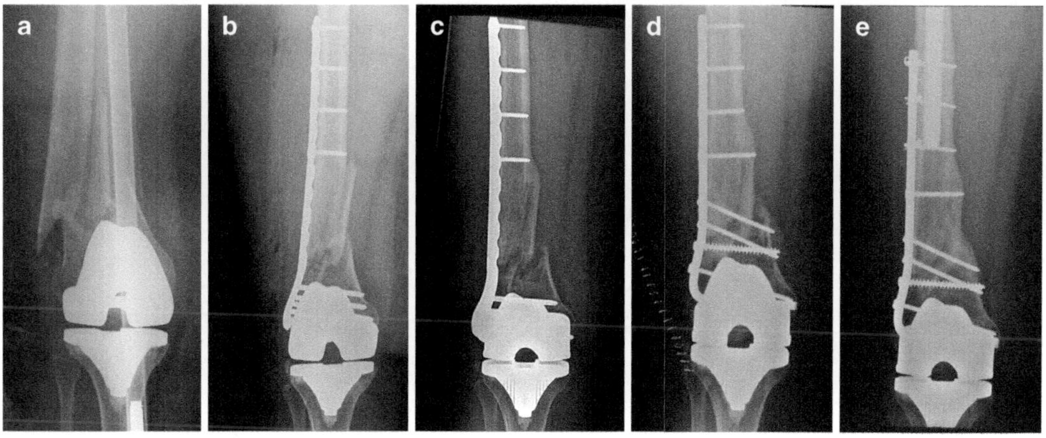

Fig. 11.5 (**a**) Periprosthetic distal femur fracture. (**b**) Same fracture treated with a locking plate. (**c**) 5 month post-repair, the fracture remains ununited. (**d**) Distal femur nonunion was reconstructed with a 95-degree angled blade plate and autografting. (**e**) Final Xray demonstrating union 6 mos. after nonunion repair

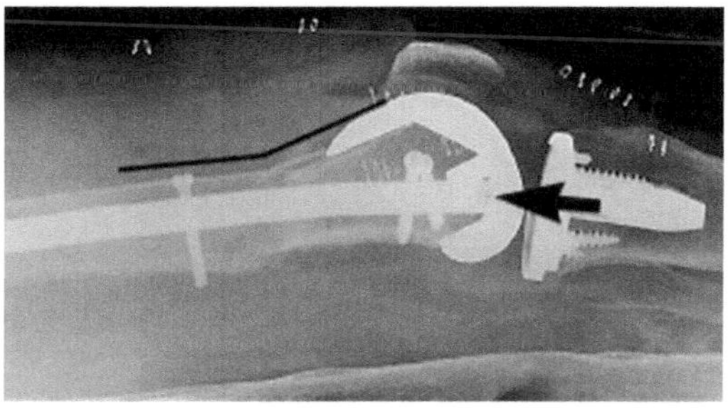

Fig. 11.6 Posterior entry point (arrow) and nail deflection in the intercondylar notch of the femoral implant can force the fracture into extension (angled lines). A nail with more distal bend might have been selected

Tips, Tricks, and Avoiding Pitfalls

Surgical Planning and Technique

Due to the large spectrum of periprosthetic distal femur fractures, no single implant or approach will be optimal for every case. The method of fixation should be based on a preoperative plan that incorporates the fracture pattern, soft-tissue injury, patient factors, surgeon preference/familiarity, and hospital resources (Fig. 11.7). As such, thorough assessment of the patients must be performed and plain radiographs must be scrutinized to assess the "personality" of the fracture. Quality images must be obtained (Fig. 11.8a) and occasionally advanced imaging with computed tomography (CT) is helpful. The sequential steps in the surgical management of periprosthetic distal femoral fractures include: (1) restoration of the articular surface, if needed, (2) stable internal fixation, (3) grafting of bone loss (rare), (4) impaction of the fracture in severely osteoporotic elderly patients, (5) early range of motion of the knee, and (6) delayed protected weight-bearing.

The vast majority of periprosthetic distal femur fractures are best treated with internal fixation. We recommend either locked plating or closed retrograde intramedullary nailing. Regardless of the implant used, the goal is anatomic reduction of the joint surface and stable internal fixation, which will allow early range of knee motion. In isolated closed fractures, internal fixation should be performed within the first 24 to 48 h. If surgery must be delayed for more than 24 to 36 h, a temporary external fixator or tibial pin traction should be considered.

While the basic principles of treatment are similar with both a plate and an intramedullary nail, the devices achieve fixation differently, and thus, have different technical methods of application and risks of usage. Restoration of alignment and preservation of fracture biology are two basic principles of treatment that cannot be over-emphasized. A predictably good long-term outcome is certainly less or not at all likely if these surgical priorities are not heeded. The specific usage of locked plates or nails, as well as an algorithm for fracture reduction, should be well thought out as part of the preoperative treatment plan. Some tips on avoiding complications are presented in Table 11.3.

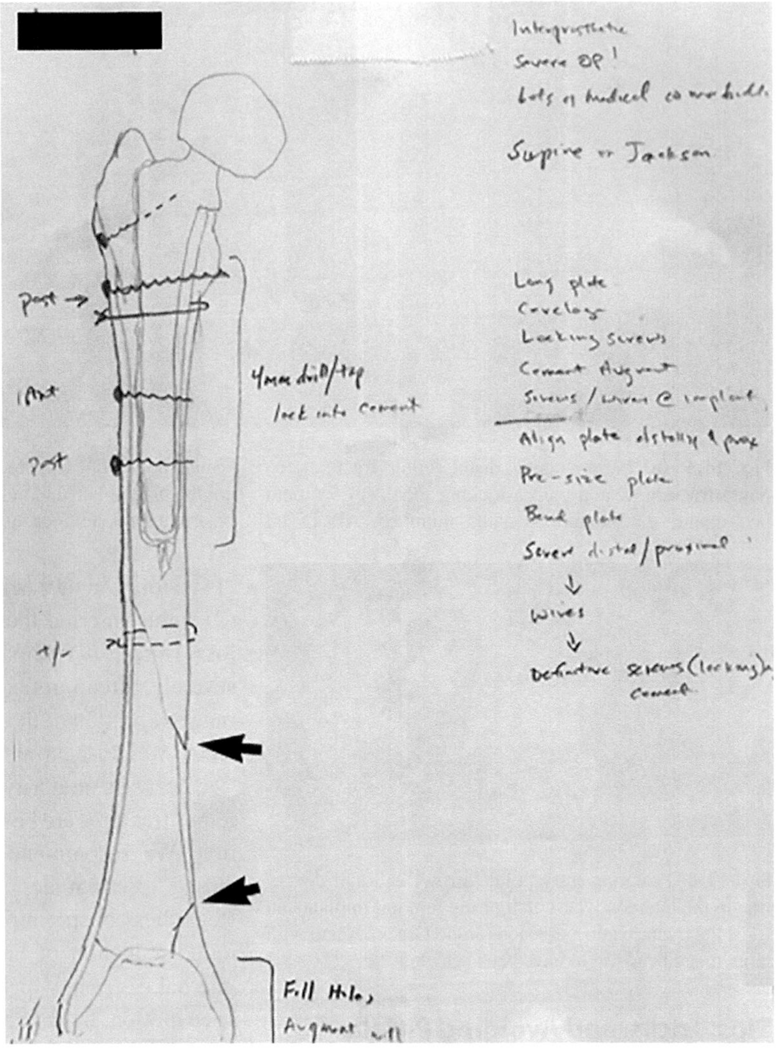

Fig. 11.7 Preoperative planning for periprosthetic fracture

A biology preserving procedure should be done. We see little biologic cost in terms of fracture healing from a thoughtful parapatellar arthrotomy or lateral approach to the distal femur as long as good technique is used, including avoiding soft-tissue stripping, preserving perforators if possible, debriding the fracture site (including hematoma), etc. We will also frequently use of radiolucent guides for percutaneous plate application, but the objectives of fracture reduction and bridge-plating must be successfully attained.

The preoperative plan should also take into consideration how intraoperative imaging will be used. High-quality radiographs are absolutely critical for proper implant placement into the femoral condyles, and preventable errors may adversely affect outcomes. C-arm is brought in from the contralateral "well" side (Fig. 11.8b, c). Before draping, the C-arm should be brought in to confirm that correct views can be obtained, unhindered by overlap of the contralateral limb. A quality image of the opposite "well" limb is often useful as a template for repair.

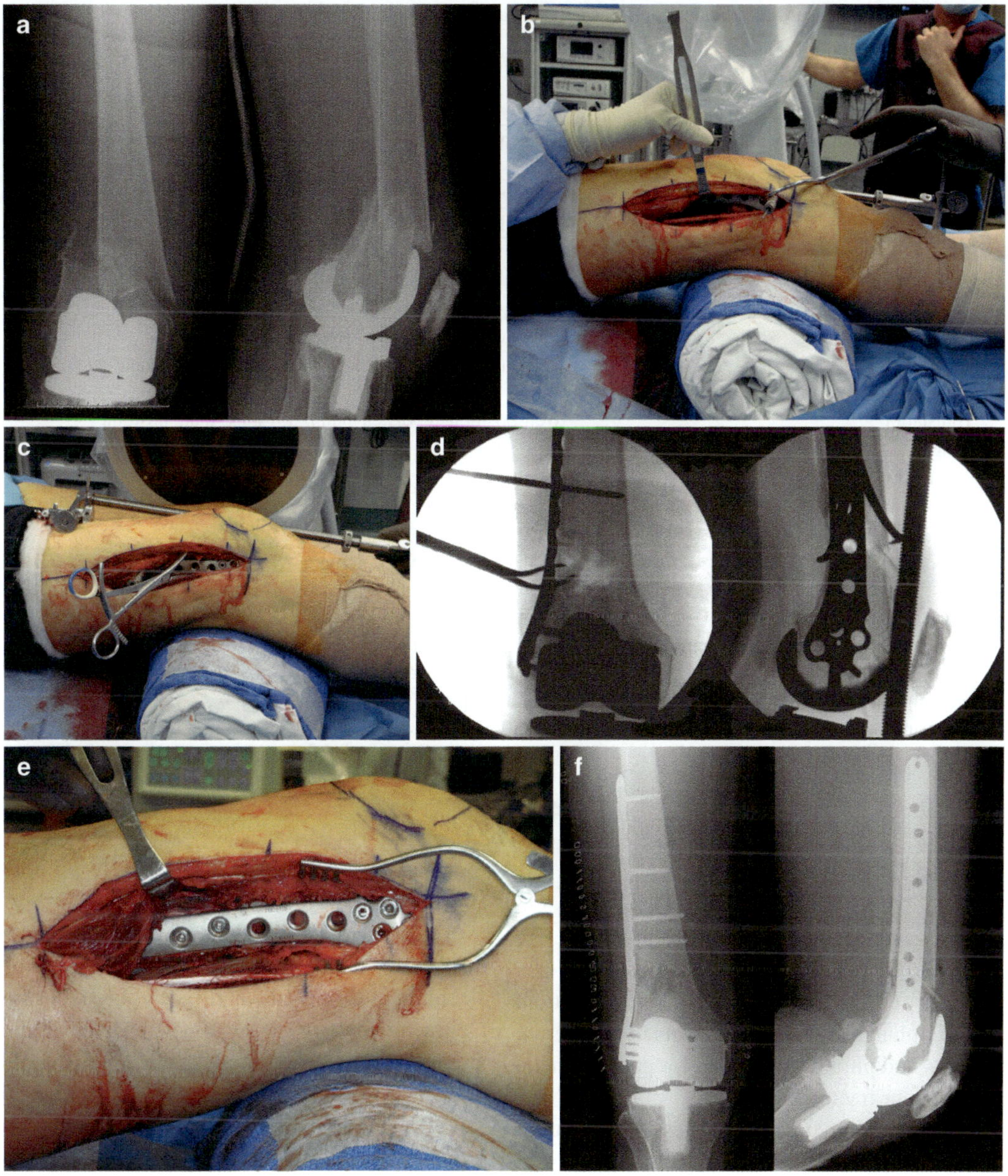

Fig. 11.8 Case of periprosthetic distal femur fracture undergoing locked plating. (**a**) Fracture. (**b**) Set-up with C-arm on opposite side, knee on a bump/ bolster to elevate and flex, and biologically friendly lateral approach to the distal femur (**c**) Reduction aids include positioning of the bump (flexion-extension), Weber clamp (translation/compression), and femoral distractor (length and rotation) (**d**) intraoperative fluoroscopic AP and lateral images exhibiting appropriately positioned lateral locked plate with temporizing K wire and clamp holding reduction (**e**) intraoperative clinical photo exhibiting laterally based minimally invasive approach with plate placement (**f**) postoperative AP and lateral xrays with appropriate length alignment rotation and implant placement

General endotracheal anesthesia is preferred to allow for complete muscle paralysis; however, spinal or other regional techniques are occasionally indicated. The patient is positioned supine on a radiolucent flat-top (Jackson) table. The anesthesia team should understand that complete muscle paralysis is necessary to help regain length and overcome the powerful deforming muscle forces crossing the fracture. The entire limb is draped free into the field to allow manipulation of the extremity, which will also assist intraoperative fluoroscopy.

Table 11.3 Technical tips for planning periprosthetic distal femur fracture surgery

Prevent medical complications	Medical clearance/risk assessment
Assess bone quality	Assess plain X-rays, history
Assess for implant stability	Quality plain X-rays
Assess for compatibility with intramedullary nailing, if chosen	Medical records, joint replacement staff, online database
Malalignment:	Intraoperative diligence is key!
	Contralateral side is a good guide
	Pharmacologic paralysis with anesthesia.
Varus-valgus	Intraoperative guides, Bovie-cord
Flexion-extension	Quality lateral fluoroscopy, well-positioned bolster/bump, posterior cortical read ("constant fragment")
Rotational	Cortical reads, rotational profiles (compared to contralateral side)
Translation	Well-positioned bolster/-bump, joystick, plate position
Length	Cortical reads, radiolucent ruler
Construct decisions	
Mechanical environment	More comminuted, osteoporotic fractures > bridging plate construct
Stability	Long plates, increased number, well-spaced and/or locked screws
Balanced fixation	Similar "density" of fixation proximal and distal to fracture
Augmentation of standard implants	Combine nail and plate, add cements for screw augmentation ($CaPO_4$ or PMMA)
Interfacing with pre-existing implants	Overlap implants where possible
Avoid irritable implants	Avoid long screws around knee, roll-over view
Avoid knee stiffness	Stable repair (pain control), early range of motion

Locked Plating

When using plate fixation, accurate fracture reduction is a vital component in restoring normal function and allowing for early mobilization. Each implant and technique has its own inherent benefits and pitfalls when used for periprosthetic distal femur fractures.

Anatomically contoured plates must be used thoughtfully, as a number of pitfalls are possible. Not all patients match the plate anatomy, and this mismatch can impart deformity. Plates may occasionally need to be bent or applied off the bone to allow for anatomic reduction. If the plate does fit, it must be applied in the proper position on the bone, as misapplication also leads to deformity. For example, a plate applied in an overly distal or posterior manner will push the condyles medially, thereby resulting in the "golf-club" deformity: in general, a plate secured to the condyles in a non-anatomic position is likely to promulgate deformity across the fracture.

Indirect reduction of the metaphyseal or metadiaphyseal portion of the fracture is achieved by a combination of methods (Fig. 11.8b–d). In simple fracture patterns, reduction using manual longitudinal traction alone may suffice. A well-placed pointed reduction forceps or "King Tong" clamp can also aid reduction by holding the fracture in proper position. The authors have found the universal (femoral) distractor to be a valuable tool. Placed anteriorly into the femoral shaft proximally and anchored in the proximal tibia, distraction usually restores overall length and alignment. Initial overdistraction permits gentle teasing of comminuted fracture fragments into near-anatomic position. A large or medium sterile towel roll or bump can be effective at controlling sagittal alignment; moving it distally or proximally even a few centimeters may be very helpful. Finally, if correctly applied, periarticular plates can fine-tune the reduction by pulling the bone to the anatomically contoured plate using conventional screws. Combining standard cortical screws to lag the bone to the plate followed by locked screws to aid in construct stability is a useful tactic and employs benefits of both screw types. It is important to remember that if a combination of non-locked screws and locked screws is used in any given fracture fragment, the non-locked screws must be inserted first in that fragment before any locking screws are inserted ("lag before you lock"), or the fixation of the non-locked screws can be compromised.

Plate application has become more complex with the introduction of locked implants, but also potentially more effective with multiple options for screw placement. Screws can be standard or locked, cannulated or noncannulated, bicortical or unicortical, and plates can be inserted open or through minimally invasive approaches. The variety of screw options has become especially useful for periprosthetic distal femur fracture because of the limited bone stock and distal femoral prosthesis. When using most plates (not polyaxial) as a reduction tool, it is important to align the most distal locked screws or their guidewires parallel to the knee joint to ensure that the 5 to 8 degrees or so of valgus built into the plate is achieved. Plates with polyaxial screws also have similar alignment guides to ensure restoration of the appropriate valgus alignment, but these and subsequent condylar screws must be applied thoughtfully. All non-locked screws must be inserted into the proximal or distal segment before any locked screws are placed. If a periprosthetic fracture is well reduced and has particularly good bone quality, compression could be applied to increase stability, promote primary bone healing, and allow for earlier weight-bearing. Nonetheless, *only* when the medial cortex is restored can the plate be effectively loaded. Properly done, the plate is placed under tension and in theory subject to load sharing, rather than load bearing. Much more typically, in cases with comminution, the plate is fixed to the proximal and distal fracture, bridging the zone of comminution (Fig. 11.8e, f). In this environment, the plate acts as an internal splint. However, the fracture fragments spanned by the plate are left undisturbed and capable of rapid consolidation if their soft-tissue attachments have been respected. In cases of severe osteoporosis where the patient is non-ambulatory or must bear weight immediately, acute shortening with compression across the metaphyseal fracture may be chosen. While this may maximize bone-to-bone contact, the surgeon should still be aware that the fracture stability may soon be lost by resorption and further "settling" of fragments with micromotion.

In comminuted fracture patterns, reduction can be achieved with the aid of a femoral distractor or an external fixator. Most of the reduction methods used for simple fractures are applicable to comminuted fractures. We have found that it is often easier to reduce the fracture to the plate rather than the plate to the fracture in complex fracture patterns. In this situation, the plate must be used to aid reduction. It is important to re-emphasize that the most distal locked screws must be parallel to the joint surface as assessed on AP image as a guide for restoring limb alignment.

The length of the plate and the number and placement of screws are based on the preoperative plan. In general, we favor treating comminuted and osteoporotic fractures with less soft-tissue dissection, longer plates, more screws in each segment, and more locked screws. In general, a longer plate with spaced screws provides better mechanical stability compared with shorter plates and clustered screws. When selecting plate length, eight cortices of fixation above and below the fracture site are recommended to provide adequate stability to prevent early torsional and axial failure. Subjective "balance" in the fixation proximally and distally is suggested. This may not always be possible in the distal segment because of the femoral prosthesis. The use of longer plates with well-spaced cortical screws limits implant stiffness and encourages secondary bone healing. If a locked construct is chosen, a plate of sufficient length to allow no more than 50% of screw holes to be filled is required to prevent stress concentration and premature implant breakage. If the fracture is located between prostheses, the proximal femoral component should be spanned in order to prevent stress riser between the junction of the implants. The plate is centered on the lateral aspect of the femur and a K-wire is applied in a wire hole in the plate (if available) or cannulated wire guide. With the plate centered on the distal diaphyseal fracture fragment, it is provisionally fixed close to the fracture. Intraoperative fluoroscopy is used to confirm fracture alignment and implant position. The guide pin closest to the joint is typically designed to restore varus–valgus alignment if placed parallel to the joint axis. A series of cortical screws followed by locked screws (hybrid technique) allows the benefits of both screw types to be realized. The condylar segment is stabilized predominately with locked screws.

Retrograde Intramedullary Nailing

The main potential advantage of retrograde nailing over plating is that they may be inserted through smaller, potentially less invasive surgical approaches than plates, and the devices are centrally placed so that bending forces may be better resisted. Keys to successful nailing in the distal femur as well as elsewhere are (1) optimizing the starting point and initial reamer pass and (2) obtaining and maintaining a quality reduction during the procedure.

There are several *potential* advantages of nailing over plating: it is a load-sharing device compared with a plate and has the potential to stabilize complex fractures with less soft-tissue dissection. Modern nailing systems now allow multiple distal screws in different planes and rigid locking capability to improve stabilization of the condylar block compared to a decade ago. These screws have "locking" capability just as modern plating systems do, and "plate/washers" linking a plate on the lateral cortex with additional condylar screws outside the nail are available. Most surgeons currently favor full-length nails inserted beyond the isthmus of the femur to the level or just above the lesser trochanter to prevent residual instability or fractures above short nails.

Potential disadvantages of retrograde nailing include knee sepsis, stiffness, patella-and-femoral pain. Additionally, the starting point may be difficult to ascertain through standard fluoroscopy due to the femoral prosthesis.

Technique of Intramedullary Nailing

The goals of intramedullary nailing remain the same as for plating restoration of axial alignment and length, fracture stabilization, and maintenance of a biologic environment conducive to healing with avoidance of infection. Surgery is done on a radiolucent table with the aid of an image intensifier.

The patient is positioned supine and the affected limb supported on a radiolucent triangle or large bump to a 20- or 30-degree angle. The C-arm unit should come in from the opposite side of the table, and the underside of the table should be clear to move the C-arm from the hip to knee without obstruction in both the AP and lateral projection. When possible, the fracture should be reduced before nailing. Many of the indirect reduction methods described in femoral plating are useful for nailing.

Intramedullary nailing is usually performed through the previous incision. The arthrotomy will usually be performed in the direction that was used for the TKA, if that can be determined. If there is knee contracture, a wider incision is made to facilitate access to the intercondylar notch. The intramedullary nail can then be inserted through the open incision. It is important to leave 5 to 6 mm of capsular tissue for a stable side-to-side repair during closure. The patella and local soft tissues should be protected from reamers and other instrumentation during nailing. A working "soft-tissue" cannula is available in most nailing sets or carefully placed right-angle retractors are effective.

Metaphyseal fracture reduction is performed manually or using the femoral distractor with pins placed eccentrically or unicortically in the shaft, a well-placed sterile towel roll, and Schanz pins attached to a T-handle chuck (joysticks) in the femoral shaft or condyles, to reduce the major fragments.

In a native knee, the optimal portal of entry for the nail is in the intercondylar notch at the junction of Blumensaat's line and the subchondral line of the distal femoral trochlea. Obviously the standard technique to obtain the starting point is not a feasible option when a prosthesis is in place. The use of an AP and lateral view, aiming for the center of the canal, provides an adequate reference point. In addition, if the prosthesis was appropriately centered, the starting point on the AP should be the same. It may be necessary to remove cement within the canal if it is blocking the entry point. In addition, careful attention must be paid while nailing in order prevent damage to the prosthesis. A threaded tipped guide pin and cannulated drill are used to open the distal femur before nailing. The pin is carefully inserted in line with the femoral shaft to ensure restoration of coronal plane alignment on the AP image. Once the guide pin placement is confirmed with AP and lateral radiographs, the step reamer is advanced through the working channel soft-tissue sleeve over the entry wire to prepare the insertion site. Occasionally, an "open" notch femoral implant will push the nail insertion point somewhat posteriorly. We feel that few millimeters of posteriorization is quite acceptable, but one must be watchful and in the rare occasion where the starting point is significantly altered, the surgeon should consider aborting nailing in favor of plating.

A beaded tip guidewire is inserted into the intramedullary canal and advanced past the fracture site, into the proximal femur under fluoroscopic control. With the fracture reduced, the position of the guidewire should be center—center in both the AP and lateral views in both the proximal and distal fragments. An intramedullary fracture reducer or "finger" is available in most nailing sets and can be used to facilitate reduction and guide wire passage across the fracture site. Blocking screws are sometimes used to narrow the effective canal diameter of distal femur to improve alignment and prevent deformity. Although impossible in some cases, blocking screws can be placed in the distal segment to help reduce coronal or sagittal plane deformity. A rule of thumb is to apply the screws on the concave side of existing deformity.

Distal Femoral Replacement

An in-depth discussion distal femoral replacement is probably outside the scope of this chapter, but a number of general comments can be made. First, the decision for DFR should not be made without significant consideration as it is truly a salvage procedure without a good "bail out" if it should fail. Second, the principles of good knee arthroplasty surgery should be applied strictly. Limb alignment and length, implant sizing, extensor kinematics, must be considered. The implants are constrained and modular, so that an understanding of how the implants and trials work is necessary. An extensile surgical approach to the knee is used. The patella is mobilized. Resection length is estimated above the fracture and a transverse saw cut is made. The fractured distal femur and TKA are excised. Cemented and press-fit options exist for DFR. Standard orthopedic and implant specific instrumentation is used to prepare the femur and proximal tibia.

Summary

In conclusion, management of periprosthetic fractures of the femur above TKA depends on bone quality, fracture characteristics, size of distal fragment, stability of the implants, and condition, ambulatory function of the patient, and surgeon experience. If the fracture is amenable to repair and TKA is well fixed, attempts are made to fix the fracture with modern locked plates and/or intramedullary nail, whereas if implants are loose, consideration should be given to DFR surgery. Preoperative planning and an understanding of the available implants for these surgeries is central to ensuring the highest rate of success possible for the patients' outcomes.

References

1. Streubel PN. Mortality after periprosthetic femur fractures. J Knee Surg. 2013;26(1):27–30.
2. Streubel PN, Ricci WM, Wong A, Gardner MJ. Mortality after distal femur fractures in elderly patients. Clin Orthop Relat Res. 2011;469(4):1188–96.
3. Rorabeck CH, Taylor JW. Classification of periprosthetic fractures complicating total knee arthroplasty. Orthop Clin North Am. 1999;30(2):209–14.
4. Kim KI, Egol KA, Hozack WJ, Parvizi J. Periprosthetic fractures after total knee arthroplasties. Clin Orthop Relat Res. 2006;446:167–75.
5. Su ET, DeWal H, Di Cesare PE. Periprosthetic femoral fractures above total knee replacements. J Am Acad Orthop Surg. 2004;12(1):12–20.
6. Culp RW, Schmidt RG, Hanks G, Mak A, Esterhai JL Jr, Heppenstall RB. Supracondylar fracture of the femur following prosthetic knee arthroplasty. Clin Orthop Relat Res. 1987;222:212–22.
7. Merkel KD, Johnson EW Jr. Supracondylar fracture of the femur after total knee arthroplasty. J Bone Joint Surg Am. 1986;68(1):29–43.
8. Streubel PN, Gardner MJ, Morshed S, Collinge CA, Gallagher B, Ricci WM. Are extreme distal periprosthetic supracondylar fractures of the femur too distal to fix using a lateral locked plate? J Bone Joint Surg Br. 2010;92(4):527–34.
9. Taljanovic MS, Hunter TB, Miller MD, Sheppard JE. Gallery of medical devices: part 1: orthopedic devices for the extremities and pelvis. Radiographics. 2005;25(3):859–70.
10. Healy WL, Siliski JM, Incavo SJ. Operative treatment of distal femoral fractures proximal to total knee replacements. J Bone Joint Surg Am. 1993;75(1):27–34.
11. Davison BL. Varus collapse of comminuted distal femur fractures after open reduction and internal fixation with a lateral condylar buttress plate. Am J Orthop. 2003;32(1):27–30.
12. Figgie MP, Goldberg VM, Figgie HE 3rd, Sobel M. The results of treatment of supracondylar fracture above total knee arthroplasty. J Arthroplast. 1990;5(3):267–76.
13. Ricci WM, Loftus T, Cox C, Borrelli J. Locked plates combined with minimally invasive insertion technique for the treatment of periprosthetic supracondylar femur fractures above a total knee arthroplasty. J Orthop Trauma. 2006;20(3):190–6.
14. Norrish AR, Jibri ZA, Hopgood P. The LISS plate treatment of supracondylar fractures above a total knee replacement: a case-control study. Acta Orthop Belg. 2009;75(5):642–8.
15. Kolb W, Guhlmann H, Windisch C, Marx F, Koller H, Kolb K. Fixation of periprosthetic femur fractures above total knee arthroplasty with the less invasive stabilization system: a midterm follow-up study. J Trauma. 2010;69(3):670–6.
16. Hoffmann MF, Jones CB, Sietsema DL, Koenig SJ, Tornetta P 3rd. Outcome of periprosthetic distal femoral fractures following knee arthroplasty. Injury. 2012;43(7):1084–9.
17. Kregor PJ, Hughes JL, Cole PA. Fixation of distal femoral fractures above total knee arthroplasty utilizing the Less Invasive Stabilization System (L.I.S.S.). Injury. 2001;32 Suppl 3:SC64–75.
18. Raab GE, Davis CM 3rd. Early healing with locked condylar plating of periprosthetic fractures around the knee. J Arthroplast. 2005;20(8):984–9.
19. Kolb W, Guhlmann H, Windisch C, Marx F, Kolb K, Koller H. Fixation of distal femoral fractures with the less invasive stabilization system: a minimally invasive treatment with locked fixed-angle screws. J Trauma. 2008;65(6):1425–34.
20. Weight M, Collinge C. Early results of the less invasive stabilization system for mechanically unstable fractures of the distal femur (AO/OTA types A2, A3, C2, and C3). J Orthop Trauma. 2004;18(8):503–8.
21. Falck M, Hontzasch T, Krettek C. LISS (less invasive stabilization system) als minimalinvasive Alternative bei distalen Femurfrakturen. Trauma Berufskrankh. 1999;1:402–6.
22. Althausen PL, Lee MA, Finkemeier CG, Meehan JP, Rodrigo JJ. Operative stabilization of supracondylar femur fractures above total knee arthroplasty: a comparison of four treatment methods. J Arthroplast. 2003;18(7):834–9.
23. Hierholzer C, von Ruden C, Potzel T, Woltmann A, Buhren V. Outcome analysis of retrograde nailing and less invasive stabilization system in distal femoral fractures: a retrospective analysis. Indian J Orthop. 2011;45(3):243–50.
24. Anglen J, Kyle RF, Marsh JL, et al. Locking plates for extremity fractures. J Am Acad Orthop Surg. 2009;17(7):465–72.
25. Ebraheim NA, Liu J, Hashmi SZ, Sochacki KR, Moral MZ, Hirschfeld AG. High complication rate in locking plate fixation of lower periprosthetic distal femur fractures in patients with total knee arthroplasties. J Arthroplast. 2012;27(5):809–13.
26. Bong MR, Egol KA, Koval KJ, et al. Comparison of the LISS and a retrograde-inserted supracondylar intramedullary nail for fixation of a periprosthetic distal femur fracture proximal to a total knee arthroplasty. J Arthroplast. 2002;17(7):876–81.
27. Herrera DA, Kregor PJ, Cole PA, Levy BA, Jonsson A, Zlowodzki M. Treatment of acute distal femur fractures above a total knee arthroplasty: systematic review of 415 cases (1981–2006). Acta Orthop. 2008;79(1):22–7.
28. Wick M, Muller EJ, Kutscha-Lissberg F, Hopf F, Muhr G. [Periprosthetic supracondylar femoral fractures: LISS or retrograde intramedullary nailing? Problems with the use of minimally invasive technique]. Unfallchirurg 2004;107(3):181–8.
29. Cordeiro EN, Costa RC, Carazzato JG, Silva JS. Periprosthetic fractures in patients with total

knee arthroplasties. Clin Orthop Relat Res. 1990;252:182–9.

30. Pour AE, Parvizi J, Slenker N, Purtill JJ, Sharkey PF. Rotating hinged total knee replacement: use with caution. J Bone Joint Surg Am. 2007;89(8):1735–41.
31. Chen F, Mont MA, Bachner RS. Management of ipsilateral supracondylar femur fractures following total knee arthroplasty. J Arthroplast. 1994;9(5):521–6.
32. Kassab M, Zalzal P, Azores GM, Pressman A, Liberman B, Gross AE. Management of periprosthetic femoral fractures after total knee arthroplasty using a distal femoral allograft. J Arthroplast. 2004;19(3):361–8.
33. Saidi K, Ben-Lulu O, Tsuji M, Safir O, Gross AE, Backstein D. Supracondylar periprosthetic fractures of the knee in the elderly patients: a comparison of treatment using allograft-implant composites, standard revision components, distal femoral replacement prosthesis. J Arthroplast. 2014;29(1):110–4.

Revision Knee Arthroplasty in the Infectious Setting

12

Thomas L. Bernasek, Steven T. Lyons, Brian T. Palumbo, and T. Kyle Stoops

Introduction

Periprosthetic joint infection (PJI) after total knee arthroplasty (TKA) is an ever-present risk that results in substantial patient morbidity and mortality. The reported incidence of 0.39–2.18% places total knee infection as the leading cause of failure, accounting for 25% to 35% of TKA revisions [1–9]. The incidence and cost of TKA infections is projected to increase steadily. By 2020 an estimated 49,000 cases annually will cost approximately one billion dollars of healthcare spending [4].

PJI can occur at any time following primary or revision surgery but is most common in the first year after TKA [9]. PJIs can be acute or chronic in nature and understanding this is important in guiding surgical management. An acute PJI is defined as an infection that occurs within the first 4 to 6 weeks following a TKA, whereas a chronic infection is a delayed, often indolent infection that occurs months to years after undergoing a TKA [10–12].

Diagnosis and treatment of an infected TKA can be challenging. The most commonly isolated organisms associated with a PJI are Gram-positive cocci including *Staphylococcus Aureus (S. Aureus)* and Coagulase-negative *Staphylococcus (S. Epidermidis)*. However, infections are not limited to these organisms and may include Gram-negative bacteria and polymicrobial infections [2, 8, 9]. Drug resistance is on the rise with organisms such as Methicillin-resistant *S. Aureus (MRSA)* now responsible for 30–60% of PJIs following TKA [9, 10]. *MRSA* infections have increased the economic burden of treatment through longer hospital stays, poorer outcomes, and increased morbidity compared to PJIs caused by other organisms [10, 13–15]. The surgeon can anticipate a fivefold increase in mortality at 1 year for infected revision TKR compared to aseptic revisions [16].

The increase in TKR and infections has increased scrutiny on prevention. Much of this translates into careful patient selection, starting with identification of modifiable risk factors and implementing appropriate methods to reduce them. Two of the most common modifiable risk factors are obesity and uncontrolled diabetes. The odds ratio for PJI infection after TKA is increased to nine in morbidly obese patients (BMI > 40) compared to non-morbidly obese patients [17]. In 2013, the American Academy of Orthopaedic Surgeons (AAOS) released guidelines recommending that patients with a BMI >25 undergo a weight reduction of 5% total body weight using diet and exercise before receiving a TKA [18]. The American Association of Hip and

T. L. Bernasek (✉) · S. T. Lyons · B. T. Palumbo
T. K. Stoops
Florida Orthopaedic Institute, Tampa, FL, USA
e-mail: tbernasek@floridaortho.com;
slyons@floridaortho.com;
bpalumbo@floridaortho.com

R. S. Yoon et al. (eds.), *Trauma and Infection Control in Revision Hip and Knee Arthroplasty*,
https://doi.org/10.1007/978-3-031-71971-4_12

Knee Surgeons (AAHKS) observed a BMI of 40 as the threshold for increased perioperative complications and recommends "strong consideration" of weight reduction before considering a TKA [19]. Obese (BMI 30–39) diabetic patients have a seven times increase in odds ratio of developing a PJI [17]. Further, evidence suggests that uncontrolled diabetes (glycosylated hemoglobin (HbA1c) >7) is an independent risk factor for developing a PJI after TKA [8, 17, 20]. Many surgeons have implemented analysis of glycemic markers (e.g., HbA1c, fasting blood glucose (FBG), postprandial glucose (PPG2)) into their pre-operative regime for diabetic patients.

This chapter addresses the management of the infected total knee replacement including infection work-up, diagnostic criteria, and surgical management with the goal of optimizing patient outcomes.

Clinical Evaluation of the Infected Total Knee Arthroplasty

Clinical History and Physical Exam

Methods for diagnosing the infected TKA have advanced significantly over the past several decades. Despite improvements, an accurate diagnosis requires the surgeon's expertise, combining patient history and physical exam, with interpretation of basic laboratory and radiographic findings. Often the surgeon must synthesize several clinical and diagnostic details to prepare the patient for definitive treatment. Keen suspicion and preparation are crucial and cannot be overemphasized.

PJI has been defined by the Musculoskeletal Infection Society [21]:

1. A sinus tract communicating with the prosthesis.
2. A pathogen is isolated by culture from two or more separate tissue or fluid samples obtained from the affected prosthetic joint.
3. Four of the following six criteria exist:
   (a) Elevated serum erythrocyte sedimentation rate (ESR) and serum C-reactive protein (CRP) concentration
   (b) Elevated synovial white blood cell count (WBC)
   (c) Elevated synovial polymorphonuclear percentage (PMN %)
   (d) Presence of purulence in the affected joint
   (e) Isolation of a microorganism in one culture of periprosthetic tissue or fluid
   (f) Greater than five neutrophils per high-power field in five high-power fields observed from histologic analysis of periprosthetic tissue at ×400 magnification

Despite forming an accurate definition of PJI, the Musculoskeletal Infection Society panel acknowledges that an infection may be present if less than four criteria are met. Fastidious (e.g., *Tuberculosis*) or low-grade organisms (e.g., *Propionibacterium Acnes*, a slow-growing aerotolerant bacterium) can be present with minimal diagnostic evidence. A high level of suspicion includes making infection a diagnosis of exclusion for all painful TKA cases to avoid a missed diagnosis.

A general history including patient demographics and medical comorbidities (i.e., obesity, diabetes, rheumatoid arthritis, malignancy, physiologic age, nutritional status, etc.) obtained during evaluation of a painful TKA help stratify the patient's risk of active infection. In the acute infection, defined as six or fewer weeks after the primary TKA, findings include excessive pain, erythema, persistent drainage, induration, and lymphadenopathy. Recent illness (e.g., upper respiratory or urinary tract infection) or invasive procedures (e.g., dental) followed by a painful and symptomatic TKA can be etiologic for hematogenous bacterial seeding resulting in periprosthetic infection. Differentiation of acute from chronic infection can alter the treatment algorithm and outcome. The acute period is the optimal time for early surgical intervention with irrigation, debridement, and modular component exchange [22]. Findings such as peri-incisional

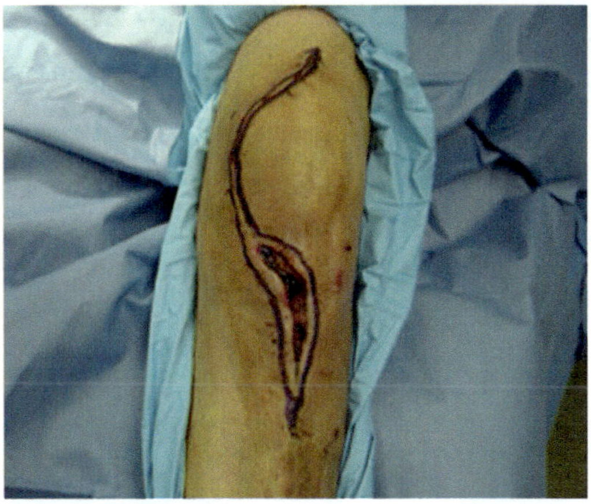

Fig. 12.1 This dehiscence began as distal wound drainage which was ignored

cellulitis, persistent drainage postoperatively, or wound dehiscence are findings that require immediate evaluation and possibly surgical treatment. Wound dehiscence or drainage of the distal wound is especially troubling due to thin soft-tissue coverage with limited blood supply providing an area of ready access for bacterial inoculation (Fig. 12.1). Wound drainage, dehiscence or signs of infection distally requires immediate evaluation and aggressive treatment to prevent deep infection. Plastic surgery consultation for early flap coverage may be necessary to achieve a stable wound.

In the chronically infected TKA, the patient's history can aid diagnosis, especially when the treating surgeon is not the primary surgeon. A history of perioperative complications such prolonged wound drainage and/or dehiscence are potential clues to the infection's genesis. Unexpected or early re-operations such as irrigation and debridement and/or modular component exchanges can be indicators of infection. Septic TKA pain is often present soon after the initial surgery and increases with time. Pain is often constant throughout the day and can occur with or without activity and at night. Episodic fever and chills, nausea and vomiting are not requisite for the diagnosis of periprosthetic infection but may indicate systemic involvement and should raise the concern for sepsis requiring emergent

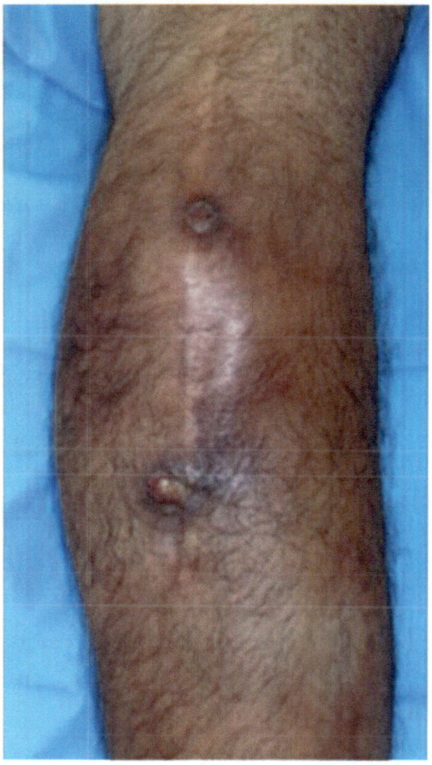

Fig. 12.2 An example of a chronically draining sinus at the superior and inferior aspects of the incision several years after TKA

treatment. Physical exam findings in the chronically infected TKA are usually less apparent with the exception of a chronically draining sinus tract, which is pathopneumonic for a periprosthetic infection [21] (Fig. 12.2). In the chronic setting, a broad spectrum of physical exam findings can exist. The knee's appearance can be completely innocuous with little evidence of infection to the extreme of severe swelling, erythema, induration, and active drainage. In cases with few or no physical findings, laboratory markers and advanced imaging have increased relevance (Fig. 12.3).

Laboratory Evaluation: Serologic Studies

Serum ESR and CRP markers are routine and cost-effective measures to detect an infection or

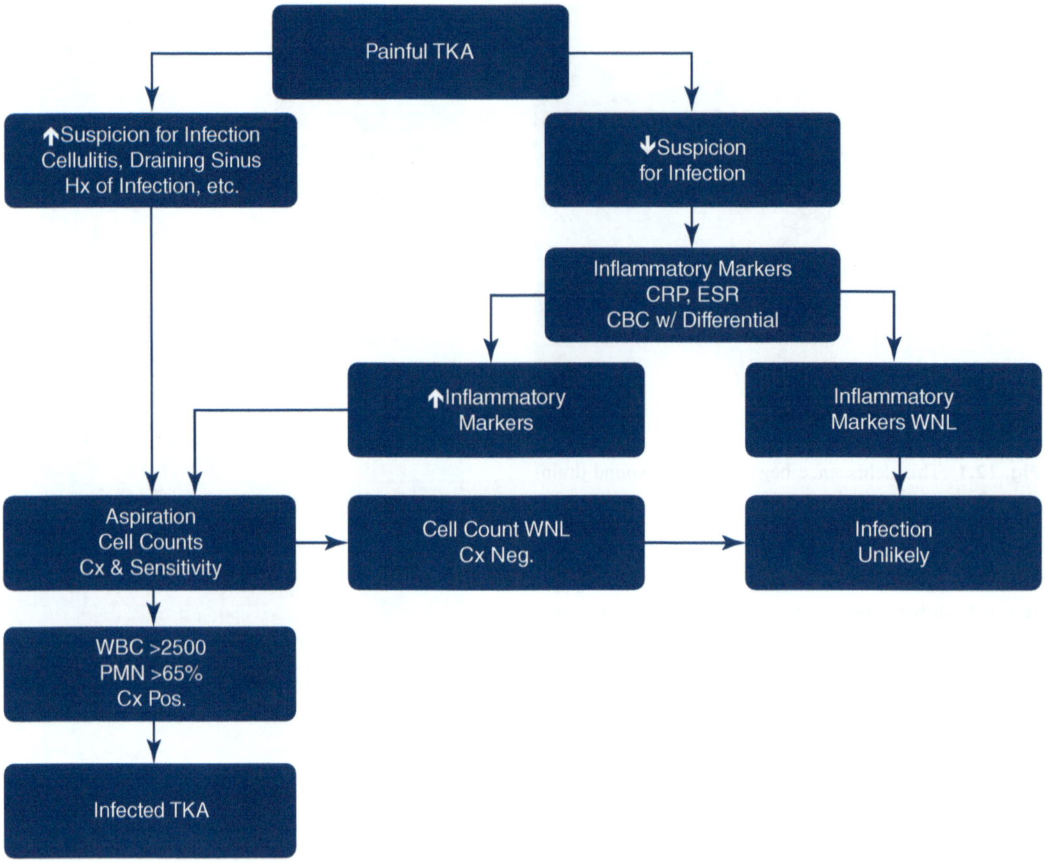

Fig. 12.3 Infected TKA Work-up Algorithm

acute inflammatory process [23]. CRP is an acute phase reactant protein synthesized by the liver which is increased in the presence of tissue injury, infection, or inflammation and is measured in mg/L. ESR is the rate at which anticoagulated erythrocytes sediment within 1 h and is measured in mm/h. These serologic studies have been demonstrated to have high sensitivity and negative predictive value (NPV) [24]. They reported an ESR of greater than 30 mm/h to have a sensitivity of 0.91 and NPV of 0.93. A CRP of greater than 10 mg/L had a sensitivity and NPV for infection of 0.94 and 0.95, respectively [24]. The optimal positivity criterion for ESR and CRP for infection was reported to be 22.5 mm/h and 13.5 mg/L, respectively [25]. With these values they reported sensitivities of 0.93 and 0.91 and specificities of 0.83 and 0.86 for infection for the two tests, respectively. Importantly, in the acute postoperative periods after primary TKA acute phase reactants may be elevated as long as 30 to 60 days [26, 27]. Therefore in the acute postoperative period, monitoring suspected PJI requires baseline acute phase reactants and periodic testing increasing or decreasing trends. Current AAOS Guidelines on the Diagnosis of Periprosthetic Joint Infections of the Hip and Knee recommend all painful TKAs be screened for infection with serum CRP and ESR due to their low cost and high sensitivity [23]. These guidelines should be reviewed by all arthroplasty surgeons diagnosing and managing periprosthetic joint infections.

Laboratory Evaluation: Synovial Fluid Aspiration and Infectious Markers

Standard synovial fluid analysis (Fig. 12.4) should include a cell count with differential, aerobic, and anaerobic cultures with sensitivities in those cases suspicious for infection. This includes the painful TKA with elevated inflammatory markers and cases of known infection to obtain accurate cultures for an optimal antibiotic regimen. Prior to aspiration the patient should be off all antibiotics for at least 3 weeks to avoid a false negative result [28]. Meticulous sterile technique during aspiration avoids iatrogenic infection and mitigates the risk of culture contamination. Avoid using bacteriostatic local anesthetics as they can affect culture results. If only scant (a drop) fluid is obtained from the joint, prioritize culture and sensitivity.

Recent consensus recommendations suggest that acid-fast bacillus or mycobacterial and fungal cultures only be obtained in high suspicion scenarios [21]. However, we suggest obtaining cultures for such organisms routinely to improve one's chance for an accurate diagnosis and to better direct antibiotic therapy. Isolation of low-virulence organisms such as coagulase-negative *Staphylococcus*, *Propionibacterium* acnes, or *Corynebacterium*, in the absence of clinical or laboratory evidence of infection, can represent culture contamination [21]. In such scenarios, we recommend disclosure to the patient and close observation for clinical symptoms. Gram stain has been shown to have poor sensitivity and NPV in diagnosing PJI and its routine use functions primarily to expedite culture medium inoculation [29].

The most sensitive and specific synovial fluid test is the cell count with differential. Mason et al. reported a recommended synovial WBC count of 2500 cells/mL with greater than 60% polymorphonuclear leukocytes (PMNs) based on 86 pre-operative aspirates of aseptic and septic TKAs prior to revision [30]. In 2008, Ghanem et al. reported synovial aspiration results in 429 revision TKAs and recommended a threshold of 1100 leukocytes/mL with greater than 64% neutrophils. Further, they reported a positive predictive value (PPV) of 98.6% when both tests surpassed these thresholds and an NPV of 98.25% when both tests were below these values [31]. The acutely infected TKA less than 3 months

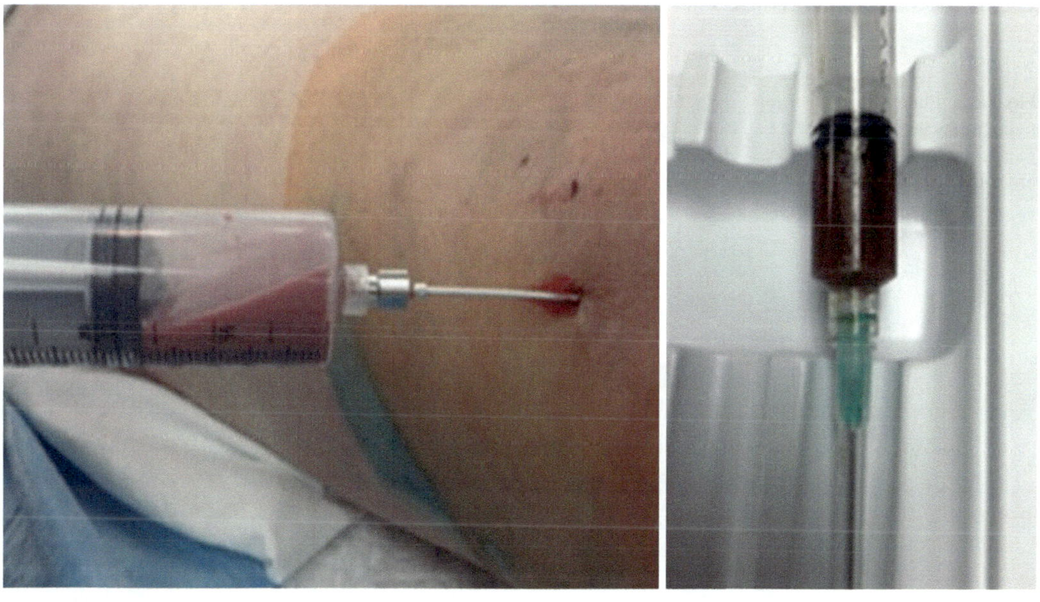

Fig. 12.4 Aspiration of purulent fluid from an infected TKA

postop shows significantly higher leukocytes and PMNs (27,000 cells/μL and 89%) compared to the uninfected TKA (4200 cells/μL and 76.9%) [32]. Values approaching these thresholds should raise the suspicion of an infection with the purpose to initiate patient discussion and formulation of a treatment strategy.

Other biomarkers have been shown to be effective in the detection of PJIs. Synovial leukocyte esterase assay using colorimetric or urine test strips demonstrated a sensitivity of 80.6% and 100% specificity, a 100% PPV and 93.3% NPV [33]. The testing strips are inexpensive, readily available and results are immediate making this test a potentially valuable tool in the surgeon's armamentarium.

Synovial CRP and alpha-defensin levels have been shown effective in detection of PJIs. Parvizi et al. demonstrated a statistically significant difference in synovial CRP levels of 40 and 2 mg/L for septic and aseptic failures, respectively [34]. Further, there was an 85% sensitivity and 95% specificity for detection of PJI when synovial CRP was elevated in this series [34]. Alpha-defensin is a protein secreted by synovial neutrophils in a septic environment. Several studies have demonstrated excellent sensitivity and specificity for detection of periprosthetic infections in the presence of this protein [35–37]. Combined synovial CRP and alpha-defensin testing has been shown to be superior to previous methods discussed even in the setting of concomitant inflammatory arthropathy and ongoing antibiotic treatment [36, 37].

Radiologic Evaluation and Advanced Imaging: Radiography

Posterior-anterior radiographs of bilateral knees with anterior, lateral, and merchant radiographs of the affected knee are the routine radiographic work-up for any painful TKA. Fluoroscopically guided images improve detection of implant interface radiolucencies which define loosening or infection. In the acute setting, radiographic findings rarely exist to help in the diagnosis. In the chronic setting, implant interface radiolucencies or the pathognomonic marginal erosions alert the surgeon to the possibility of periprosthetic infection (Fig. 12.5). In chronic infections, large radiolucencies in the distal femur and proximal tibial represent bone loss which is often greater than expected from plain radiographs. Femoral or tibial component migration and subsidence indicates loosening which can be associated with marked bone loss (Fig. 12.6).

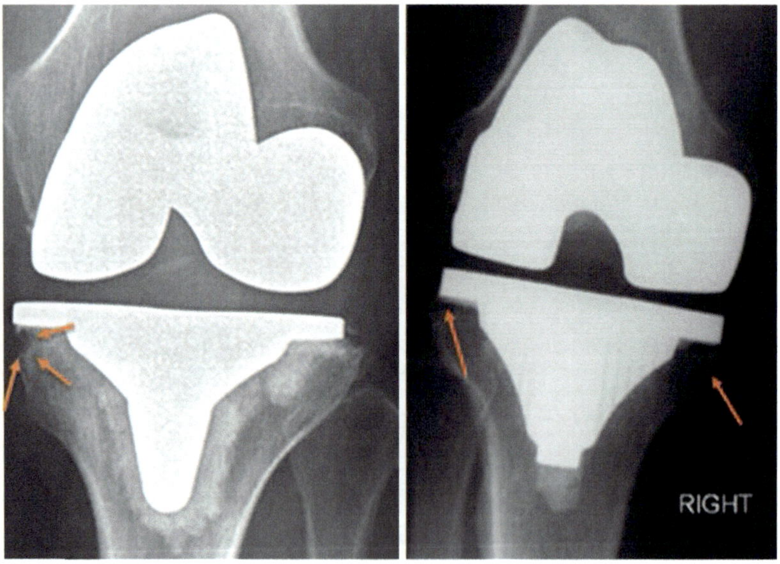

Fig. 12.5 Plain film radiographs with arrows identifying marginal erosions/radiolucencies)

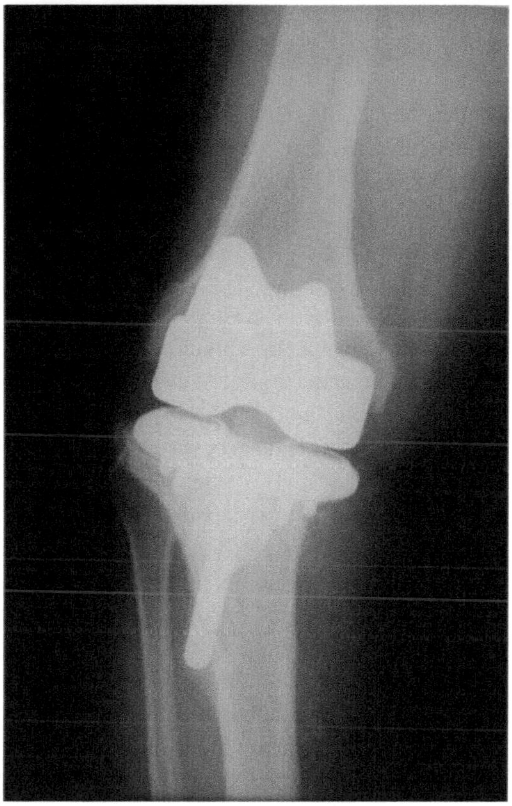

Fig. 12.6 Varus tibial component migration and severe proximal tibial bone loss in a chronically infected TKA

Radiologic Evaluation and Advanced Imaging: Nuclear Medicine

Radionuclear studies may be helpful in difficult to diagnose cases when clinical, serological, and synovial tests are equivocal. Levitsky reported only 33% sensitivity and 86% specificity using triple-phase technetium-99 bone scans to detect periprosthetic joint infections [38]. However, when combined with an indium-111 leukocyte scan, diagnostic accuracy was improved to 100% specificity and 46% sensitivity [39]. Routine use of radionuclear studies is not recommended until all other clinical and laboratory methods have been employed.

Intraoperative Evaluation: Frozen Pathological Analysis

Frozen-section analysis of joint tissue is recommended as an intraoperative step to confirm or rule out infection. While recommendations regarding cells per high-powered field (HPF) exist, this test serves only as a guide. The accuracy of frozen-section analysis can vary, including false positives or negatives, due to sampling errors, the pathology department's team experience and the presence of focal infection. It is useful to simultaneously send some of the harvested tissue for aerobic and anaerobic culture as well. In patients already treated with antibiotics, swabbing areas of the prosthesis isolated from intra-articular fluid (e.g., polyethylene liner-baseplate interface) might improve the isolation and culture of organisms.

Both 5 and 10 PMNs/HPF have been reported as thresholds for the diagnosis of periprosthetic infection [40–42]. Feldman et al. reported a 100% sensitivity and 96% specificity in the detection of infection of 33 THA and TKAs when greater than 5 PMNs/HPF in five specimens [40]. Increasing the threshold to 10 PMNs/HPF increased specificity with little impact on sensitivity. Lonner et al. showed that using 10 versus 5 PMNs/HPF had the same sensitivity of 84% but with an increased specificity of from 96% to 99% [41]. Zhao compared thresholds of 5 versus 10 PMNs/HPF and reported the same sensitivity but improved specificity with 10PMNs/HPF [42]. The authors recommend three to five specimens for analysis to improve the yield for detection of infectious foci and to determine consistency of results. For example, detection 5 or 10 PMNs/HPF at one site with all other specimens demonstrating no acute inflammation may not be indicative of infection. The contrary is true as well, detection of four PMNs/HPF at all sites may be indicative of septic failure even though this value does not cross the traditional threshold of 5 or 10 cells.

Treatment of the Infected TKA

Each patient with a periprosthetic TKA infection is unique and treatment should be tailored to meet that individual's circumstance. Patient age, medical comorbidities, soft-tissue quality, organism virulence, prior functional status and patient expectations guide the treatment plan.

Non-operative and Suppressive Therapy

Non-operative treatment with suppressive antibiotic therapy is relegated to patients of low function and unacceptable surgical risk. In some cases, surgery is not technically feasible (severe bone loss, severe soft-tissue deficiencies, etc.) or the patient simply refuses to have additional surgery. The well-informed patient should understand that suppressive therapy *is not* curative that the organism can become resistant and that antibiotic treatment will likely be managed by the infectious disease physician.

Occasionally, intraoperative cultures may be positive without evidence of infection perioperatively. These results are often reported several days after surgery and may be the result of contamination. The condition of the surgical bed, the presence of acute inflammation on frozen section, virulence of the cultured organism, and the number of positive cultures should be taken into account when considering treatment options. There are no established guidelines for these scenarios; therefore, the surgeon should use best judgment to monitor for clinical infection. Acute debridement and modular exchange is usually unwarranted and should only be considered when clinical evidence suggests acute infection. If a single positive culture without other clinical evidence of infection, an IV antibiotics for up to 2 weeks is usually recommended by the authors. In the presence of two or more cultures for the same organism, we recommend a 6-week course of IV antibiotic therapy managed by the infectious disease team and close observation. If any clinical evidence for acute infections arises, prompt surgical debridement and modular component exchange is recommended.

Debridement, Component Retention with Modular Component Exchange

Debridement with retention of TKA components is generally relegated to acute hematogenous infections, early acute postoperative infections, and patients unable or unwilling to tolerate a more complicated surgery. Advantages of this approach include modest physiologic impact in the frail patient, quicker recovery, and preservation of bone stock. The extent of the surgical debridement and bio-burden reduction is likely the most important factor for success but also the most subjective and poorly controlled variable with this treatment pathway. Removal, debridement, and replacement of the polyethylene insert should be performed when possible to decrease bacteria and biofilm on the component. This also increases access to the posterior joint for removal of necrotic and inflamed tissue. Have polyethylene inserts available including thicker sizes to compensate for increased ligamentous laxity after soft-tissue debridement.

Variable success has been reported with component retention and modular component exchange. In 2003, Rao et al. reported an 82% survivorship in 32 patients treated with acute debridement and long-term suppressive therapy at a mean follow-up of 60 months [43]. Tintle et al. established criteria for long-term suppressive therapy that included poor surgical candidates, refusal of surgery, arthrodesis or resection arthroplasty patients, documented sensitive organism, ability to tolerate oral antibiotics and good patient compliance. They reported an implant retention protocol and no revisions required at an average 37 months follow-up [44].

Deirmengian et al. reported only 35% infection-free 10-year outcomes for acute Gram-positive TKA infections in 31 knees. Also reported was an 8% eradication rate in *Staphylococcus aureus* infections compared with a 56% eradication rate with *Staphylococcus epi-*

dermidis or Streptococcus [45]. Bradbury et al. reported 16% Methicillin-Resistant *Staphylococcus Aureus* (MRSA) eradication in 19 acutely infected TKAs treated with debridement and component retention [13].

Arthroscopic debridement has a limited role in management of periprosthetic infections. Chung reported 16 early acute infected TKA cases initially treated with arthroscopic debridement. Eradication of infection occurred in 63% of cases at 2 years follow-up. Cases that failed arthroscopic debridement subsequently underwent open debridement with modular component exchange and retention of components resulting in a 100% eradication rate [46]. Arthroscopic debridement is limited due to exposure and inability to remove modular components for residual infection debridement.

Pre-operative Preparation and General Techniques of the Staged Revision

Preparation begins with patient counseling on surgical options and final plan, expected outcomes of those options, associated risks and the plan in the event of treatment failure. Preoperative radiographs guide surgical planning. Identify current components in preparation for explantation and request compatible polyethylene inserts for possible exchange. Define osseous deficiencies and template for reconstruction with an articulating spacer or final implantation. Request an experienced pathologist for frozen-section analysis. Order essential equipment such as reverse curettes and flexible osteotomes. A micro-sagittal saw, Lambotte osteotomes and knee impactors can be helpful in disrupting the bone-cement interfaces and component extraction. A high-speed carbide tip burr can facilitate removal of incarcerated implants or internal fixation hardware. Heat stable antibiotic powder (i.e., vancomycin, tobramycin, gentamycin) should be available as well as your preferred cement.

Surgical Exposure

When multiple skin incisions are present, use the most lateral skin incision and maximize the distance between incisions. Dissect deep to Scarpa's fascia to develop full-thickness fascio-cutaneous skin flaps. If a muscle flap reconstruction is present, elevate the flap and preserve its vascular pedicle (Plastic surgery consultation and assistance is warranted if uncertain).

We recommend an extensile arthrotomy such as the medial parapatellar approach if practical. In cases of ankylosis or inflamed and friable periarticular soft tissues, extensile measures such as a quadriceps snip [47] (Fig. 12.7) or tibial tubercle osteotomy (TTO) [48, 49] (Fig. 12.8a, b) can achieve exposure while reducing the need for forceful retraction and the possibility of collateral ligament and/or extensor injury.

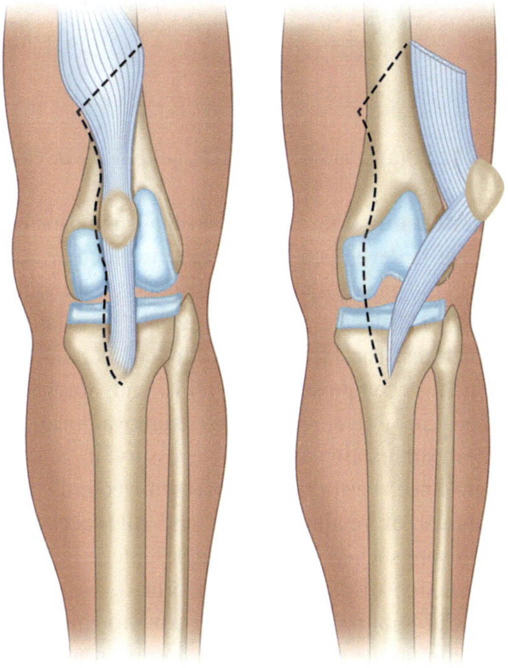

Fig. 12.7 Illustrates the use of the quadriceps snip to gain additional exposure

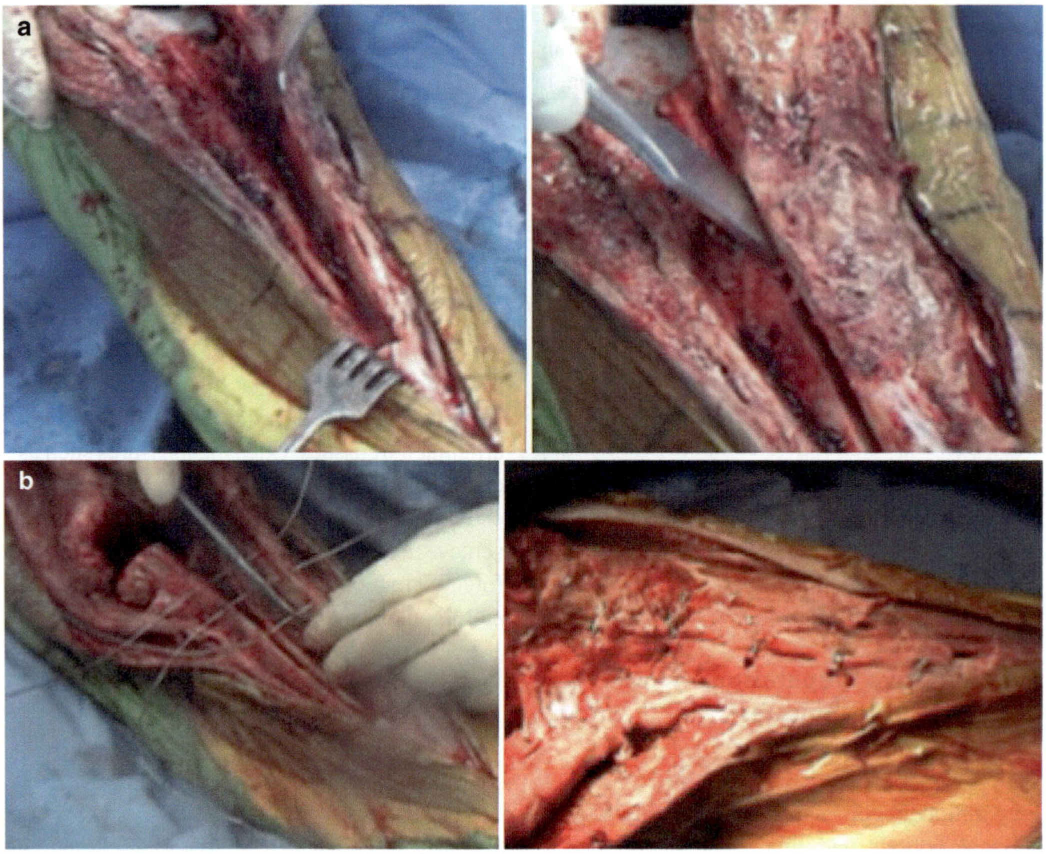

Fig. 12.8 (**a**) Demonstrates a TTO, utilizing a wire closure (**b**)

After arthrotomy, a medial tibial subperiosteal sleeve is developed to the posterior-medial corner. This release should be adequate to allow the tibia to dislocate and pivot around the lateral structures. The exposed polyethylene is removed which decompresses the joint and improves exposure. Polyethylene insert removal prior to tibial subluxation may be necessary in a very tight knee. Perform complete synovectomy and removal of retained debris and all accessible hardware such as ligament staples, etc.

Flexion of the knee is performed; we prefer patellar subluxation (not eversion) to minimize tension on the patellar tendon insertion to avoid avulsion. Knee flexion facilitates removal of the femoral component which is performed with maximal bone preservation in mind. Break the implant-cement or implant-bone interfaces with thin osteotomes prior to impacting the component off of the femur.

The tibia is subluxed anteriorly, maximally flexed and removal of the tibial component proceeds by breaking the implant-cement or implant-bone interfaces with thin osteotomes then impacting the component out.

Patellar component removal is performed last to decrease the risk of inadvertent patella fracture. During the above steps, careful retractor placement is important to avoid injury to exposed patellar bone. Be aware of the bone which protrudes distally beyond the component and avoid retraction other than on the component.

Following component removal, the knee and soft tissues are generally more pliable allowing full exposure of the joint. Completion of synovectomy and second-look debridement of all

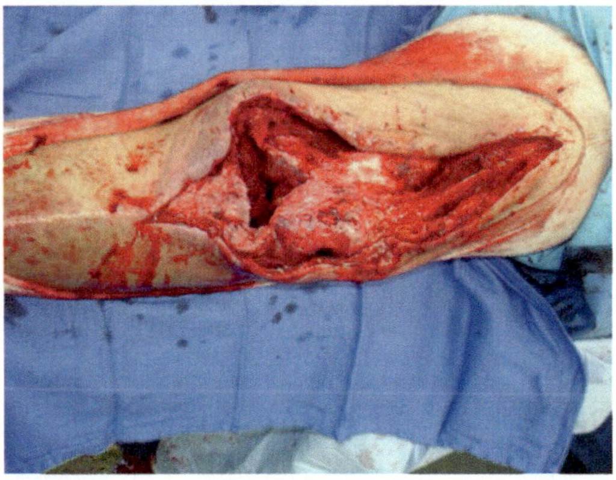

Fig. 12.9 Infected TKA post-implant removal and irrigation and debridement)

inflamed pseudo-capsule, necrotic tissue, cement debris, and foreign material is performed at this juncture. A drill or high-speed burr is helpful in removing small-embedded cement fragments such as found in peg holes in the distal femur. Expose fresh bone by removal of a very thin layer. Avoid thinning the patella to minimize the risk of fracture. Remove the canal membrane and potential bacterial foci by reaming, reverse curetting, and canal brushing. Visualize and debride the posterior capsule and femoral condyles which can harbor inflamed or necrotic tissue. Next pulse lavage the knee with a large volume (e.g., 9 L) of sterile saline, including irrigation of the intramedullary canals followed by repeat inspection and final debridement as warranted (Fig. 12.9).

Upon completion of irrigation and debridement, we recommend all operating personnel change their gloves, apply sterile sleeves or a new gown, remove the contaminated instruments, place a new sterile drape underneath the knee in preparation for the reconstruction and bring sterile instruments into the field. More extensive preparation for the final procedure have been described by Haddad et al. including serially soaking the wound with betadine and hydrogen peroxide solutions followed by pulsatile saline lavage. The skin edges are then loosely approximated, the surgical team re-gowns and an entirely new set of surgical instruments and drapes are used after the room is cleaned. The re-implantation of the final implant then takes places [50].

Single-Stage Revision Arthroplasty

Controversy persists regarding the most effective strategy for staged TKA management. While many consider two-staged reconstruction the gold standard, one-stage revision has gained popularity. Advantages of a single-stage revision include: avoiding a second surgery [51, 52], improved function, ease of rehabilitation, decreased cost [53], and improved outcomes in quality-adjusted years [54].

Regardless of the technique, the primary goals are to eradicate infection and restore a functional, painless, and stable knee. Several European centers have demonstrated single-stage revision results that approach those for two-stage TKA and THA reconstructions [54–58]. Careful patient selection, attention to patient comorbidities and soft-tissue quality is paramount to a successful single-stage revision. Also important to the success of single-stage revision is bacterial sensitivity and the bone stock quality [59] The 2014 International Consensus Group suggested five factors that negatively influenced the success of a single-stage revision including: (1) the presence of systemic sepsis, (2) the presence of drug-resistant bacteria, (3) culture-negative infection (4) peri-articular soft-tissue deficiency, and (5) the presence of a sinus tract [60]. The Consensus considers single-stage revisions in the absence of these factors. Still crucial to proper patient selection is consideration of comorbidities including obesity, immunosuppression, diabetes, tobacco use, renal insufficiency or failure, active malignancy, and cardiac disease which can compromise outcomes and should be optimized if possible. Relative contraindications include the multiply-revised TKA, multiple incisions surrounding the joint and/or compromised peri-articular soft-tissue envelope. The authors perform single-stage revisions in otherwise healthy patients with an initial infection with an identified bacterium sensitive to most antibiotics.

Two-Stage Reconstruction

Two-stage reconstruction includes implant removal, debridement, and irrigation with or without placement of an articulating or static spacer. Eradication of infection can require more than one procedure. The second-stage surgery completes reconstruction of the joint. Despite the increasing popularity of single-stage revisions, two-stage remains the treatment standard in North America. The 2014 International Consensus Group Conference recommended two-stage reconstructions be performed on the more challenging infected TKA patient [60]. Examples include resistant bacteria, culture-negative infections, systemic sepsis, peri-articular soft-tissue deficiencies, the need for rotational muscle flaps, and the presence of a sinus tract [60].

Controversy persists as to whether two-stage spacers should be static or articulating [61–63]. Static spacer advantages include simplicity of implantation, greater cement surface area for antibiotic elution and fewer exposed and untreated surfaces for bacterial growth. Disadvantages include patient dissatisfaction between surgeries, peri-articular bone loss and fracture, decreased range of motion after final implantation and a longer, more complex second reconstruction if severe stiffness of the knee develops. Advantages of articulating spacers include greater function and satisfaction between reconstructions, improved final range of motion and greater ease of second-stage reconstruction [64].

Static Spacers

A static spacer can be defined as a mass of antibiotic-impregnated cement implanted between the femur and tibia (Fig. 12.10). We recommend using some form of endoskeleton (intramedullary nail, Steinmann pins, Rush rod, etc.) for antibiotic dowels in the femur and tibia to improve strength and stability of the construct. This can prevent bone loss from fracture or extensor mechanism and skin erosion from spacer displacement [65, 66] (Fig. 12.11). The 2014 Consensus Group [60] strongly agreed (89%) that either static or articulating spacers improve eradication of infection. The Consensus panel agreed that a static spacer is best suited for massive bone loss, lack of ligamentous restraint, or soft-tissue incompetence. Benefits of the static spacer include ease of initial implantation and preservation of the joint space with distraction of the joint. Drawbacks include decreased final range of motion (Emerson et al. observed ROM of 93.7 degrees and 107.8 degrees with static and mobile spacers, respectively) [67]; increased complexity of final reconstruction due to stiffness after months of knee immobilization (e.g., increased risk of ligament avulsion and/or extensor mechanism disruption during the second-stage re-implantation). The threshold to perform extensile procedures such as a quadriceps snip or tibial tubercle osteotomy should be lowered in these circumstances to prevent untoward complications. The potential for bone loss is also a con-

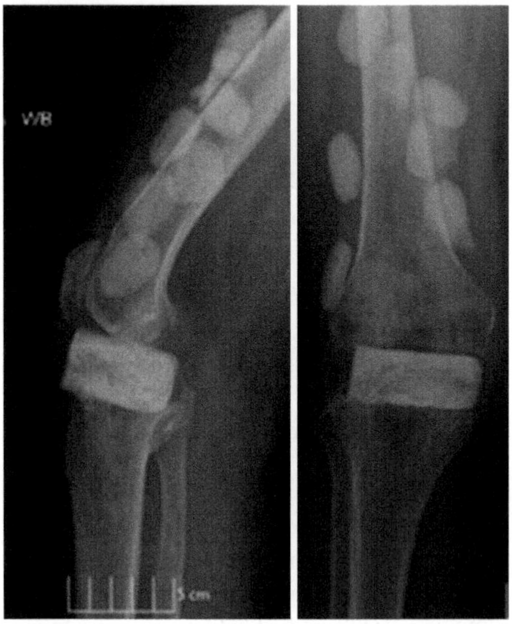

Fig. 12.10 Static spacer with antibiotic impregnated cement augmented with antibiotic cement beads

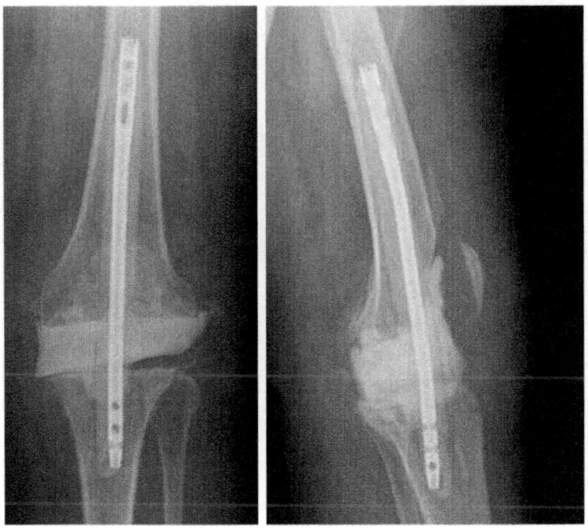

Fig. 12.11 Static spacer utilizing an endoskeleton antibiotic-coated rod

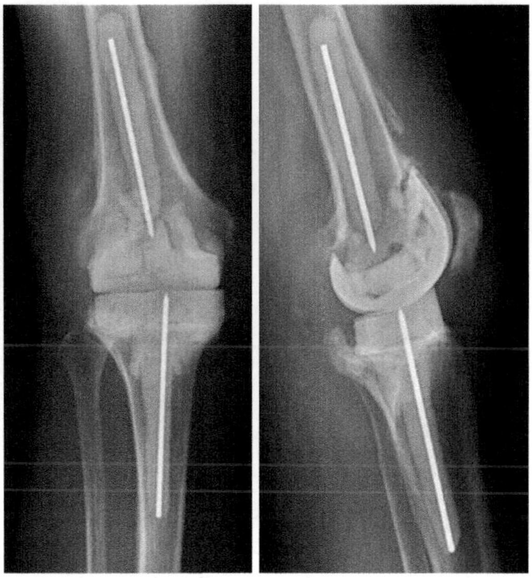

Fig. 12.12 Preformed cement (Interspace) articulating spacer with dowels

cern with use of static spacers. Fehring et al. evaluated 25 TKA periprosthetic infections treated with static spacers compared to 15 articulating spacers. They noted that 60% patients with static spacers had unexpected bone loss between surgeries compared to no instances of unexpected bone loss with articulated spacers [61].

The appropriate heat stable antibiotics to which the bacteria are most susceptible should be utilized in the cement for spacer fabrication. A wide variation of combinations and dosages of antibiotics has been reported and little consensus exists [67–70]. Both "high dose" and "low dose" constructs have been shown to be effective [71, 72]. Antibiotic elution from the cement is dependent on factors including surface area of the cement, cement porosity, the type of cement, and antibiotic dosing. Generally, elution is known to peak within the first 24–72 h followed by prolonged lower levels of elution over the following weeks [73, 74].

High-Friction Articulating Spacer (Preformed Antibiotic Cement Implants)

Preformed antibiotic cement implants are high-friction articulating spacers fabricated or molded in the shape of traditional TKA prostheses that are cemented using higher dose antibiotic cement. They can be pre-fabricated or fabricated intraoperatively. Examples of pre-fabricated spacers include the Interspace (Exactech, Gainsville, Florida) or the Spacer-K (Tecres, Verona Italy) (Fig. 12.12). Concerns exist regarding the cement antibiotic dosing in pre-fabricated constructs which may impact their effectiveness. Gentamycin doses in the Interspace implant range from 0.8 to 1.7 g which is below recommended dosing for bactericidal activity. These implants lack an endoskeleton pre-disposing them to fracture, especially in large patients (Fig. 12.13). The high-friction nature of the articulating surface may cause seizing and transfer of strain to the bone-implant interface leading to loosening and possible dislocation [75]. Despite legitimate deficiencies, good clinical success has been reported with this construct. Durbhakula et al. reported their results with custom cement molded spacers for two-staged reconstructions in 24 patients with an average follow-up of 33 months. There were two failures to eradicate infection, no cases of reinfection and a 92% long-term survivorship. The average range of motion at final follow-up was 104° [68]. Ha et al. fabricated custom molds from explanted components for articulating spacers in two-staged reconstruc-

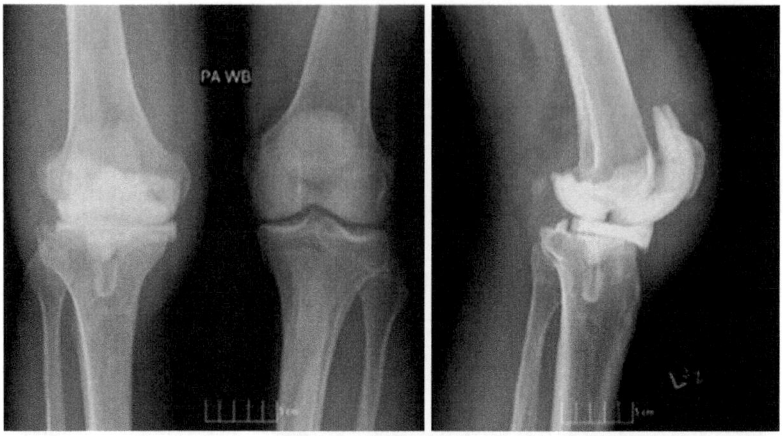

Fig. 12.13 Demonstrates a fractured (Interspace) preformed cement spacer

tions and reported excellent mean ROM of 100° and no cases of reinfection [76]. Kohl et al. reported 100% success and no infection recurrence in 16 custom fabricated high-friction spacers at minimum 2-year follow-up in 16 patients. Final range of motion was 102° of flexion [77]. They concluded this was an efficient and inexpensive compared to other methods. Pitto et al. reported 100% infection eradication at 2 years follow-up in 21 infected TKA cases. The average ROM was 77° during treatment and 94° at final follow-up after re-implantation [78].

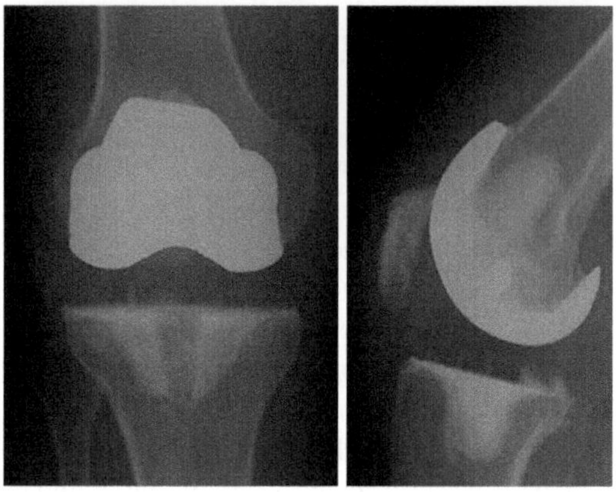

Fig. 12.14 Autoclaved femoral component with all-polyethylene tibial component (low friction) articulating spacer

Low-Friction Articulating Spacers (Cobalt-Chrome on Polyethylene)

A low-friction spacer consists of a cobalt-chromium femur and all-polyethylene tibial component fixed with high-dose antibiotic-impregnated bone cement (Fig. 12.14). Advantages include maintenance of joint space, ligament tensioning, and preserved range of motion while eradicating infection. At re-implantation, surgical exposure is facilitated decreasing surgical time, blood loss, and patient recuperation. First described by Hofmann et al. in 1995 the technique recycles the explanted femoral component by sterilizing and re-implanting it with a new all-polyethylene insert [79]. Components are fixed by bone cement mixed with 4.8 g of Tobramycin per 40-g batch of cement. Various iterations of this technique have developed including the use of new femoral components (rather than a recycled one) with an all-polyethylene tibial baseplate. The use of stems and Steinmann pins pre-coated with high-dosed antibiotic cement to act as antibiotic dowels may improve elution of antibiotics into infected canals (Fig. 12.15a–c).

Although metal component recycling has been shown to be cost-effective, many hospitals and hospital systems have not allowed this technique for fear of reinfection and possible liability [80]. This fear persists despite several reports indicating equivalent infection eradication and recurrence rates [79–81]. Lyons et al. recently reported histological results after sterilization of explanted, previously infected femoral components in an

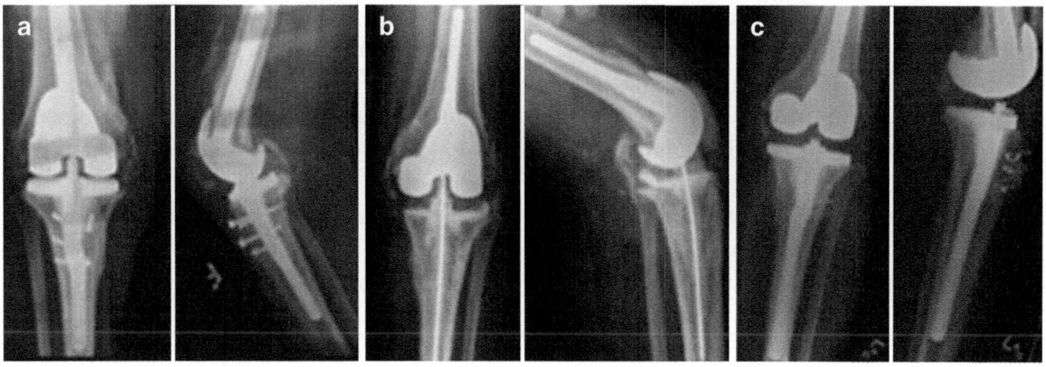

Fig. 12.15 (**a**) Displays a radiograph of a chronically infected TKA, followed by (**b**). Demonstrating implantation of a low-friction articulating spacer with (**c**) capturing final revision TKA with concomitant allograft extensor reconstruction

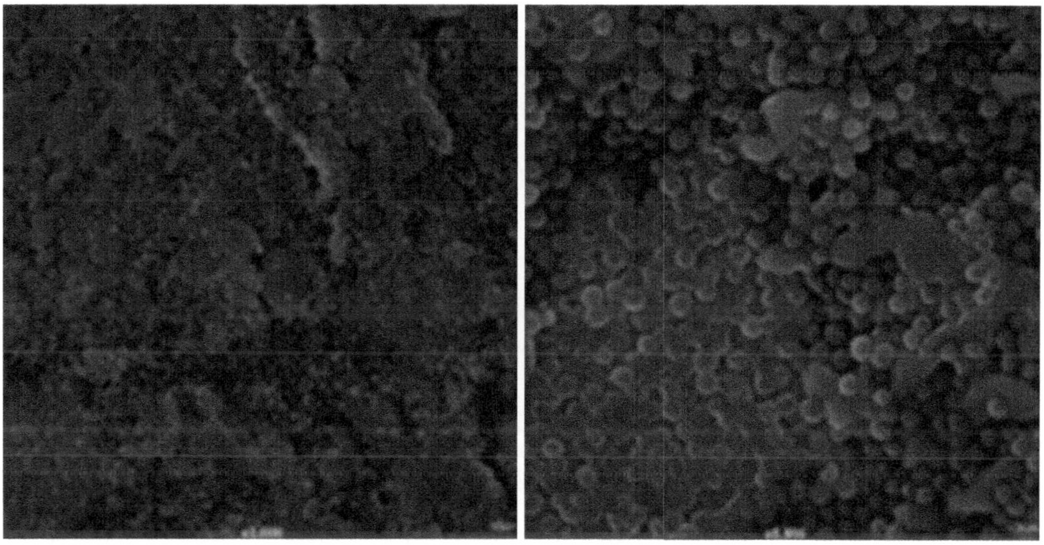

Fig. 12.16 Electron microscopy showing biofilm on implant surface

autoclave. They confirmed 100% bacterial eradication of intentionally contaminated in vitro specimens and in vivo specimens from grossly purulent TKA infections. All femoral implants were rendered bacteria-free based on final cultures of femoral implants as well as with electron microscopy evaluating for both bacteria and biofilm on implant surfaces [80] (Fig. 12.16).

Eradication of infection using low-friction articulating knee spacers has been reported by several authors [67, 69, 78, 81, 82]. Hofmann reported a 100% success rate with no reinfections at 30 months and achieved a mean arc of motion of 5–106° post re-implantation with high patient satisfaction (mean modified HSS Score- 87) [78]. A follow-up study 10 years later reported 88% infection eradication rate at a mean of 73 months. The arc of motion before re-implantation was 6–91°and 4–104° after re-implantation and the mean modified HSS Knee Score was 89 points. Emerson et al. reported a 91% infection eradication rate and a 7.7% rate of recurrence in 26 infected TKAs at 36 months [67]. Low-friction articulating spacers demonstrated greater flexion compared with high-friction or static spacers at final follow-up.

Some patients are satisfied with the low-friction articulating spacer and elect to postpone or even decline second-stage reconstruction [82–85]. It may be difficult and unnecessary to proceed with re-implantation if the infection has been eradicated, minimal pain exists, and motion and function are adequate. Obvious candidates for this approach include low-demand, elderly patients with multiple medical comorbidities. In 2013, Choi et al. reported seven cases in which high-friction TKA spacers were retained. At a mean follow-up of 44 months, the average Knee Society score was 92. Two knees were revised for loosening and one for recurrence. The remaining spacers continued to function well at 6 years without further surgical intervention [86]. Lyons et al. reported excellent functional improvement and ROM in 55 low-friction spacers in 49 patients for TKA periprosthetic infection. The low-friction spacer was left in place in 42.6% patients. In these patients, the mean KSS increased from 52 to 80 and the mean ROM was 86° [87].

Author's Preferred Two-Stage Reconstruction Technique

After implant removal and meticulous debridement is performed, a freshening resection of the proximal tibia is performed perpendicular to the long axis of the tibia. In cases of severe proximal tibial bony deficiencies, preserve bone by not over resecting the proximal tibia to make the "perfect" perpendicular cut. Resection of 1–2 mm of the distal femoral surface is performed. The knee is grossly sized and trialed with femoral and tibial trial components. Flexion and extension gaps are balanced by altering femoral size and/or tibial trial thickness. Defects are filled with cement thereby preserving bone for future procedures. If appropriate balancing is not impossible due to severe bone and/or ligamentous deficiency or lack of implant options, consider aborting the spacer and performing a resection arthroplasty. Femoral component recycling may not be permitted by certain hospitals and hospital systems therefore individual hospital by-laws or policies should be checked to determine if this is an option. When recycling the femoral component completely remove all debris and cement, brush, and sterilize (settings = 132 °C at 27 PSIG) for 10 min in an autoclave. If the femoral component cannot be recycled, a new femur component is used. In cases of severe distal femur bone loss, a revision femoral component with stem extension offers added mechanical stability. The stem should be coated with antibiotic-impregnated cement which acts as an antibiotic dowel for the femoral canal. Similarly, for tibial stability, the stem of an all-polyethylene baseplate or antibiotic-coated Steinmann pins can be utilized (Fig. 12.15b). After bone preparation, the tourniquet is deflated to flush remaining debris and deep-seated bacteria from the cancellous bed. The cementation strategy is to capture gross surface topography of bone, not pressurized cancellous interdigitation. Score the undersurface of the tibial insert cementation a burr or saw to improve cement adherence. Antibiotic selection varies with the bacterial culture. We prefer 4.8 g of Tobramycin or 4 g of Vancomycin per 40-g batch of cement used for fixation. In polymicrobial TKA infections with varying resistances or in culture negative cases we mix 2.4 g of Tobramycin and 2 g of Vancomycin per 40-g batch of cement. Tuberculosis infections are often resistant to Vancomycin and Tobramycin and therefore an effective heat stable antibiotic such as Amikacin should be used. Many arthroplasty surgeons have their own spacer techniques, antibiotic combinations, and doses without evidence of superiority of one methodology over the other [72]. We recommend doughy cement. The tibia positioning should consider appropriate depth, rotation, varus and valgus, and posterior slope. Control component orientation during cement curing. Careful retraction by the surgeon and assistants avoids component displacement by stiff, non-compliant tissues. Tibial and femoral cementation is usually performed separately to facilitate ligament tensioning as the knee is extended. Extruded antibiotic cement is allowed at the bone-implant margins, removing enough to avoid soft-tissue irritation. Closure is with monofilament suture and no drain. Unless severe bony deficiencies exist, full weight bearing is permitted and physi-

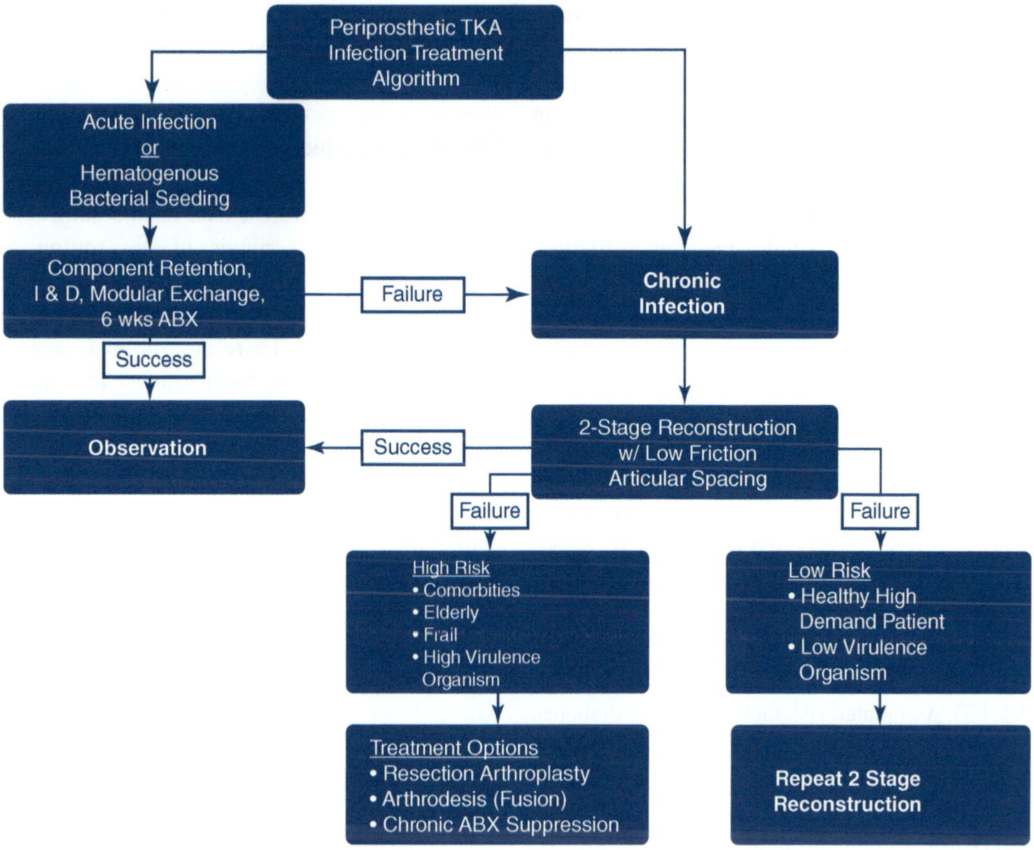

Fig. 12.17 Infected TKA Treatment Algorithm

cal rehabilitation is performed early in the hospital stay. A 6-week course of intravenous antibiotics directed by the Infectious Disease team is followed by a 2- to 6-week antibiotic holiday and consideration of re-implantation. If the patient has no clinical or laboratory evidence of infection, final reconstruction may be considered. If positive for infection, the above steps are repeated (Fig. 12.17).

Author's Single-Stage Reconstruction or Re-implantation Technique

The current author's preferred technique is to cement the femur and tibial metaphyseal bone-implant interfaces and engages the diaphysis with a long cementless stem in a single-stage reconstruction. A completely cemented short, metaphyseal stem is also acceptable but may necessitate more bone loss during cement removal in the case of septic failure. The tibia is rigidly reamed until intramedullary contact is achieved. The proximal tibial resection performed using an intramedullary jig and is made perpendicular to the long axis of the tibia in neutral slope. The proximal tibia is prepared for the appropriately sized tibial baseplate in the correct rotational alignment. Since anatomic landmarks may be obliterated, the medial one-third of the tibial tubercle is often used to approximate correct rotational alignment. The femur is then prepared with rigid reamers until intramedullary contact achieved. Intramedullary jigs are again used to perform a distal femoral resection carefully assessing the position of the joint line both intraoperatively as well as based on pre-operative films. Spacer blocks or balancing jigs are used to approximate the correct flexion and extension balance. Trial components are implanted and stability assessed. Appropriate corrections are made to improve the flexion and extension balance at this time. Final implantation is performed with either 1.2 g of Tobramycin or 1.0 g of Vancomycin per 40-g batch. Polyethylene inserts that provide coronal constraint should always be available in the case of ligamentous laxity.

In the case of a single-stage reconstruction appropriate antibiotics are continued for 6 weeks intravenously under the direction of the infectious disease service.

Extensor Mechanism Disruption

Concomitant TKA infection and extensor mechanism failure is a double catastrophe with a poor prognosis for patient function and overall outcome. The incidence of patellar tendon disruption ranges from 0.17% to 1.4% [88–90] and quadriceps rupture ranges from 0.1% to 1.1% [91, 92]. Associated risk factors include diabetes, immunosuppression (malignancy, rheumatoid arthritis, HIV, etc.), obesity, and renal disease [89, 93, 94]. The multiply operated knee has been shown a consistent and significant risk factor [91, 93, 95–97]. Intraoperative iatrogenic injury to the patellar tendon is a common method of injury during surgical exposure of the ankylosed TKA [97]. Prevention of extensor injury requires patience during exposure and a thorough understanding of extensile techniques. Patellar subluxation rather than eversion reduces tension and the risk of tendon avulsion or rupture. Patellar eversion creates a rotational strain on the patella tendon insertion increasing the risk of avulsion from the tibial tubercle or an intrasubstance tear during exposure. Extensile options to improve exposure include the quadriceps snip, tibial tubercle osteotomy, and the V-Y turndown. The tibial tubercle osteotomy and quadriceps snip techniques have predictable on recovery and long-term outcome. A V-Y turndown is rarely performed because of substantial morbidity, the likelihood of postoperative extensor lag [98, 99], and the need for postoperative bracing. Extensor mechanism disruption observed at the time of initial infection debridement indicates a two-stage reconstruction, resection arthroplasty, or fusion.

Extensor Repair

A paucity of literature exists on the subject of extensor disruption repair in the setting of infected TKA. Several studies have reported poor outcomes for primary repair of TKR extensor disruptions [90, 92]. Therefore, surgical repair is typically augmented by reconstructive techniques including autograft, allograft, or synthetic material incorporated to increase the strength of the extensor reconstructions [91, 100]. The authors recommend primary repair during first-stage debridement, then augmented repair after the infection is eradicated.

Allograft Reconstruction

Since first-stage extensor reconstruction is not recommended due to the risk of introducing nonviable tissue to an infected bed knee immobilization is necessary. The authors prefer a static spacer or resection arthroplasty (KAFO required) due to the risk of articulating spacer dislocation in the absence of an extensor mechanism. Augmented extensor mechanism repair is performed at the second-stage revision.

Our preferred technique for patella or quadriceps tendon disruption is augmentation with fresh-frozen Achilles tendon allograft with calcaneal bone block [94, 101]. This technique has been employed in the acute or chronic setting with reliable results [94, 95, 101]. The surgical technique achieves bone to allograft healing of Achilles tendon calcaneal bone block to the proximal tibia. The female trough is created just distal to the tibial tubercle leaving a proximal bone with any salvageable patellar tendon attachment. The calcaneal bone block is fashioned to mate with the female tibial trough in a dovetail fashion (Fig. 12.18) which provides inherent stability when performed correctly. The allograft bone block is secured to the tibia by cerclage of heavy

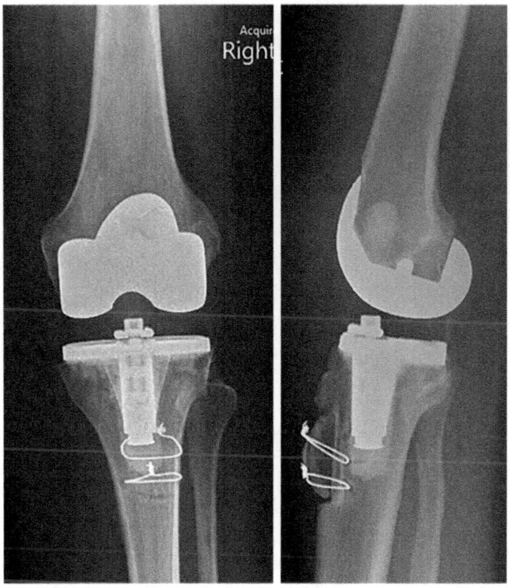

Fig. 12.18 Plain film radiograph of an extensor mechanism repair utilizing an Achilles allograft with a calcaneal bone block

suture (e.g., 3 mm cottony Dacron) or 18 gauge cerclage stainless steel wires passed through tibial drill holes. Screws should be avoided as the small avascular allograft fragment is vulnerable to fracture. The native extensor mechanism is the pulled distally to an anatomic position and held in place with clamps or preliminary sutures while the allograft is pulled proximally under maximum tension and secured with numerous non-resorbable sutures. The knee should be fully extended. The allograft is sutured to the native tendon with a Krackow stitch. Any remnants of the native patellar tendon can be sutured to the allograft to further improve its viability. In the case of a quadriceps disruption (typically avulsed from the proximal pole of the patella), the tendon is secured with heavy non-absorbable sutures (e.g., 3 mm cottony dacron, Deknatel) passed through tunnels in the patella. If patellectomy or poor patellar bone stock is encountered, perform a heavy suture repair of the allograft to the quadriceps and patellar tendons under maximum tension.

In cases of severe compromise of the proximal tibia and tubercle (Fig. 12.19), use of a complete extensor mechanism allograft may be necessary [94]. This includes an allograft proximal tibia, patellar tendon, patella, and quadriceps tendon attached in continuity. This can be used similar to the previously described Achilles tendon allograft. The tibial allograft bone functioning in place of the calcaneal bone block (Fig. 12.20a–d) Implant availability at the time of surgery should include Varus/Valgus constraint and hinge options with stems and augments.

Postoperative rehabilitation requires an extended period of immobilization using double uprights incorporated into a shoe with a knee hinge locked in full extension and a custom thigh cuff (KAFO) (Fig. 12.21). The authors prefer 6 months KAFO immobilization. Specific instructions: include KAFO locked in extension 0 to 3 months; 3–6 months: KAFO knee hinge unlocked to allow gentle self-directed flexion BID, the KAFO is locked in extension for walking and at all other times; after 6 months wean out of the KAFO, continue working on ROM and gait training. The goal of a strong extension mechanism requires significant healing in a relatively avascular bed, therefore extensive healing time and effective immobilization is critical. In the final result, the goal of strong extension strength is often at the cost of decreased flexion—an acceptable compromise.

Autograft

In 1992, Cadambi and Engh [88] described use of the semitendinosus tendon as an augment to a primary tendon repair or to augment reconstructions of extensor disruptions. Use of this technique has been limited and sparsely reported in the literature with generally dismal results [90]. The technique involves harvesting the semitendinosis subcutaneously, freeing it at the proximal musculotendinous junction and tunneling it through a 5 mm drill hole in the patella. The tendon is then passed distally on the patella surface and secured with non-resorbable suture. The authors have utilized this technique in the rarest of circumstances, find it difficult to execute and have had limited clinical success.

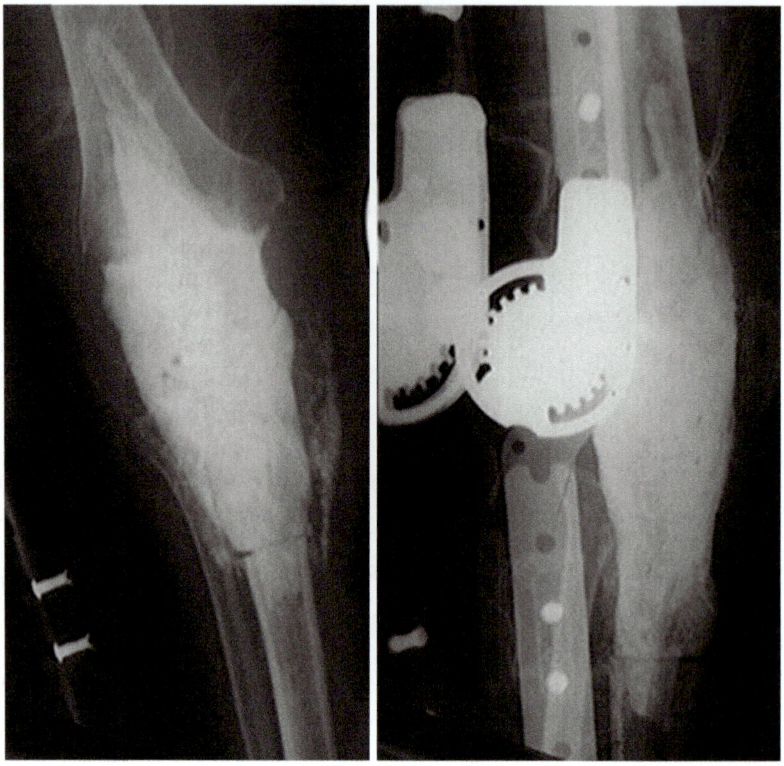

Fig. 12.19 Radiograph of a segmental tibial defect utilizing a static cement spacer with hinged a knee brace

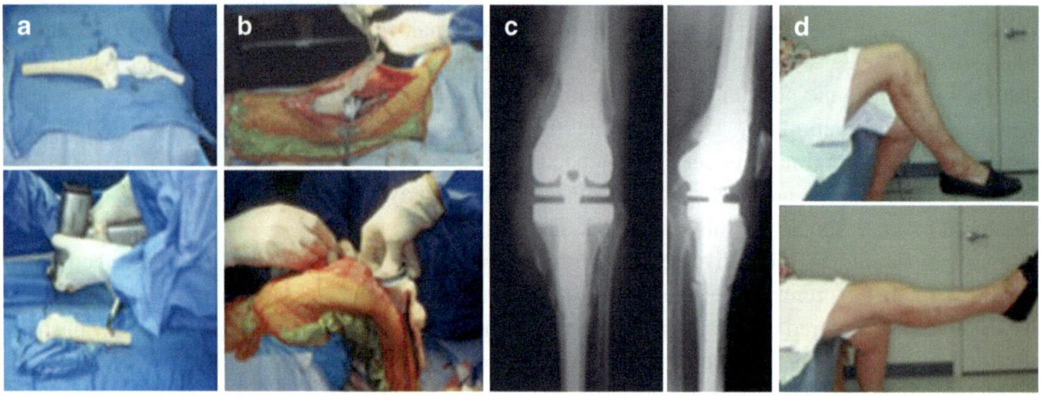

Fig. 12.20 (**a**) Preparation of proximal tibia allograft. (**b**) Insertion of tibial allograft. (**c**) Postoperative radiographs demonstrating proximal tibial allograft, with (**d**) showing the restoration of the extensor mechanism following tibial allograft

Synthetic Graft

Reconstruction with a synthetic material was first described by Browne and Hanssen [100]. This technique uses Marlex mesh (C.R. Bard) which is used in place of allograft or autograft. It is secured distally in a trough made in the proximal tibia and augmented with screws and cement. It is then brought proximally and tensioned through and around what remains of the patient's extensor mechanism. Browne and Hanssen have shown promising clinical results in one series [91].

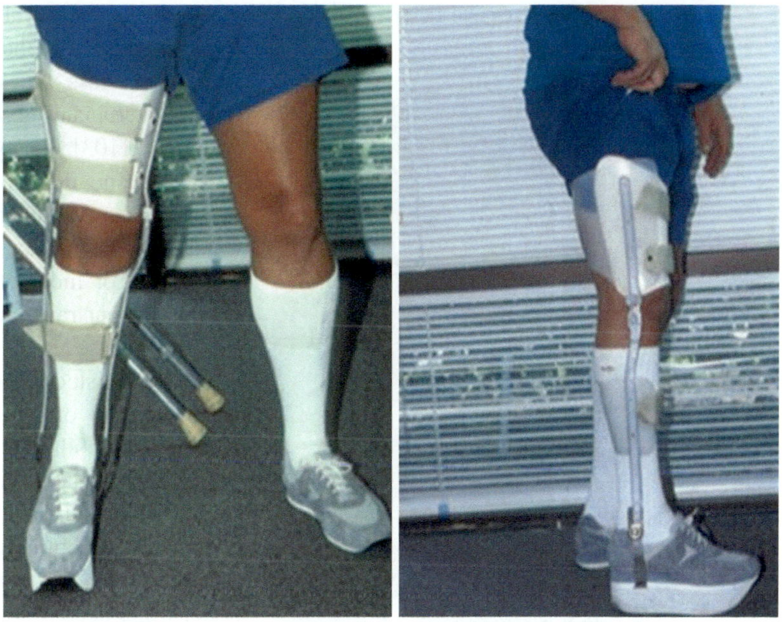

Fig. 12.21 Example of a patient using a KAFO to achieve knee immobilization

Bone Defect Management

Bone defects are commonly encountered in RTKA in the setting of an eradicated PJI. The Anderson Orthopaedic Research Institute (AORI) classification system (Table 12.1) described by Engh and Ammeen was set forth to define femoral and tibial defects and is the most widely used system today [102]. The goal when managing knees with bone defects is to restore bone stock, obtain an anatomic joint line, and provide stability to improve mobility and function. Surgeons have several options to employ, with management determined by the location and severity of defect.

Table 12.1 Anderson Orthopaedic Research Institute classification of bone defects

Type	Severity
1	Minimal femoral or tibial defect with intact metaphyseal bone
	Able to obtain good stability and alignment of revision component
2	Damaged metaphyseal bone requiring reconstruction (cement, bone graft, prosthetic augment)
	2A: Defect of one femoral or one tibial condyle
	2B: Defect of both femoral or tibial condyles
3	Deficient metaphyseal bone that compromises a significant portion of the condyles or plateau
	May be associated with soft tissue incompetence

Implant Selection

Bone defects arising from PJI necessitate careful implant selection to facilitate knee stability. Constraints and stems are available to provide maximum knee stability in the setting of bone and soft-tissue defects. When choosing constraint, select the least constraint needed to obtain the appropriate stability. General constraint options include posterior stabilized (PS), varus-valgus constraint (VVK), and rotating hinged constraint (RHK) knee implants. VVK provide increased coronal and sagittal plane stability through a tall tibial post (Fig. 12.22), differing from the RHK implants which are mechanically linked (Fig. 12.23a, b). Implant constraint selection is influenced by bone defect severity, compe-

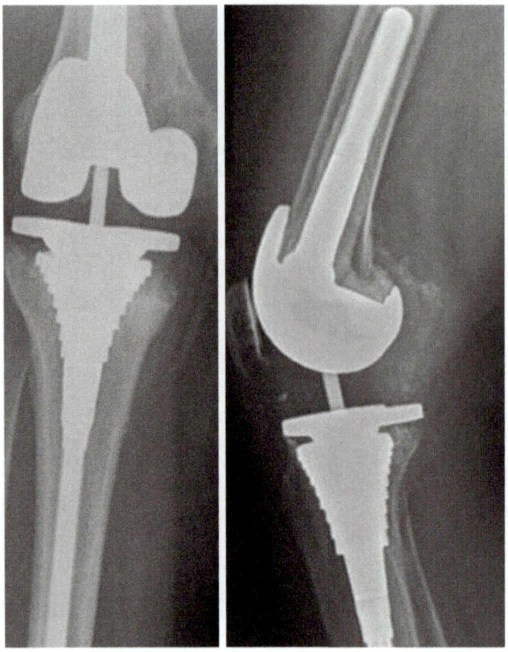

Fig. 12.22 Increased stability is obtained with the tall tibial post of a VVK

tency of the collateral ligaments, and posterior capsule integrity. In the setting of minimal, AORI type 1 bone loss with intact and competent collaterals, a cruciate substituting PS design may be sufficient [103]. In patients with large bone defects causing incompetent or complete absence of the collateral ligaments, increased constraint is required. VVK implants are often reserved for less severe or moderate bone defects requiring increased constraint and should be avoided in patients with severe posterolateral laxity, as stabilizer post dislocations may occur (Fig. 12.24). In the setting of large AORI type 3 defects, incompetent collaterals, or knees with severe posterior capsular insufficiency, RHK is a reasonable selection.

Stems are routinely used in the setting of RTKR and serve to bypass and offload deficient bone, while decreasing interface stresses arising from damaged bone at the tibiofemoral joint. Fixation can be achieved through fully cemented and cementless stems. Some controversy exists

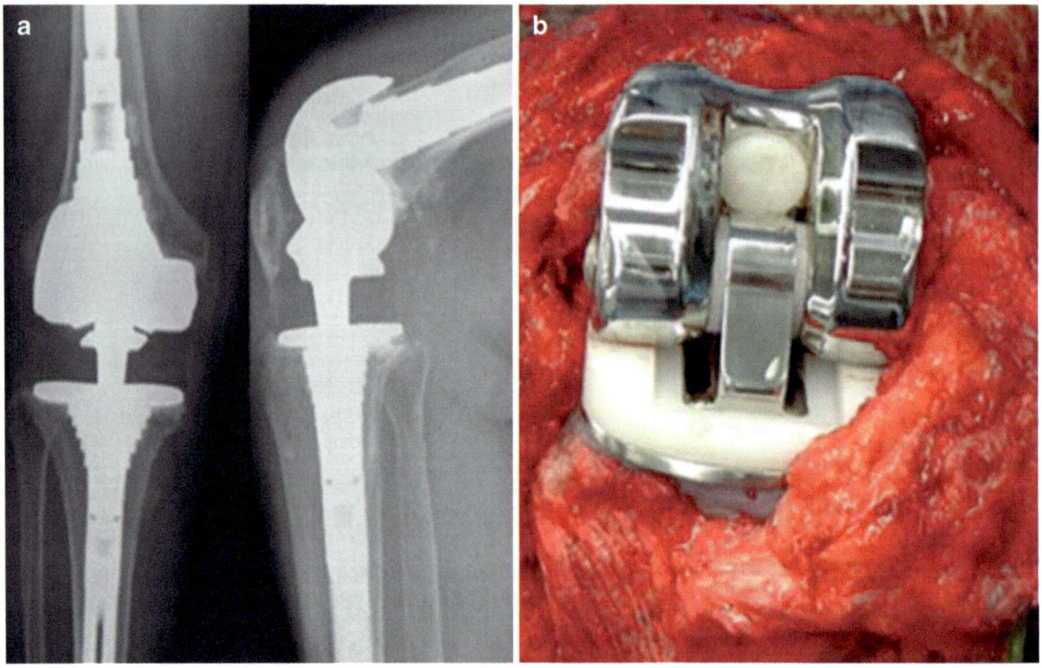

Fig. 12.23 Increased stability is obtained with the tall tibial post of a VVK as seen in Fig. 12.20

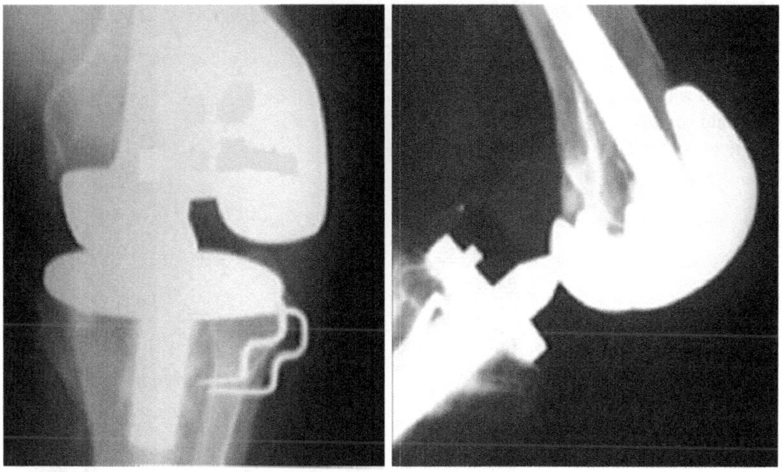

Fig. 12.24 Plain film radiographs demonstrating a stabilizer post dislocation in a patient with posterolateral laxity

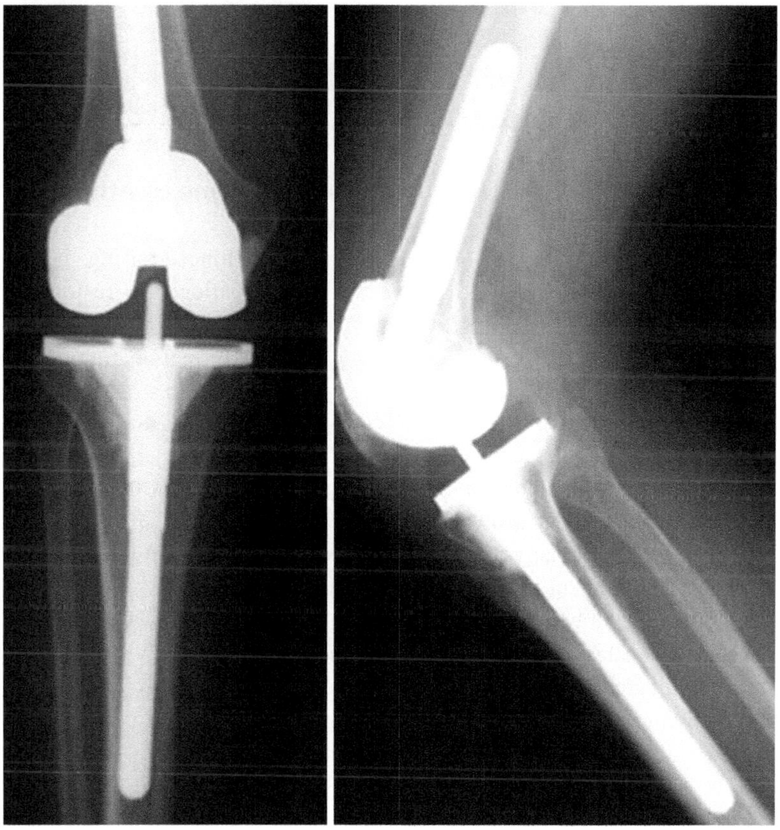

Fig. 12.25 Plain radiographs of a diaphyseal press-fit stem utilizing cement fixation in the metaphysis

on the preferred method of stem fixation. Several studies have shown good to excellent survivorship of cemented stems [104–106]. The advantage of using a fully cemented stem is immediate fixation. The disadvantage of a distally cemented stem is the increased potential for stress shielding of the metaphyseal bone. The hybrid technique of using a diaphyseal press-fit stem with metaphyseal cement fixation can also be utilized and is the authors preferred method (Fig. 12.25). Wood

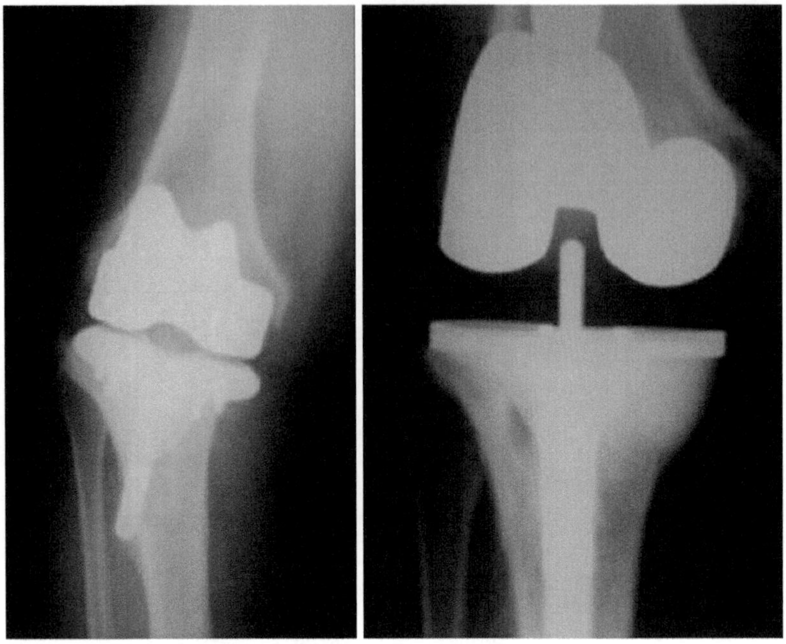

Fig. 12.26 Demonstrates a tibial defect (left) that was managed with a revision stem and cement augment (right)

et al. found that this technique provided similar functional and clinical results comparatively with fully cemented stems [107].

Cement

Once appropriate implants are selected, augments are generally used to restore bone stock when bone defects are present. Cement augmentation with or without screws may be utilized (Fig. 12.26). Additionally, in patients with a history of a PJI, cement can be impregnated with antibiotics. The drawback to cement filling is its poor mechanical support. Brooks et al. found that there was increased deflection of the tibial tray when relying solely on cement filling to augment bone defects [108]. Cement filling should be reserved for small AORI type 1 defects or small type 2 defects with minimal cortical rim involvement. Additional stability may be achieved by adding rebar screws (Fig. 12.27) to cement augmentation. Ritter reported on 57 patients with cement filing reinforced with screws and had zero failures at 3 years [109].

Bone Grafting

Bone grafting is a viable option for some patients to restore bone stock and offers the ability for intraoperative contouring to obtain optimal anatomic placement. Grafts can be utilized in structural or moralized form. Autografts may be used in cases of small defects but have limited utility in the revision setting, as large defects often require more augmentation than autologous graft available. Allograft is more commonly used in RTKR to manage large defects. Structural mass allograft provides an avenue to restore bone stock in large defects and may be optimal for young patients if secondary procedures are required.

Engh et al. reported excellent results with no cases of graft collapse at a mean follow-up of 9–7 months [110]. Clatworthy et al. also published encouraging mid- to long-term results with a 72% allograft survival rate at 10 years [111]. Despite good reported results, patients and surgeons may have reservations receiving and using allografts as allografts pose a small theoretical risk of disease transmission. However, extensive

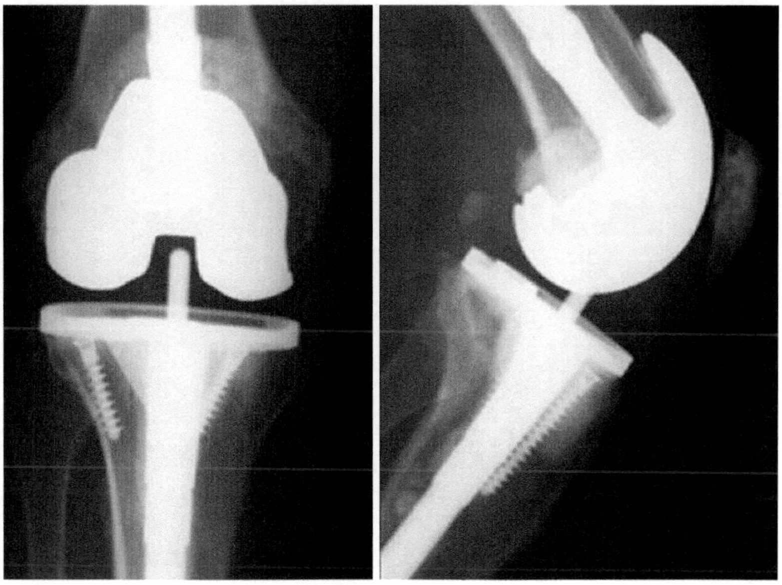

Fig. 12.27 AP and lateral radiographs depicting the use of rebar screws to add stability to the cement augment

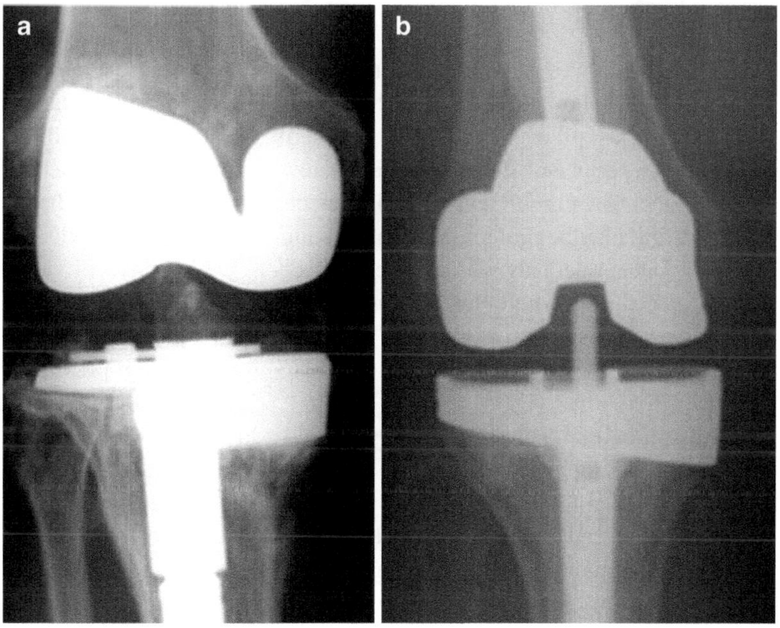

Fig. 12.28 (**a**) Is an AP radiograph of metal block augmentation, (**b**) demonstrate an AP radiograph of a metal wedge augment

measures are in place to reduce these risks and can still be used with confidence as a reasonable option for bone stock restoration [112].

Metal Augmentation

Metal block and wedge augmentation is another countermeasure for bone defects (Fig. 12.28a, b). These augments offer some advantages over bone grafting, as these augments need not incorporate into host bone and do not pose a risk for non-union and collapse. Some debate exists as to the superiority of block augmentation as compared to wedge augments [113]. Ferhing et al. reported that block augmentation offers a better strain distribution in comparison to wedge augments [114]. While Rand et al. reported good and excel-

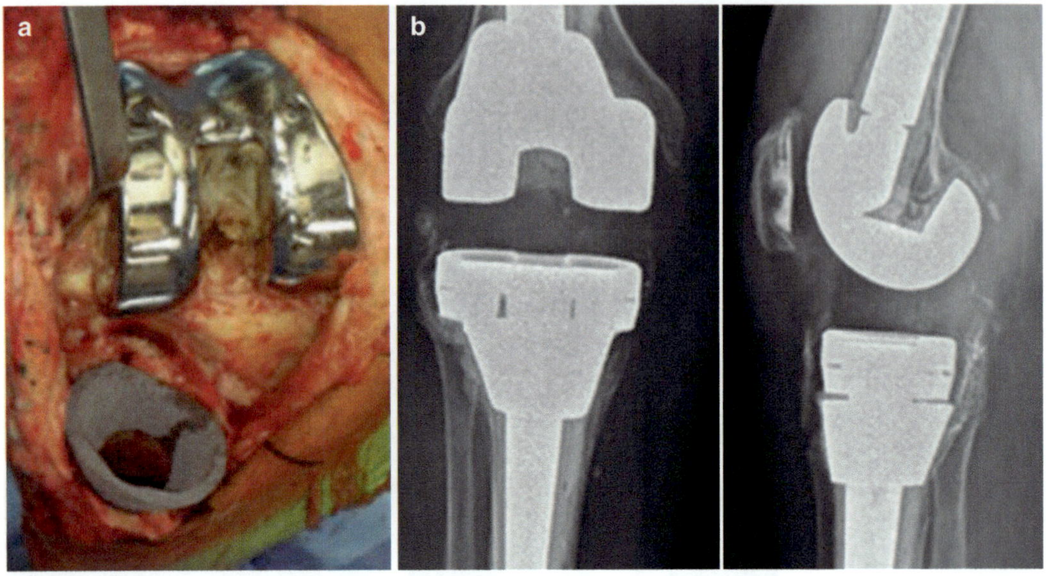

Fig. 12.29 (**a**) The tantalum metaphyseal cone achieves a press-fit, (**b**) the revision stem is cemented inside the tantalum press-fit metaphyseal cone

lent results with wedge augmentation with no failures at latest follow-up [115]. Metal block and wedge augments offer a reasonable option in patients with peripheral defects in elderly low-demand patients with AORI type 1 and 2 defects. Bone grafting may be preferred over metal augments in younger patients who may require secondary procedures, where restoration of bone stock is a possibility [115, 116].

Tantalum Metaphyseal Cones and Sleeves

Large (AORI 2b and 3) defects are challenging to manage and often require more coverage and stability than can be achieved with cement filling, bone grafts, and metal augments. Tantalum metaphyseal cones and sleeves offer a solution. Tantalum cones increase contact area between prosthesis and host bone. Reportedly, this will ultimately decrease stress shielding of adjacent bone [117]. The tantalum cone utilizes metaphyseal press-fit fixation with the tibial component cemented into the metal cone (Fig. 12.29a, b). Tantalum cones have good reported short-term results [118, 119].

Metaphyseal sleeves are a relatively newer concept. These sleeves can be cemented or noncemented. Bernasek et al. reported good success using press-fit metaphyseal sleeves for large AORI type 2b and type 3 defects [118–120] (Fig. 12.30). Press-fit sleeves may be used to obtain biologic fixation. This can be achieved by using a Morse taper to fix the sleeve to the tibial component [120]. Press-fit sleeves offers an advantage by avoiding the potential complications of the cemented metal block and wedge augments, as well as graft complications such as fracture, resorption, and disease transmission in the case of bulk allografts.

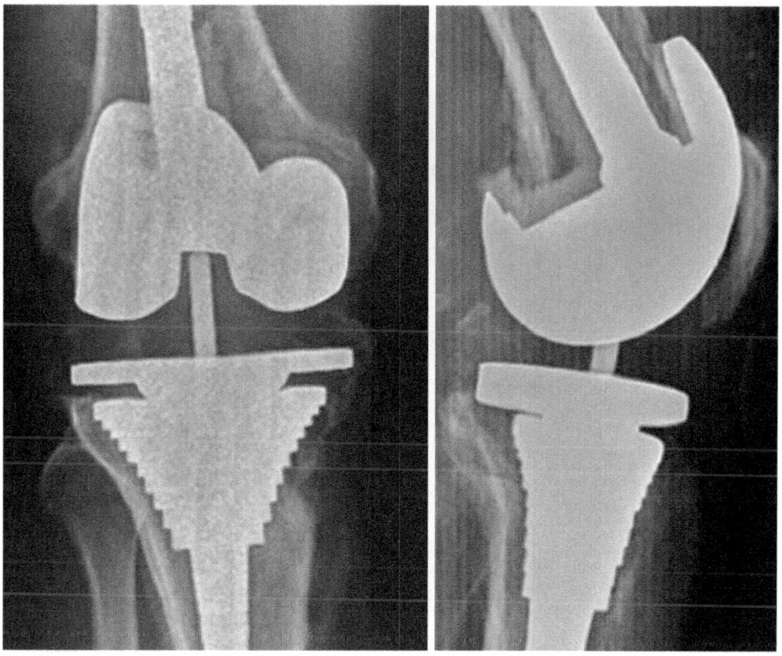

Fig. 12.30 Plain film AP and lateral radiographs of a large peripheral defect managed with a press-fit metaphyseal sleeve

The Unimplantable Knee

In some infected total knees, re-implantation has little or no likelihood of success and carries unacceptable medical risks. Re-implantation may not be possible due to inadequate bone or soft tissue for reconstruction, or is best avoided to obviate additional surgery. This section covers treatment options for the un-implantable patient.

Resection Arthroplasty

Total knee resection arthroplasty successfully eradicates infection in 50–89% of patients [121, 122]. Resection as definitive treatment (Fig. 12.31) is indicated in several patient scenarios including recurrent infections after re-implantation, inadequate bone for re-implantation, an incompetent extensor mechanism, wheelchair patients that are debilitated with low functional demands, patients unable to tolerate multiple surgeries, or where fusion is not possible or acceptable to the patient.

The technique for resection arthroplasty includes incision and debridement (I&D) with removal of all infected tissue, any protruding bone which might compromise the skin, cement, and implants followed by bracing. Immediately postoperatively the joint is immobilized by brace or cast and range of motion is allowed as tolerated by the patient. After initial postoperative swelling subsides, the patient is converted to a permanent brace using a KAFO which includes double-uprights incorporated into the shoe, a knee hinge locked in full extension with a quick-release hinge and a custom-fit thigh cuff (Fig. 12.32). A shoe lift is almost always required and can be up to a few inches in height. Patients undergoing resection will have functional limitations and in some cases can lose the ability to walk independently [122], but this is minimized with early mobilization and physical therapy for rapid progression to ambulation and range of motion.

Arthrodesis

Knee arthrodesis (fusion) can alleviate pain, stabilize the knee, and in most cases preserve ambulatory function. Loss of knee motion can make

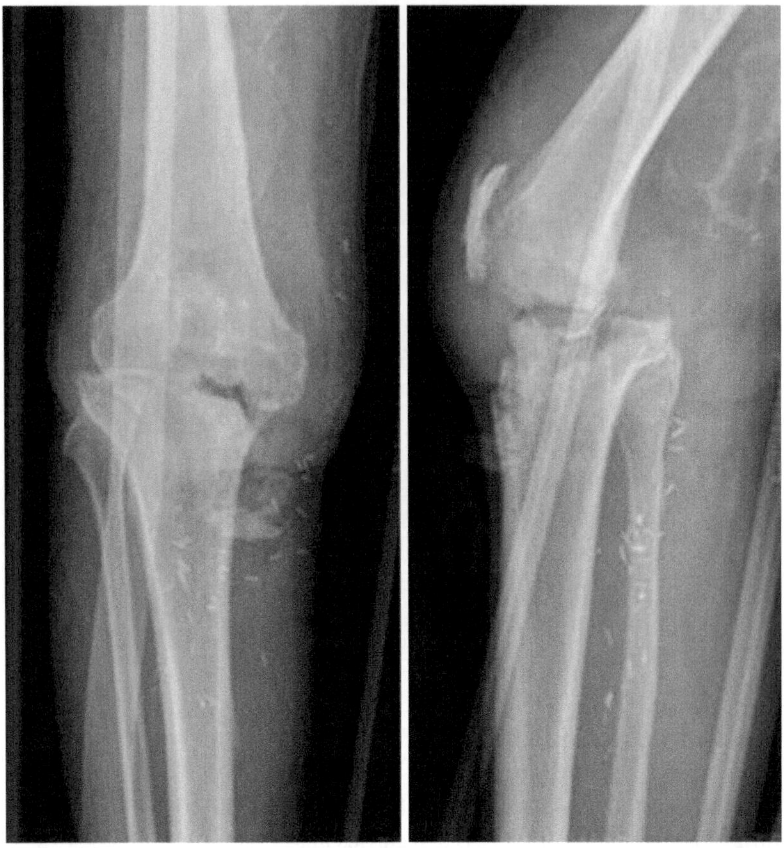

Fig. 12.31 Plain film radiographs of resection arthroplasty

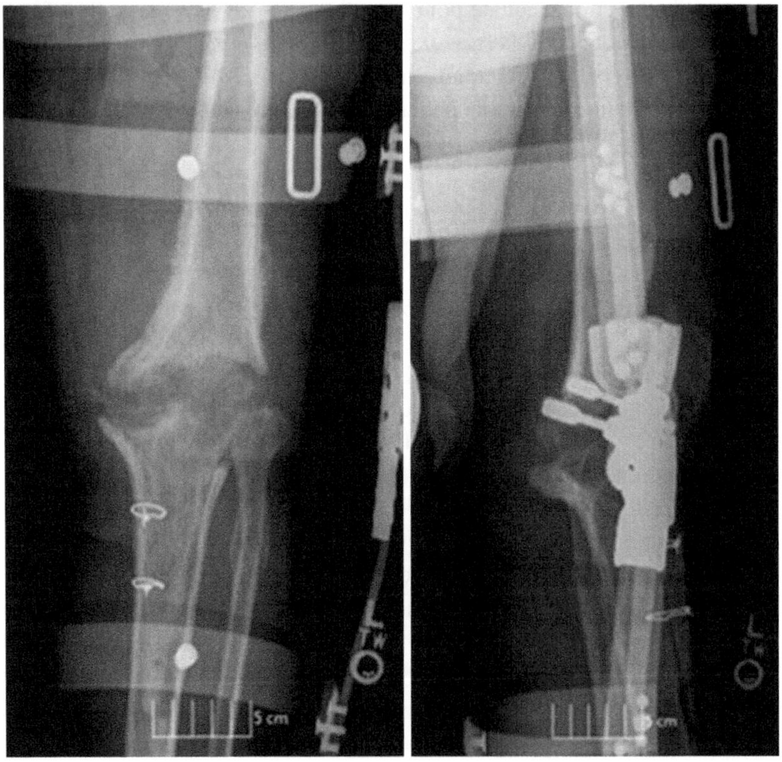

Fig. 12.32 Plain film radiographs displaying the utilization of a KAFO post resection arthroplasty

sitting, stairs and other activities challenging and requires increased energy requirements to complete daily activities and ambulation. Elderly or debilitated patients might lose the ability to ambulate or not regain ambulation after fusion [123]. In physiologically young, higher demand patients, fusion can allow return to work and some leisure activities [124, 125]. Primary contraindications for knee fusion are ipsilateral hip and ankle arthritis, contralateral extremity amputation, and contralateral knee fusion [126] and persistent infection.

Knee fusion has a reported success rate ranging from 58% to 100%, depending on technique [127–134]. Fusion is indicated when the patient has adequate bone stock for femur to tibia healing and when unable to reimplant after removal of an infected TKR. Associated findings often include extensor mechanism disruption, extensive soft-tissue defects, an immunocompromised patient, infection with resistant bacteria or pathogens that require toxic antibiotic doses [123, 135–137]. While Gram negative and mixed infections are particularly detrimental to the goal of fusion, eradication of any infection is necessary for its success [136, 138]. Therefore, arthrodesis is usually a two-stage procedure in which stage one requires elimination of infection and stage two involves rigid fixation.

Knee fusion is achieved through one of three general fixation methods: (1) external fixation, (2) IM nail fixation, (3) compression plating. With all techniques, healing requires adequate vascularity and rigid fixation that achieves stable tibiofemoral bone contact, compression, and alignment [138–140]. Patients with extensive bone loss may have limited capacity to achieve fusion even using adjunctive techniques such as vascularized fibular rotation grafts [141] and autogenous bone grafts from intramedullary reaming's [142] or the iliac crest. These patients are often best served by resection arthroplasty and KAFO bracing.

Fusion after removal of total knee explantation results in significant limb shortening. Therefore, knee fusion in full extension is desirable. The foot progression angle should be anatomic, matching the contralateral side (typically 0 to 15 degrees external), but avoid internal rotation. Postoperatively, a shoe lift will be necessary in most cases.

External Fixation

External fixation can provide rigid support and compression, while minimizing infection risks that accompany internal fixation. External fixation may be a better choice in the presence of an active infection or one-stage treatments. Mabry et al. reported deep infection rates of 4.9% and 8.3% for patients fused with external fixation and IM nails, respectively [130]. Additionally, external fixation affords the surgeon the ability to effectively adjust knee alignment to accommodate optimal coronal and sagittal plane position [143].

Disadvantages of using external fixation for knee fusion are pin site infections [128, 129, 144], pin loosening, cumbersome frame, transient nerve palsy's [128], and overall lower union rates when compared to internal fixation [129, 130]. Options for external fixation constructs include uniplanar, biplanar, and circular frames.

The use of uniplanar and biplanar external fixators have reported fusion rates ranging from 58% to 71% [129, 138, 145]. Uniplanar fixators generally do not provide the same rigidity as other fixation methods and lower fusion rates are observed. External fixators with circular or horseshoe frames (Fig. 12.33) such as the Ace-Fisher (Zimmer-Biomet, Warsaw, IN) or Ilizarov (Smith & Nephew, Memphis, TN) control the joint in three planes, permit compression, provide stable resistance to torsional and shear stress and have union rates between 93% and 100% [132, 144, 146]. When rigid fixation is achieved, early weight bearing is permissible. Although a rare consideration, patients with significant bone loss and limb shortening can undergo simultaneous lengthening using the Ilizarov technique [147].

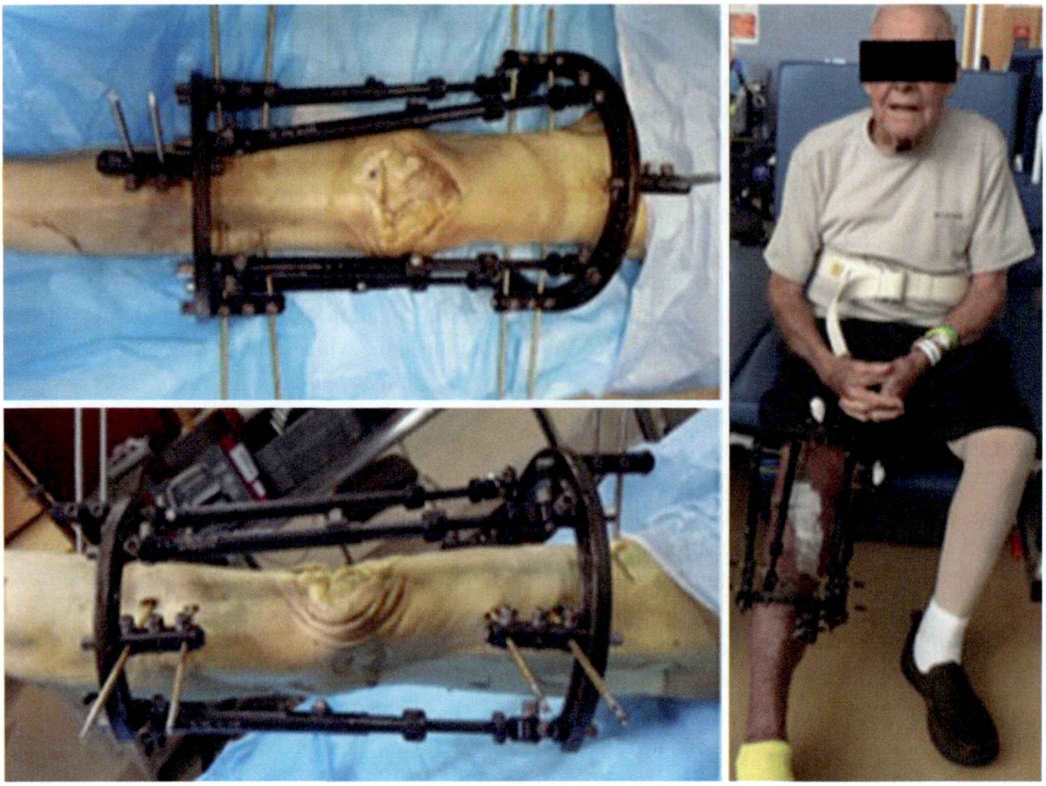

Fig. 12.33 Ace-Fischer horseshoe external fixator

Intramedullary Nail Fixation

This procedure is the second stage of a two-stage procedure as infection must be eradicated prior to intramedullary rodding for knee fusion. Many orthopedic surgeons are familiar with IM nail fixation and prefer this technique due to favorable union rates [130], the ability for early weight bearing which facilitates dynamic compression [148], the ease of intercalary graft placement for extensive bone loss, and avoidance of external hardware [143]. Fusion can be accomplished using a long IM nail or a short modular IM nail (Fig. 12.34a, b). In both techniques, eradication of infection is necessary prior to internal fixation.

The long IM nail is most commonly inserted antegrade with a piriformis fossa starting point, and traverses the length of the femur across the knee into the distal tibia. The long IM nail has reported union rates between 83% and 100% with mean time to union of 5.5–6.5 months [127, 130, 131, 133]. Despite the success possible with long IM nailing, active infection, if present, can disseminate throughout the femur and tibia. Reported complications include tibial and femoral fracture, nail breakage, proximal nail migration, painful hardware, and trochanteric bursitis [136, 138, 149].

Modular nail intramedullary fixation has the advantage of placement through the knee incision. The femoral component of the nail is placed retrograde into the femoral canal and the tibial component is placed antegrade into the tibial canal. Both tibial and femoral rods are secured with locking screws. Following insertion, the nail is connected at the knee joint and compressed. Two examples of a short modular IM nail are the Wichita Fusion Nail (Stryker, Kalamazoo, MI) and the Neff Fusion Nail (Zimmer, Warsaw, IN). Union rates for modular nails range from 75% to 100% with mean time to union being 3–9 months

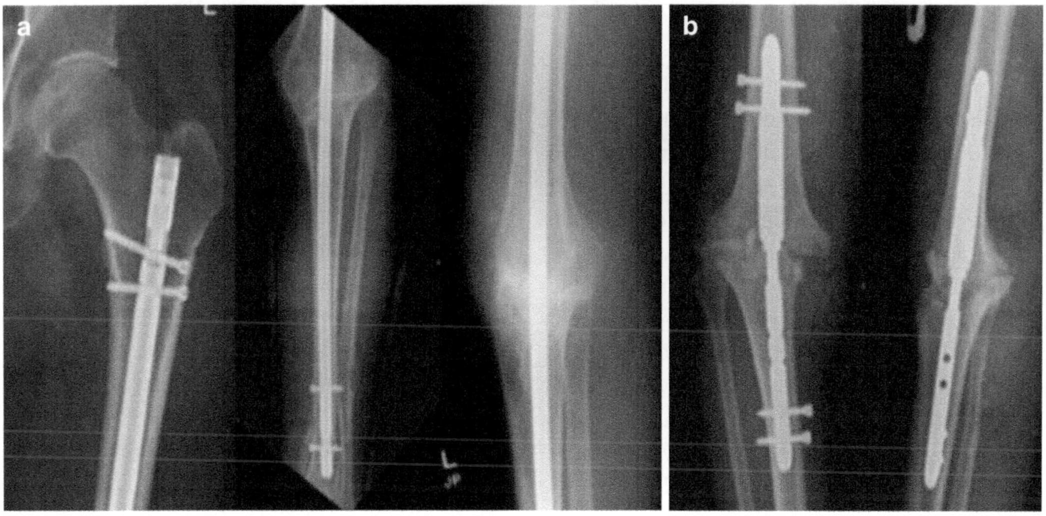

Fig. 12.34 (**a**) Long IM nail. (**b**) Short modular IM nail

[131, 134, 150]. The short modular IM nail has gained in popularity because it offers multiplanar rigidity, rotational stability, allows for immediate postoperative weight bearing, and is effective in tibial and femoral canal size mismatch [148]. The short modular nail has a high failure rate when stable bone contact in the desired alignment cannot be achieved due to bone deficiency and can be difficult to remove if failed [128, 134, 148].

Compression Plate Osteosynthesis

Compression plate osteosynthesis (Fig. 12.35) offers another avenue for fusion. This method utilizes one or two internal fixation plates across the knee joint which fix and compress the distal femur and proximal tibia to achieve fusion. Nichols et al. reported on 11 patients undergoing fusion using duel compression plating followed by casting and found that all patients in this group achieved fusion with mean time to union of 5.6 months [151]. Immediately following surgery patients are able to be partial weight bearing [143, 152] or weight bearing as tolerated with casting or bracing until knee has united [151]. Compression plating may also be used in conjunction with IM nailing to add compression across the joint.

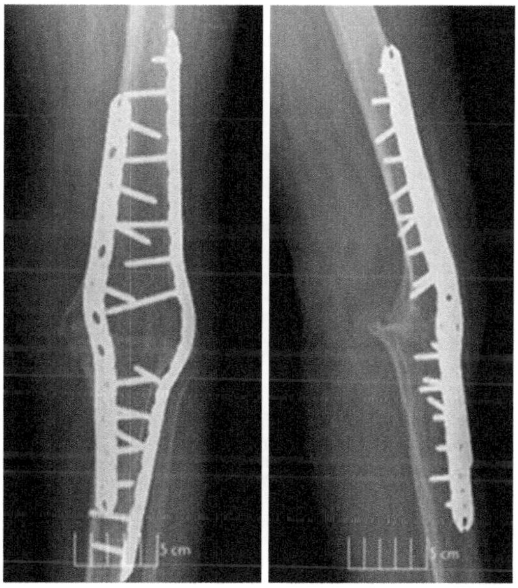

Fig. 12.35 Radiographs of a completely fused knee following duel compression plate osteosynthesis

This technique requires absence of infection and adequate bone stock for stable internal fixation, alignment, and compression of the knee joint. Large fragment 4.5 mm plates are often contoured and applied using compression technique to internally fix the freshened tibial and femoral bone ends.

Complications of Knee Fusion

Knee fusions have reported complication rates from 40% to 84%, regardless of fixation method, which are treated non-operatively in most cases [129, 130, 148, 153]. Potential complications include recurrent or recalcitrant infection, nonunion, delayed union, and periprosthetic and/or implant fracture (Fig. 12.36). However, challenging patients with nonunion and recurrent sepsis often lead to a return trip to the operating room.

Leg length discrepancy (LLD) will occur in all patients undergoing knee fusion after removal of a TKR. The affected extremity will be shortened an average 3.5–5.5 cm [126, 127, 132, 144, 146]. Shortening of the fused extremity can be desirable as it allows foot clearance when walking. Non-operative management with shoe lifts can be used to treat LLD of 5 cm [135] or greater. LLD requiring operative intervention such lengthening procedures are rare in our experience. Rozbruch et al. retrospectively reviewed four patients with septic knees and significant bone loss who underwent fusion and simultaneous leg lengthening with the Ilizarov method, reporting that all four patients achieved union while lengthening an average 5.4 cm [147]. Other alternatives include lengthening around an existing IM nail with a distal femur or proximal tibia osteotomy and external fixation distraction osteogenesis or exchange nailing with an expandable IM nail [154].

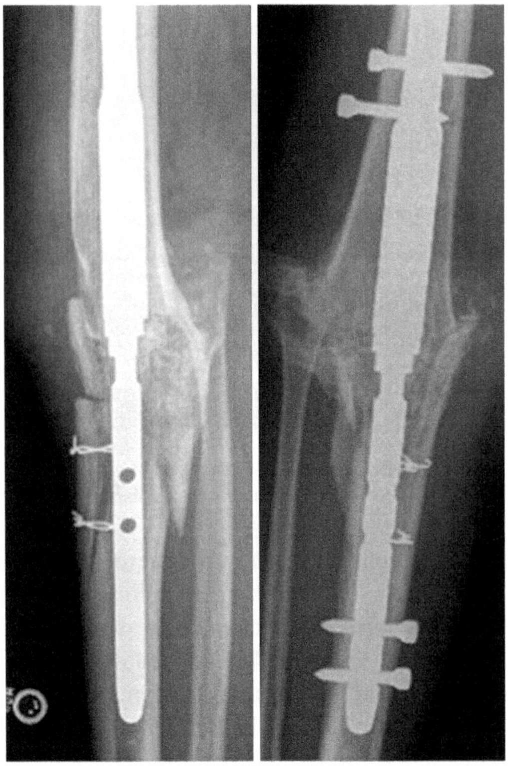

Fig. 12.36 Peri-prosthetic fracture of a short modular fusion nail

Reported nonunion rates are highly variable and dependent on fixation method and patient comorbidities. Nonunion following attempted fusion are often asymptomatic for several months and often can be treated non-operatively unless clinically indicated [154]. In the event of a symptomatic aseptic nonunion or implant failure, circular external fixation [155], exchange IM nailing [156, 157], and supplemental plate fixation [154] with and without bone graft are the mainstays for treatment.

Patients with a septic nonunion require internal hardware removal, I&D, antibiotics, and external fixation [155]. Patients with a recalcitrant infection and those who have exhausted all attempts at fusion, or are poor candidates for limb salvage, may require resection arthroplasty and bracing or an above knee amputation (AKA).

Amputation

Amputation of an infected TKR is the last resort in patients with life-threatening systemic sepsis, multiple failed attempts at fusion or resection, and recalcitrant infections [123]. Reports that approximately 5% of infected TKR's result in amputation provide the sobering consequence of unsuccessfully treated TKR infection [158]. Although potentially lifesaving, AKA is associated with increased energy expenditure for ambulation and a significant decrease or complete loss of ambulation in elderly patients [123, 159, 160]. Fedorka et al. observed that only half of post TKR above knee amputees were able to be fitted for a prosthesis and of those fitted 53% remained independent outside their home environment

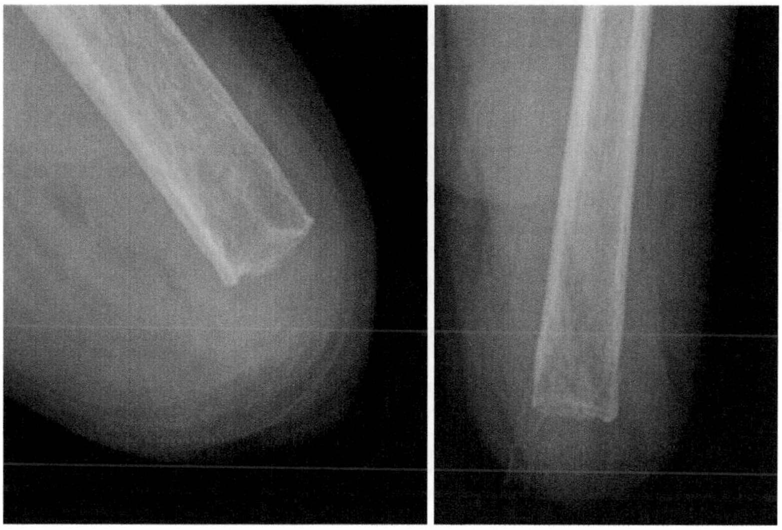

Fig. 12.37 Plain film radiographs of an AKA

[159]. Despite the significant functional limitations and impact on quality of life, an AKA can be lifesaving and the best option available to effectively eradicate the infection (Fig. 12.37).

Summary

The infected TKA is a challenging problem requiring diagnostic precision, thoughtful pre-operative preparation, and meticulous surgical technique. The host's nutritional and medical state is crucial to infection eradication and must be addressed to achieve a successful outcome. Irrigation and debridement with component retention, single-stage and two-stage reconstructions all have roles TKA infection management but are dependent on the health of the host, bacterial virulence, and the surgeon's experience and preference. While diagnostic, medical and surgical techniques will almost certainly change with time, the surgeon should adapt appropriately to continue to render expert care in TKA infection management.

References

1. Blom AW, Brown J, Taylor AH, Pattison G, Whitehouse S, Bannister GC. Infection after total knee arthroplasty. J Bone Joint Surg Br. 2004;86(5):688–91.
2. Chesney D, Sales J, Elton R, Brenkel IJ. Infection after knee arthroplasty a prospective study of 1509 cases. J Arthroplast. 2008;23(3):355–9. https://doi.org/10.1016/j.arth.2007.05.052.
3. Crowe B, Payne A, Evangelista PJ, Stachel A, Phillips MS, Slover JD, et al. Risk factors for infection following total knee arthroplasty: a series of 3836 cases from one institution. J Arthroplast. 2015;30(12):2275–8. https://doi.org/10.1016/j.arth.2015.06.05.
4. Kurtz SM, Lau E, Schmier J, Ong KL, Zhao K, Parvizi J. Infection burden for hip and knee arthroplasty in the United States. J Arthroplast. 2008;23(7):984–91. https://doi.org/10.1016/j.arth.2007.10.017.
5. Kurtz SM, Lau E, Watson H, Schmier JK, Parvizi J. Economic burden of periprosthetic joint infection in the United States. J Arthroplast. 2012;27(8 Suppl):61–5. e61. https://doi.org/10.1016/j.arth.2012.02.022.
6. Kurtz SM, Ong KL, Lau E, Bozic KJ, Berry D, Parvizi J. Prosthetic joint infection risk after TKA in the Medicare population. Clin Orthop Relat Res. 2010;468(1):52–6. https://doi.org/10.1007/s11999-009-1013-5.
7. Mahomed NN, Barrett J, Katz JN, Baron JA, Wright J, Losina E. Epidemiology of total knee replacement in the United States Medicare population. J Bone Joint Surg Am. 2005;87(6):1222–8. https://doi.org/10.2106/JBJS.D.02546.
8. Peersman G, Laskin R, Davis J, Peterson M. Infection in total knee replacement: a retrospective review of 6489 total knee replacements. Clin Orthop Relat Res. 2001;392:15–23.
9. Pulido L, Ghanem E, Joshi A, Purtill JJ, Parvizi J. Periprosthetic joint infection: the incidence, timing, and predisposing factors. Clin Orthop Relat Res. 2008;466(7):1710–5. https://doi.org/10.1007/s11999-008-0209-4.
10. Siddiqui MM, Lo NN, Ab Rahman S, Chin PL, Chia SL, Yeo SJ. Two-year outcome of early deep MRSA infections after primary total knee arthroplasty: a

joint registry review. J Arthroplast. 2013;28(1):44–8. https://doi.org/10.1016/j.arth.2012.04.007.
11. Toms AD, Davidson D, Masri BA, Duncan CP. The management of peri-prosthetic infection in total joint arthroplasty. J Bone Joint Surg Br. 2006;88(2):149–55.
12. Tsukayama DT, Estrada R, Gustilo RB. Infection after total hip arthroplasty. A study of the treatment of one hundred and six infections. J Bone Joint Surg Am. 1996;78(4):512–23.
13. Bradbury T, Fehring TK, Taunton M, Hanssen A, Azzam K, Parvizi J, Odum SM. The fate of acute methicillin-resistant Staphylococcus aureus periprosthetic knee infections treated by open debridement and retention of components. J Arthroplast. 2009;24(6 Suppl):101–4. https://doi.org/10.1016/j.arth.2009.04.028.
14. Kilgus DJ, Howe DJ, Strang A. Results of periprosthetic hip and knee infections caused by resistant bacteria. Clin Orthop Relat Res. 2002;404:116–24.
15. Parvizi J, Pawasarat IM, Azzam KA, Joshi A, Hansen EN, Bozic KJ. Periprosthetic joint infection: the economic impact of methicillin-resistant infections. J Arthroplast. 2010;25(6 Suppl):103–7. https://doi.org/10.1016/j.arth.2010.04.011.
16. Zmistowski B, Karam JA, Durinka JB, Casper DS, Parvizi J. Periprosthetic joint infection increases the risk of one-year mortality. J Bone Joint Surg Am. 2013;95(24):2177–84. https://doi.org/10.2106/JBJS.L.00789.
17. Dowsey MM, Choong PF. Obese diabetic patients are at substantial risk for deep infection after primary TKA. Clin Orthop Relat Res. 2009;467(6):1577–81. https://doi.org/10.1007/s11999-008-0551-6.
18. American Academy of Orthopaedic Surgeons. Treatment of osteoarthritis of the knee. 2nd edition: summery of recommendations. AAOS; 2013.
19. Workgroup of the American Association of Hip and Knee Surgeons Evidence Based Committee. Obesity and total joint arthroplasty: a literature based review. J Arthroplast. 2013;28(5):714–21. https://doi.org/10.1016/j.arth.2013.02.011.
20. Bozic KJ, Lau E, Kurtz S, Ong K, Berry DJ. Patient-related risk factors for postoperative mortality and periprosthetic joint infection in medicare patients undergoing TKA. Clin Orthop Relat Res. 2012;470(1):130–7. https://doi.org/10.1007/s11999-011-2043-3.
21. Workgroup Convened by the Musculoskeletal Infection Society. New definition for periprosthetic joint infection. J Arthroplast. 2011;26(8):1136–8. https://doi.org/10.1016/j.arth.2011.09.026.
22. Scott RD, Siliski JM. The use of a modified V-Y quadricepsplasty during total knee replacement to gain exposure and improve flexion in the ankylosed knee. Orthopedics. 1985;8(1):45–8.
23. American Academy of Orthopaedic Surgeons. Diagnosis of periprosthetic hip and knee infections. AAOS; 2010.
24. Austin MS, Ghanem E, Joshi A, Lindsay A, Parvizi J. A simple, cost-effective screening protocol to rule out periprosthetic infection. J Arthroplast. 2008;23(1):65–8. https://doi.org/10.1016/j.arth.2007.09.005.
25. Greidanus NV, Masri BA, Garbuz DS, Wilson SD, McAlinden MG, Xu M, Duncan CP. Use of erythrocyte sedimentation rate and C-reactive protein level to diagnose infection before revision total knee arthroplasty. A prospective evaluation. J Bone Joint Surg Am. 2007;89(7):1409–16. https://doi.org/10.2106/jbjs.d.02602.
26. Bilgen O, Atici T, Durak K, Karaeminogullari, Bilgen MS. C-reactive protein values and erythrocyte sedimentation rates after total hip and total knee arthroplasty. J Int Med Res. 2001;29(1):7–12.
27. Larsson S, Thelander U, Friberg S. C-reactive protein (CRP) levels after elective orthopedic surgery. Clin Orthop Relat Res. 1992;275:237–42.
28. Moyad TF, Thornhill T, Estok D. Evaluation and management of the infected total hip and knee. Orthopedics. 2008;31(6):581–8; quiz 589–90.
29. Morgan PM, Sharkey P, Ghanem E, Parvizi J, Clohisy JC, Burnett RS, Barrack RL. The value of intraoperative Gram stain in revision total knee arthroplasty. J Bone Joint Surg Am. 2009;91(9):2124–9. https://doi.org/10.2106/jbjs.h.00853.
30. Mason JB, Fehring TK, Odum SM, Griffin WL, Nussman DS. The value of white blood cell counts before revision total knee arthroplasty. J Arthroplast. 2003;18(8):1038–43.
31. Ghanem E, Parvizi J, Burnett RS, Sharkey PF, Keshavarzi N, Aggarwal A, Barrack RL. Cell count and differential of aspirated fluid in the diagnosis of infection at the site of total knee arthroplasty. J Bone Joint Surg Am. 2008;90(8):1637–43. https://doi.org/10.2106/jbjs.g.00470.
32. Bedair H, Ting N, Jacovides C, Saxena A, Moric M, Parvizi J, Della Valle CJ. The Mark Coventry Award: diagnosis of early postoperative TKA infection using synovial fluid analysis. Clin Orthop Relat Res. 2011;469(1):34–40. https://doi.org/10.1007/s11999-010-1433-2.
33. Parvizi J, Jacovides C, Antoci V, Ghanem E. Diagnosis of periprosthetic joint infection: the utility of a simple yet unappreciated enzyme. J Bone Joint Surg Am. 2011;93(24):2242–8. https://doi.org/10.2106/jbjs.j.01413.
34. Parvizi J, McKenzie JC, Cashman JP. Diagnosis of periprosthetic joint infection using synovial C-reactive protein. J Arthroplast. 2012;27(8 Suppl):12–6. https://doi.org/10.1016/j.arth.2012.03.018.
35. Bingham J, Clarke H, Spangehl M, Schwartz A, Beauchamp C, Goldberg B. The alpha defensin-1 biomarker assay can be used to evaluate the potentially infected total joint arthroplasty. Clin Orthop Relat Res. 2014;472(12):4006–9. https://doi.org/10.1007/s11999-014-3900-7.

36. Deirmengian C, Kardos K, Kilmartin P, Cameron A, Schiller K, Parvizi J. Combined measurement of synovial fluid alpha-defensin and C-reactive protein levels: highly accurate for diagnosing periprosthetic joint infection. J Bone Joint Surg Am. 2014a;96(17):1439–45. https://doi.org/10.2106/jbjs.m.01316.
37. Deirmengian C, Kardos K, Kilmartin P, Cameron A, Schiller K, Parvizi J. Diagnosing periprosthetic joint infection: has the era of the biomarker arrived? Clin Orthop Relat Res. 2014b;472(11):3254–62. https://doi.org/10.1007/s11999-014-3543-8.
38. Levitsky KA, Hozack WJ, Balderston RA, Rothman RH, Gluckman SJ, Maslack MM, Booth RE Jr. Evaluation of the painful prosthetic joint. Relative value of bone scan, sedimentation rate, and joint aspiration. J Arthroplast. 1991;6(3):237–44.
39. Joseph TN, Mujtaba M, Chen AL, Maurer SL, Zuckerman JD, Maldjian C, Di Cesare PE. Efficacy of combined technetium-99m sulfur colloid/indium-111 leukocyte scans to detect infected total hip and knee arthroplasties. J Arthroplast. 2001;16(6):753–8. https://doi.org/10.1054/arth.2001.24446.
40. Feldman DS, Lonner JH, Desai P, Zuckerman JD. The role of intraoperative frozen sections in revision total joint arthroplasty. J Bone Joint Surg Am. 1995;77(12):1807–13.
41. Lonner JH, Desai P, Dicesare PE, Steiner G, Zuckerman JD. The reliability of analysis of intraoperative frozen sections for identifying active infection during revision hip or knee arthroplasty. J Bone Joint Surg Am. 1996;78(10):1553–8.
42. Zhao X, Guo C, Zhao GS, Lin T, Shi ZL, Yan SG. Ten versus five polymorphonuclear leukocytes as threshold in frozen section tests for periprosthetic infection: a meta-analysis. J Arthroplast. 2013;28(6):913–7. https://doi.org/10.1016/j.arth.2012.10.015.
43. Rao N, Crossett LS, Sinha RK, Le Frock JL. Long-term suppression of infection in total joint arthroplasty. Clin Orthop Relat Res. 2003;414:55–60. https://doi.org/10.1097/01.blo.0000087321.60612.cf.
44. Tintle SM, Forsberg JA, Potter BK, Islinger RB, Andersen RC. Prosthesis retention, serial debridement, and antibiotic bead use for the treatment of infection following total joint arthroplasty. Orthopedics. 2009;32(2):87.
45. Deirmengian C, Greenbaum J, Lotke PA, Booth RE Jr, Lonner JH. Limited success with open debridement and retention of components in the treatment of acute Staphylococcus aureus infections after total knee arthroplasty. J Arthroplast. 2003;18(7 Suppl 1):22–6.
46. Chung JY, Ha CW, Park YB, Song YJ, Yu KS. Arthroscopic debridement for acutely infected prosthetic knee: any role for infection control and prosthesis salvage? Arthroscopy. 2014;30(5):599–606. https://doi.org/10.1016/j.arthro.2014.02.008.
47. Garvin KL, Scuderi G, Insall JN. Evolution of the quadriceps snip. Clin Orthop Relat Res. 1995;321:131–7.
48. Dolin MG. Osteotomy of the tibial tubercle in total knee replacement. A technical note. J Bone Joint Surg Am. 1983;65(5):704–6.
49. Whiteside LA. Exposure in difficult total knee arthroplasty using tibial tubercle osteotomy. Clin Orthop Relat Res. 1995;321:32–5.
50. Haddad FS, Sukeik M, Alazzawi S. Is single-stage revision according to a strict protocol effective in treatment of chronic knee arthroplasty infections? Clin Orthop Relat Res. 2015;473(1):8–14. https://doi.org/10.1007/s11999-014-3721-8.
51. De Man FH, Sendi P, Zimmerli W, Maurer TB, Ochsner PE, Ilchmann T. Infectiological, functional, and radiographic outcome after revision for prosthetic hip infection according to a strict algorithm. Acta Orthop. 2011;82(1):27–34. https://doi.org/10.3109/17453674.2010.548025.
52. Ure KJ, Amstutz HC, Nasser S, Schmalzried TP. Direct-exchange arthroplasty for the treatment of infection after total hip replacement. An average ten-year follow-up. J Bone Joint Surg Am. 1998;80(7):961–8.
53. Klouche S, Sariali E, Mamoudy P. Total hip arthroplasty revision due to infection: a cost analysis approach. Orthop Traumatol Surg Res. 2010;96(2):124–32. https://doi.org/10.1016/j.rcot.2010.02.005.
54. Wolf CF, Gu NY, Doctor JN, Manner PA, Leopold SS. Comparison of one and two-stage revision of total hip arthroplasty complicated by infection: a Markov expected-utility decision analysis. J Bone Joint Surg Am. 2011;93(7):631–9. https://doi.org/10.2106/JBJS.I.01256.
55. Bejon P, Berendt A, Atkins BL, Green N, Parry H, Masters S, et al. Two-stage revision for prosthetic joint infection: predictors of outcome and the role of reimplantation microbiology. J Antimicrob Chemother. 2010;65(3):569–75. https://doi.org/10.1093/jac/dkp469.
56. Gehrke T, Kendoff D. Peri-prosthetic hip infections: in favour of one-stage. Hip Int. 2012;22(Suppl 8):S40–5. https://doi.org/10.5301/HIP.2012.9569.
57. Gulhane S, Vanhegan IS, Haddad FS. Single stage revision: regaining momentum. J Bone Joint Surg Br. 2012;94(11 Suppl A):120–2. https://doi.org/10.1302/0301-620X.94B11.30746.
58. Kordelle J, Frommelt L, Kluber D, Seemann K. [Results of one-stage endoprosthesis revision in periprosthetic infection cause by methicillin-resistant Staphylococcus aureus]. Z Orthop Ihre Grenzgeb. 2000;138(3):240–4. https://doi.org/10.1055/s-2000-10143.
59. Silva M, Tharani R, Schmalzried TP. Results of direct exchange or debridement of the infected total knee arthroplasty. Clin Orthop Relat Res. 2002;404:125–31.

60. Lichstein P, Gehrke T, Lombardi A, Romano C, Stockley I, Babis G, et al. One-stage versus two-stage exchange. J Orthop Res. 2014;32(Suppl 1):S141–6. https://doi.org/10.1002/jor.22558.
61. Fehring TK, Odum S, Calton TF, Mason JB. Articulating versus static spacers in revision total knee arthroplasty for sepsis. The Ranawat Award. Clin Orthop Relat Res. 2000;380:9–16.
62. Guild GN 3rd, Wu B, Scuderi GR. Articulating vs. static antibiotic impregnated spacers in revision total knee arthroplasty for sepsis. A systematic review. J Arthroplasty. 2014;29(3):558–63. https://doi.org/10.1016/j.arth.2013.08.013.
63. Romano CL, Gala L, Logoluso N, Romano D, Drago L. Two-stage revision of septic knee prosthesis with articulating knee spacers yields better infection eradication rate than one-stage or two-stage revision with static spacers. Knee Surg Sports Traumatol Arthrosc. 2012;20(12):2445–53. https://doi.org/10.1007/s00167-012-1885-x.
64. Jacobs C, Christensen CP, Berend ME. Static and mobile antibiotic-impregnated cement spacers for the management of prosthetic joint infection. J Am Acad Orthop Surg. 2009;17(6):356–68.
65. Calton TF, Fehring TK, Griffin WL. Bone loss associated with the use of spacer blocks in infected total knee arthroplasty. Clin Orthop Relat Res. 1997;345:148–54.
66. Pietsch M, Hofmann S, Wenisch C. Treatment of deep infection of total knee arthroplasty using a two-stage procedure. Oper Orthop Traumatol. 2006;18(1):66–87. https://doi.org/10.1007/s00064-006-1163-5.
67. Emerson RH Jr, Muncie M, Tarbox TR, Higgins LL. Comparison of a static with a mobile spacer in total knee infection. Clin Orthop Relat Res. 2002;404:132–8.
68. Durbhakula SM, Czajka J, Fuchs MD, Uhl RL. Antibiotic-loaded articulating cement spacer in the 2-stage exchange of infected total knee arthroplasty. J Arthroplast. 2004a;19(6):768–74.
69. Hofmann AA, Goldberg T, Tanner AM, Kurtin SM. Treatment of infected total knee arthroplasty using an articulating spacer: 2- to 12-year experience. Clin Orthop Relat Res. 2005;430:125–31.
70. Masri BA, Duncan C, Beauchamp CP. The modified two staged exchange arthroplasty in the treatment of infected total knee replacement: the prostalac system and other articulated spacers, vol. 13. 20th ed. Baltimore: WIlliams and Wilkins; 1998a.
71. Joseph TN, Chen AL, Di Cesare PE. Use of antibiotic-impregnated cement in total joint arthroplasty. J Am Acad Orthop Surg. 2003;11(1):38–47.
72. Nettrour JF, Polikandriotis JA, Bernasek TL, Gustke KA, Lyons ST. Articulating spacers for the treatment of infected total knee arthroplasty: effect of antibiotic combinations and concentrations. Orthopedics. 2013;36(1):e19–24. https://doi.org/10.3928/01477447-20121217-13.
73. Bertazzoni Minelli E, Caveiari C, Benini A. Release of antibiotics from polymethylmethacrylate cement. J Chemother. 2002;14(5):492–500. https://doi.org/10.1179/joc.2002.14.5.492.
74. Masri BA, Duncan CP, Beauchamp CP. Long-term elution of antibiotics from bone-cement: an in vivo study using the prosthesis of antibiotic-loaded acrylic cement (PROSTALAC) system. J Arthroplast. 1998b;13(3):331–8.
75. Struelens B, Claes S, Bellemans J. Spacer-related problems in two-stage revision knee arthroplasty. Acta Orthop Belg. 2013;79(4):422–6.
76. Ha CW. A technique for intraoperative construction of antibiotic spacers. Clin Orthop Relat Res. 2006;445:204–9. https://doi.org/10.1097/01.blo.0000201161.52196.c5.
77. Kohl S, Evangelopoulos DS, Kohlhof H, Krueger A, Hartel M, Roeder C, Eggli S. An intraoperatively moulded PMMA prostheses like spacer for two-stage revision of infected total knee arthroplasty. Knee. 2011;18(6):464–9. https://doi.org/10.1016/j.knee.2010.09.002.
78. Pitto RP, Castelli CC, Ferrari R, Munro J. Preformed articulating knee spacer in two-stage revision for the infected total knee arthroplasty. Int Orthop. 2005;29(5):305–8. https://doi.org/10.1007/s00264-005-0670-6.
79. Hofmann AA, Kane KR, Tkach TK, Plaster RL, Camargo MP. Treatment of infected total knee arthroplasty using an articulating spacer. Clin Orthop Relat Res. 1995;321:45–54.
80. Lyons ST, Wright CA, Krute CN, Rivera FE, Carroll RK, Shaw LN. Confirming sterility of an autoclaved infected femoral component for use in an articulated antibiotic knee spacer: A pilot study. J Arthroplast. 2015;31(1):245–9. https://doi.org/10.1016/j.arth.2015.06.068.
81. Cuckler JM. The infected total knee: management options. J Arthroplast. 2005;20(4 Suppl 2):33–6.
82. Jamsen E, Sheng P, Halonen P, Lehto MU, Moilanen T, Pajamaki J, et al. Spacer prostheses in two-stage revision of infected knee arthroplasty. Int Orthop. 2006;30(4):257–61. https://doi.org/10.1007/s00264-006-0102-2.
83. Durbhakula SM, Czajka J, Fuchs MD, Uhl RL. Spacer endoprosthesis for the treatment of infected total hip arthroplasty. J Arthroplast. 2004b;19(6):760–7.
84. Regis D, Sandri A, Magnan B, Bartolozzi P. Six-year follow-up of a preformed spacer for the management of chronically infected total hip arthroplasty. Arch Orthop Trauma Surg. 2010;130(9):1111–5. https://doi.org/10.1007/s00402-009-0984-8.
85. Wentworth SJ, Masri BA, Duncan CP, Southworth CB. Hip prosthesis of antibiotic-loaded acrylic cement for the treatment of infections following total hip arthroplasty. J Bone Joint Surg Am. 2002;84-A(Suppl 2):123–8.
86. Choi HR, Freiberg AA, Malchau H, Rubash HE, Kwon YM. The fate of unplanned retention of

prosthetic articulating spacers for infected total hip and total knee arthroplasty. J Arthroplast. 2014;29(4):690–3. https://doi.org/10.1016/j.arth.2013.07.013.
87. Lyons S, Stanat S. Articulating antibiotic spacers for septic Total hip and knee arthroplasty. Longevity, function and economics. Paper presented at the FORE research day, Tampa; 2012.
88. Cadambi A, Engh GA. Use of a semitendinosus tendon autogenous graft for rupture of the patellar ligament after total knee arthroplasty. A report of seven cases. J Bone Joint Surg Am. 1992;74(7):974–9.
89. Lynch AF, Rorabeck CH, Bourne RB. Extensor mechanism complications following total knee arthroplasty. J Arthroplast. 1987;2(2):135–40.
90. Rand JA, Morrey BF, Bryan RS. Patellar tendon rupture after total knee arthroplasty. Clin Orthop Relat Res. 1989;244:233–8.
91. Aracil J, Salom M, Aroca JE, Torro V, Lopez-Quiles D. Extensor apparatus reconstruction with Leeds-Keio ligament in total knee arthroplasty. J Arthroplast. 1999;14(2):204–8.
92. Dobbs RE, Hanssen AD, Lewallen DG, Pagnano MW. Quadriceps tendon rupture after total knee arthroplasty. Prevalence, complications, and outcomes. J Bone Joint Surg Am. 2005;87(1):37–45. https://doi.org/10.2106/JBJS.D.01910.
93. Schoderbek RJ Jr, Brown TE, Mulhall KJ, Mounasamy V, Iorio R, Krackow KA, et al. Extensor mechanism disruption after total knee arthroplasty. Clin Orthop Relat Res. 2006;446:176–85. https://doi.org/10.1097/01.blo.0000218726.06473.26.
94. Springer BD, Della Valle CJ. Extensor mechanism allograft reconstruction after total knee arthroplasty. J Arthroplast. 2008;23(7 Suppl):35–8. https://doi.org/10.1016/j.arth.2008.06.016.
95. Crossett LS, Sinha RK, Sechriest VF, Rubash HE. Reconstruction of a ruptured patellar tendon with achilles tendon allograft following total knee arthroplasty. J Bone Joint Surg Am. 2002;84-A(8):1354–61.
96. Jaureguito JW, Dubois CM, Smith SR, Gottlieb LJ, Finn HA. Medial gastrocnemius transposition flap for the treatment of disruption of the extensor mechanism after total knee arthroplasty. J Bone Joint Surg Am. 1997;79(6):866–73.
97. Nazarian DG, Booth RE Jr. Extensor mechanism allografts in total knee arthroplasty. Clin Orthop Relat Res. 1999;367:123–9.
98. Barrack RL, Smith P, Munn B, Engh G, Rorabeck C. The Ranawat Award. Comparison of surgical approaches in total knee arthroplasty. Clin Orthop Relat Res. 1998;356:16–21.
99. Trousdale RT, Hanssen AD, Rand JA, Cahalan TD. V-Y quadricepsplasty in total knee arthroplasty. Clin Orthop Relat Res. 1993;286:48–55.
100. Browne JA, Hanssen AD. Reconstruction of patellar tendon disruption after total knee arthroplasty: results of a new technique utilizing synthetic mesh. J Bone Joint Surg Am. 2011;93(12):1137–43. https://doi.org/10.2106/JBJS.J.01036.
101. Barrack RL, Stanley T, Allen Butler R. Treating extensor mechanism disruption after total knee arthroplasty. Clin Orthop Relat Res. 2003;416:98–104. https://doi.org/10.1097/01.blo.0000092993.90435.69.
102. Engh G, Ammeen D. Bone loss with revision total knee arthroplasty: defect classification and alternatives for reconstruction. Instr Course Lect. 1999;48:167.
103. Vasso M, Beaufils P, Schiavone Panni A. Constraint choice in revision knee arthroplasty. Int Orthop. 2013;37(7):1279–84. https://doi.org/10.1007/s00264-013-1929-y.
104. Fehring TK, Odum S, Olekson C, Griffin WL, Mason JB, McCoy TH. Stem fixation in revision total knee arthroplasty: a comparative analysis. Clin Orthop Relat Res. 2003;416:217–24. https://doi.org/10.1097/01.blo.0000093032.56370.4b.
105. Mabry TM, Vessely MB, Schleck CD, Harmsen WS, Berry DJ. Revision total knee arthroplasty with modular cemented stems: long-term follow-up. J Arthroplast. 2007b;22(6 Suppl 2):100–5. https://doi.org/10.1016/j.arth.2007.03.025.
106. Whaley AL, Trousdale RT, Rand JA, Hanssen AD. Cemented long-stem revision total knee arthroplasty. J Arthroplast. 2003;18(5):592–9.
107. Wood GC, Naudie DD, MacDonald SJ, McCalden RW, Bourne RB. Results of press-fit stems in revision knee arthroplasties. Clin Orthop Relat Res. 2009;467(3):810–7. https://doi.org/10.1007/s11999-008-0621-9.
108. Brooks PJ, Walker PS, Scott RD. Tibial component fixation in deficient tibial bone stock. Clin Orthop Relat Res. 1984;184:302–8.
109. Ritter MA. Screw and cement fixation of large defects in total knee arthroplasty. J Arthroplast. 1986;1(2):125–9.
110. Engh GA, Ammeen DJ. Use of structural allograft in revision total knee arthroplasty in knees with severe tibial bone loss. J Bone Joint Surg Am. 2007;89(12):2640–7. https://doi.org/10.2106/JBJS.F.00865.
111. Clatworthy MG, Ballance J, Brick GW, Chandler HP, Gross AE. The use of structural allograft for uncontained defects in revision total knee arthroplasty. A minimum five-year review. J Bone Joint Surg Am. 2001;83-A(3):404–11.
112. Delloye C, Cornu O, Druez V, Barbier O. Bone allografts: what they can offer and what they cannot. J Bone Joint Surg Br. 2007;89(5):574–9. https://doi.org/10.1302/0301-620X.89B5.19039.
113. Tsukada S, Wakui M, Matsueda M. Metal block augmentation for bone defects of the medial tibia during primary total knee arthroplasty. J Orthop Surg Res. 2013;8:36. https://doi.org/10.1186/1749-799X-8-36.
114. Fehring TK, Peindl RD, Humble RS, Harrow ME, Frick SL. Modular tibial augmentations in

total knee arthroplasty. Clin Orthop Relat Res. 1996;327:207–17.
115. Rand JA. Bone deficiency in total knee arthroplasty. Use of metal wedge augmentation. Clin Orthop Relat Res. 1991;271:63–71.
116. Brand MG, Daley RJ, Ewald FC, Scott RD. Tibial tray augmentation with modular metal wedges for tibial bone stock deficiency. Clin Orthop Relat Res. 1989;248:71–9.
117. Radnay CS, Scuderi GR. Management of bone loss: augments, cones, offset stems. Clin Orthop Relat Res. 2006;446:83–92. https://doi.org/10.1097/01.blo.0000214437.57151.41.
118. Long WJ, Scuderi GR. Porous tantalum cones for large metaphyseal tibial defects in revision total knee arthroplasty: a minimum 2-year follow-up. J Arthroplast. 2009;24(7):1086–92. https://doi.org/10.1016/j.arth.2008.08.011.
119. Meneghini RM, Lewallen DG, Hanssen AD. Use of porous tantalum metaphyseal cones for severe tibial bone loss during revision total knee replacement. J Bone Joint Surg Am. 2008;90(1):78–84. https://doi.org/10.2106/JBJS.F.01495.
120. Alexander GE, Bernasek TL, Crank RL, Haidukewych GJ. Cementless metaphyseal sleeves used for large tibial defects in revision total knee arthroplasty. J Arthroplast. 2013;28(4):604–7. https://doi.org/10.1016/j.arth.2012.08.006.
121. Bengtson S, Knutson K. The infected knee arthroplasty. A 6-year follow-up of 357 cases. Acta Orthop Scand. 1991;62(4):301–11.
122. Falahee MH, Matthews LS, Kaufer H. Resection arthroplasty as a salvage procedure for a knee with infection after a total arthroplasty. J Bone Joint Surg Am. 1987;69(7):1013–21.
123. Jacofsky DJ, Campbell MD. The infected total knee arthroplasty part 2: management options. Hosp Physician. 2006;36:29–32.
124. Enneking WF, Shirley PD. Resection-arthrodesis for malignant and potentially malignant lesions about the knee using an intramedullary rod and local bone grafts. J Bone Joint Surg Am. 1977;59(2):223–36.
125. Rud B, Jensen UH. Function after arthrodesis of the knee. Acta Orthop Scand. 1985;56(4):337–9.
126. Klinger HM, Spahn G, Schultz W, Baums MH. Arthrodesis of the knee after failed infected total knee arthroplasty. Knee Surg Sports Traumatol Arthrosc. 2006;14(5):447–53. https://doi.org/10.1007/s00167-005-0664-3.
127. Bargiotas K, Wohlrab D, Sewecke JJ, Lavinge G, Demeo PJ, Sotereanos NG. Arthrodesis of the knee with a long intramedullary nail following the failure of a total knee arthroplasty as the result of infection. J Bone Joint Surg Am. 2006;88(3):558–3. https://doi.org/10.2106/JBJS.E.00575.
128. Domingo LJ, Caballero MJ, Cuenca J, Herrera A, Sola A, Herrero L. Knee arthrodesis with the Wichita fusion nail. Int Orthop. 2004;28(1):25–7. https://doi.org/10.1007/s00264-003-0514-1.
129. Hak DJ, Lieberman JR, Finerman GA. Single plane and biplane external fixators for knee arthrodesis. Clin Orthop Relat Res. 1995;316:134–44.
130. Mabry TM, Jacofsky DJ, Haidukewych GJ, Hanssen AD. Comparison of intramedullary nailing and external fixation knee arthrodesis for the infected knee replacement. Clin Orthop Relat Res. 2007a;464:11–5. https://doi.org/10.1097/BLO.0b013e31806a9191.
131. McQueen DA, Cooke FW, Hahn DL. Knee arthrodesis with the Wichita Fusion Nail: an outcome comparison. Clin Orthop Relat Res. 2006;446:132–9. https://doi.org/10.1097/01.blo.0000214429.41904.82.
132. Oostenbroek HJ, van Roermund PM. Arthrodesis of the knee after an infected arthroplasty using the Ilizarov method. J Bone Joint Surg Br. 2001;83(1):50–4.
133. Panagiotopoulos E, Kouzelis A, Matzaroglou C, Saridis A, Lambiris E. Intramedullary knee arthrodesis as a salvage procedure after failed total knee replacement. Int Orthop. 2006;30(6):545–9. https://doi.org/10.1007/s00264-006-0129-4.
134. Parcel TW, Levering M, Polikandriotis JA, Gustke KA, Bernasek TL. Failure analysis of knee arthrodesis with the WichitaFusion Nail. Orthopedics. 2013;36(11):e1336–9. https://doi.org/10.3928/01477447-20131021-11.
135. Conway JD, Mont MA, Bezwada HP. Arthrodesis of the knee. J Bone Joint Surg Am. 2004;86-A(4):835–48.
136. Damron TA, McBeath AA. Arthrodesis following failed total knee arthroplasty: comprehensive review and meta-analysis of recent literature. Orthopedics. 1995;18(4):361–8.
137. Leone JM, Hanssen AD. Management of infection at the site of a total knee arthroplasty. J Bone Joint Surg Am. 2005;87(10):2335–48.
138. Knutson K, Hovelius L, Lindstrand A, Lidgren L. Arthrodesis after failed knee arthroplasty. A nationwide multicenter investigation of 91 cases. Clin Orthop Relat Res. 1984;191:202–11.
139. Hagemann WF, Woods GW, Tullos HS. Arthrodesis in failed total knee replacement. J Bone Joint Surg Am. 1978;60(6):790–4.
140. Vlasak R, Gearen PF, Petty W. Knee arthrodesis in the treatment of failed total knee replacement. Clin Orthop Relat Res. 1995;321:138–44.
141. Rasmussen MR, Bishop AT, Wood MB. Arthrodesis of the knee with a vascularized fibular rotatory graft. J Bone Joint Surg Am. 1995;77(5):751–9.
142. Herscovici D Jr, Scaduto JM. Use of the reamer-irrigator-aspirator technique to obtain autograft for ankle and hindfoot arthrodesis. J Bone Joint Surg Br. 2012;94(1):75–9. https://doi.org/10.1302/0301-620X.94B1.27690.

143. MacDonald JH, Agarwal S, Lorei MP, Johanson NA, Freiberg AA. Knee arthrodesis. J Am Acad Orthop Surg. 2006;14(3):154–63.
144. Kuchinad R, Fourman MS, Fragomen AT, Rozbruch SR. Knee arthrodesis as limb salvage for complex failures of total knee arthroplasty. J Arthroplast. 2014;29(11):2150–5. https://doi.org/10.1016/j.arth.2014.06.021.
145. Rand JA, Bryan RS, Chao EY. Failed total knee arthroplasty treated by arthrodesis of the knee using the Ace-Fischer apparatus. J Bone Joint Surg Am. 1987;69(1):39–45.
146. David R, Shtarker H, Horesh Z, Tsur A, Soudry M. Arthrodesis with the Ilizarov device after failed knee arthroplasty. Orthopedics. 2001;24(1):33–6.
147. Rozbruch SR, Ilizarov S, Blyakher A. Knee arthrodesis with simultaneous lengthening using the Ilizarov method. J Orthop Trauma. 2005;19(3):171–9.
148. Gallusser N, Goetti P, Luyet A, Borens O. Knee arthrodesis with modular nail after failed TKA due to infection. Eur J Orthop Surg Traumatol. 2015;25(8):1307–12. https://doi.org/10.1007/s00590-015-1707-1.
149. Crockarell JR Jr, Mihalko MJ. Knee arthrodesis using an intramedullary nail. J Arthroplast. 2005;20(6):703–8. https://doi.org/10.1016/j.arth.2004.10.015.
150. Waldman BJ, Mont MA, Payman KR, Freiberg AA, Windsor RE, Sculco TP, Hungerford DS. Infected total knee arthroplasty treated with arthrodesis using a modular nail. Clin Orthop Relat Res. 1999;367:230–7.
151. Nichols SJ, Landon GC, Tullos HS. Arthrodesis with dual plates after failed total knee arthroplasty. J Bone Joint Surg Am. 1991;73(7):1020–4.
152. Pritchett JW, Mallin BA, Matthews AC. Knee arthrodesis with a tension-band plate. J Bone Joint Surg Am. 1988;70(2):285–8.
153. Garberina MJ, Fitch RD, Hoffmann ED, Hardaker WT, Vail TP, Scully SP. Knee arthrodesis with circular external fixation. Clin Orthop Relat Res. 2001;382:168–78.
154. Wood JH, Conway JD. Advanced concepts in knee arthrodesis. World J Orthop. 2015;6(2):202–10. https://doi.org/10.5312/wjo.v6.i2.202.
155. Manzotti A, Pullen C, Guerreschi F, Catagni MA. The Ilizarov method for failed knee arthrodesis following septic TKR. Knee. 2001;8(2):135–8.
156. Brinker MR, O'Connor DP. Exchange nailing of ununited fractures. J Bone Joint Surg Am. 2007;89(1):177–88. https://doi.org/10.2106/JBJS.F.00742.
157. Hak DJ, Lee SS, Goulet JA. Success of exchange reamed intramedullary nailing for femoral shaft nonunion or delayed union. J Orthop Trauma. 2000;14(3):178–82.
158. Hanssen AD, Rand JA. Evaluation and treatment of infection at the site of a total hip or knee arthroplasty. Instr Course Lect. 1999;48:111–22.
159. Fedorka CJ, Chen AF, McGarry WM, Parvizi J, Klatt BA. Functional ability after above-the-knee amputation for infected total knee arthroplasty. Clin Orthop Relat Res. 2011;469(4):1024–32. https://doi.org/10.1007/s11999-010-1577-0.
160. Pring DJ, Marks L, Angel JC. Mobility after amputation for failed knee replacement. J Bone Joint Surg Br. 1988;70(5):770–1.

Index

R. S. Yoon et al. (eds.), *Trauma and Infection Control in Revision Hip and Knee Arthroplasty*, https://doi.org/10.1007/978-3-031-71971-4

GPSR Compliance

The European Union's (EU) General Product Safety Regulation (GPSR) is a set of rules that requires consumer products to be safe and our obligations to ensure this.

If you have any concerns about our products, you can contact us on ProductSafety@springernature.com

In case Publisher is established outside the EU, the EU authorized representative is:

Springer Nature Customer Service Center GmbH
Europaplatz 3
69115 Heidelberg, Germany

Batch number: 10732809

Printed by Printforce, the Netherlands